PEDIATRIC HEMATOLOGY/ ONCOLOGY SECRETS

PEDIATRIC HEMATOLOGY/ ONCOLOGY SECRETS

MICHAEL A. WEINER, M.D.
Hettinger Professor of Clinical Pediatrics
Director, Herbert Irving Child and Adolescent Oncology Center
Hope & Heroes Division of Pediatric Oncology
Columbia University College of Physicians & Surgeons
New York, New York

Children's Hospital of New York
New York Presbyterian Hospital
Columbia Presbyterian Medical Center
New York, New York

MITCHELL S. CAIRO, M.D.
Professor of Pediatrics, Medicine, and Pathology
Pediatric Oncology
Director, Blood and Marrow Transplantation
Herbert Irving Child and Adolescent Oncology Center
Columbia University College of Physicians & Surgeons
New York, New York

HANLEY & BELFUS, INC./Philadelphia

Publisher: HANLEY & BELFUS, INC.
Medical Publishers
210 South 13th Street
Philadelphia, PA 19107
(215) 546-7293; 800-962-1892
FAX (215) 790-9330
Web site: http://www.hanleyandbelfus.com

Library of Congress Cataloging-in-Publication Data

Pediatric hematology/oncology secrets / edited by Michael A. Weiner, Mitchell Cairo.
p. ; cm—(The Secrets Series®)
Includes bibliographical references and index.
ISBN 1-56053-444-3 (alk. paper)
1. Pediatric hematology—Examinations, questions, etc. 2. Tumors in children—Examinations, questions, etc. 3. Children—Diseases—Examinations, questions, etc. 4. Blood—Diseases—Examinations, questions, etc. I. Weiner, Michael A., 1946-. II. Cairo, Mitchell, 1950-. III. Series.
[DNLM: 1. Hematologic Diseases—Child—Examination Questions. 2. Neoplasms—Child—Examination Questions. WH 18.2 P371 2001]
RJ411 .P397 2002
618.92'15'0076—dc21

2001024147

PEDIATRIC HEMATOLOGY/ONCOLOGY SECRETS ISBN 1-56053-444-3

Last digit is the print number: 9 8 7 6 5 4 3 2 1

CONTENTS

CONTRIBUTORS

Mark P. Atlas, M.D.
Assistant Professor of Pediatrics, Pediatric Oncology, Columbia University College of Physicians & Surgeons, Children's Hospital of New York, New York Presbyterian Hospital, Columbia Presbyterian Medical Center, New York, New York

Julia Glade Bender, M.D.
Assistant Professor of Clinical Pediatrics, Division of Pediatric Oncology, Columbia University College of Physicians & Surgeons, Children's Hospital of New York, New York Presbyterian Hospital, Columbia Presbyterian Medical Center, New York, New York

M. Brigid Bradley, M.D.
Assistant Professor, Department of Pediatrics, Division of Pediatric Oncology, Columbia University College of Physicians & Surgeons, Children's Hospital of New York, New York Presbyterian Hospital, Columbia Presbyterian Medical Center, New York, New York

Kiery A. Braithwaite, M.D.
Resident, Department of Medicine at Inova Fairfax Hospital, Georgetown University Hospital, Washington, DC

Gary M. Brittenham, M.D.
Professor of Pediatrics and Medicine, Columbia University College of Physicians & Surgeons, Children's Hospital of New York, New York Presbyterian Hospital, Columbia Presbyterian Medical Center, New York, New York

Mitchell S. Cairo, M.D.
Professor of Pediatrics, Medicine, and Pathology, Pediatric Oncology, Director, Blood and Marrow Transplantation, Herbert Irving Child and Adolescent Oncology Center, Columbia University College of Physicians & Surgeons, New York, New York

Gustavo del Toro, M.D.
Assistant Professor, Division of Pediatric Oncology, Columbia University College of Physicians & Surgeons, Children's Hospital of New York, New York Presbyterian Hospital, Columbia Presbyterian Medical Center, New York, New York

Karen Schueler Fountain, M.D., F.A.C.R.
Associate Clinical Professor, Department of Radiation Oncology, Columbia University College of Physicians & Surgeons, Children's Hospital of New York, New York Presbyterian Hospital, Columbia Presbyterian Medical Center, New York, New York

James H. Garvin, Jr., M.D., Ph.D.
Professor of Clinical Pediatrics, Division of Pediatric Oncology, Columbia University College of Physicians & Surgeons, Children's Hospital of New York, New York Presbyterian Hospital, Columbia Presbyterian Medical Center, New York, New York

Kenneth S. Gorfinkle, Ph.D.
Assistant Clinical Professor of Psychology in Psychiatry, Psychiatry/Behavioral Medicine, Columbia University College of Physicians & Surgeons, Children's Hospital of New York, New York Presbyterian Hospital, Columbia Presbyterian Medical Center, New York, New York

Linda Granowetter, M.D.
Associate Professor of Clinical Pediatrics, Department of Pediatrics, Division of Oncology, Columbia University College of Physicians & Surgeons, Children's Hospital of New York, New York Presbyterian Hospital, Columbia Presbyterian Medical Center, New York, New York

Jessica J. Kandel, M.D.
Assistant Professor of Surgery and Pediatrics, Surgery (Division of Pediatric Surgery), Columbia University College of Physicians & Surgeons, Children's Hospital of New York, New York Presbyterian Hospital, Columbia Presbyterian Medical Center, New York, New York

Kara M. Kelly, M.D.
Assistant Professor of Pediatrics, Division of Pediatric Oncology, Columbia University College of Physicians & Surgeons, Children's Hospital of New York, New York Presbyterian Hospital, Columbia Presbyterian Medical Center, New York, New York

Margaret T. Lee, M.D.
Assistant Professor of Pediatrics, Division of Pediatric Hematology, Columbia University College of Physicians & Surgeons, Children's Hospital of New York, New York Presbyterian Hospital, Columbia Presbyterian Medical Center, New York, New York

Judith R. Marcus, M.D.
Clinical Professor of Pediatrics, Pediatric Oncology Division, Columbia University College of Physicians & Surgeons, Children's Hospital of New York, New York Presbyterian Hospital, Columbia Presbyterian Medical Center, New York, New York

Jill S. Menell, M.D.
Assistant Professor of Pediatrics, Pediatric Oncology, Columbia University College of Physicians & Surgeons, Children's Hospital of New York, New York Presbyterian Hospital, Columbia Presbyterian Medical Center, New York, New York

Tamara N. New, M.D.
Pediatric Fellow in Hematology-Oncology, Columbia University College of Physicians & Surgeons, Children's Hospital of New York, New York Presbyterian Hospital, Columbia Presbyterian Medical Center, New York, New York

Manuela A. Orjuela, M.D., Sc.M.
Assistant Professor of Clinical Public Health and Clinical Pediatrics, Department of Environmental Health Sciences/Division of Pediatric Oncology, Columbia University College of Physicians & Surgeons, Children's Hospital of New York, New York Presbyterian Hospital, Columbia Presbyterian Medical Center, New York, New York

Sergio Piomelli, M.D.
James A. Wolff Professor of Pediatrics, Director, Pediatric Hematology, Columbia University College of Physicians & Surgeons, Children's Hospital of New York, New York Presbyterian Hospital, Columbia Presbyterian Medical Center, New York, New York

Sujit S. Sheth, M.D.
Assistant Professor of Pediatrics, Pediatric Hematology, Columbia University College of Physicians & Surgeons, Children's Hospital of New York, New York Presbyterian Hospital, Columbia Presbyterian Medical Center, New York, New York

Maria Luisa Sulis, M.D.
Pediatric Hematology and Oncology Fellow, Columbia University College of Physicians & Surgeons, Children's Hospital of New York, New York Presbyterian Hospital, Columbia Presbyterian Medical Center, New York, New York

Michael A. Weiner, M.D.
Hettinger Professor of Clinical Pediatrics, Director, Herbert Irving Child and Adolescent Oncology Center, Hope & Heroes Division of Pediatric Oncology, Columbia University College of Physicians & Surgeons, New York, New York; Children's Hospital of New York, New York Presbyterian Hospital, Columbia Presbyterian Medical Center, New York, New York

Darrell J. Yamashiro, M.D., Ph.D.
Assistant Professor of Pediatrics and Pathology, Pediatric Oncology, Columbia University College of Physicians & Surgeons, Children's Hospital of New York, New York Presbyterian Hospital, Columbia Presbyterian Medical Center, New York, New York

PREFACE

Pediatric Hematology/Oncology Secrets is a new textbook targeted to physicians in training, practitioners, and other health professionals engaged in the diagnosis and care of children with blood disorders, cancer, and immune deficiencies. This book contains a comprehensive set of questions and answers to a variety of childhood disorders including hemoglobinopathies, hemolytic anemias, coagulation disorders, marrow failure syndromes, and immune dysregulation. Additionally, this text has a focused group of questions and answers dedicated to childhood malignant disorders including acute and chronic leukemias, lymphomas, and solid tumors. Furthermore, there is a state of the art discussion of molecular diagnostics and therapeutics, stem cell transplantation, emergency care, supportive care, palliative care, and psycho-social issues. This multidisciplinary and comprehensive review of pediatric hematology-oncology provides the reader with current "secrets" to the diagnosis and management of children with these specific disorders.

We trust that this book will be a valuable resource and will provide secrets that will enable our colleagues to enhance the care of children and adolescents afflicted with cancer and blood disorders.

ACKNOWLEDGMENTS

We wish to acknowledge the Herbert Irving Child and Adolescent Oncology Hope and Heroes Fund and the Pediatric Cancer Research Foundation.

Michael A. Weiner, M.D.
Mitchell S. Cairo, M.D.
Co-Editors

DEDICATION

To our patients, their families, and the entire staff at the Herbert Irving Child and Adolescent Oncology Center.

I. Hematology

1. DIAGNOSTIC APPROACH TO ANEMIA IN CHILDHOOD

Sujit Sheth, M.D.

1. Define anemia and indicate its prevalence.

Anemia is defined as a reduction in red cell mass or blood hemoglobin concentration. It results in a decrease in the oxygen-carrying capacity of the blood. A child may be said to be anemic when his or her hemoglobin is 2 standard deviations below the mean hemoglobin for that age. Therefore, 2.5% of the population is anemic at any time. The age-specific normal ranges are given in the table below.

Age-Specific Normal Hemoglobin Levels

	HEMOGLOBIN (g/dL)		MEAN CORPUSCULAR VOLUME (fL)	
AGE (yrs)	MEAN	–2 SD	MEAN	–2 SD
0.5–1.9	12.5	11.0	77.0	70.0
2–4	12.5	11.0	79.0	73.0
5–7	13.0	11.5	81.0	75.0
8–11	13.5	12.0	83.0	76.0
12–14				
Male	14.0	12.5	84.0	77.0
Female	13.5	12.0	85.0	78.0
15–17				
Male	15.0	13.0	86.0	78.0
Female	14.0	12.0	87.0	79.0
18–19				
Male	16.0	14.0	90.0	80.0
Female	14.0	12.0	90.0	80.0

2. Describe the classification of anemia.

The most precise way to classify anemia is based on its etiology, which provides a pathophysiologic approach. Two broad categories are used: first, failure of red blood cell (RBC) production and second, increased RBC destruction.

A. Disorders of red cell production
- Marrow failure syndromes
  - Aplastic anemia: congenital or acquired
  - Pure RBC aplasia: Blackfan–Diamond anemia, transient erythroblastopenia
- Marrow replacement: malignancies, osteopetrosis, myelofibrosis
- Impaired erythropoietin production: anemia of chronic disease, renal disease, malnutrition
- Erythrocyte maturation disorders: nutritional anemias, lead poisoning, erythropoietic porphyria

- Ineffective erythropoiesis: the thalassemia syndromes
- Primary dyserythropoietic anemias
- Sideroblastic anemias, myelodysplasias

B. Disorders of red cell loss or destruction
- Defects of hemoglobin: sickle cell disease, other structural mutants
- Defects in the red cell membrane: hereditary spherocytosis
- Defects in red cell metabolism: G6PD, pyruvate kinase deficiency
- Immune hemolysis
- Physical damage to red cells: mechanical (microangiopathic), thermal
- Chemical damage to red cells: oxidants, toxins
- Infectious agent–induced damage: malaria
- Paroxysmal nocturnal hemoglobinuria (PNH)
- Blood loss: acute or chronic

3. List the six critical elements of the initial work-up of a child with anemia.
- History
- Physical examination
- Complete blood count: hemoglobin/hematocrit, white blood cell count, platelets
- Mean corpuscular volume (MCV)
- Reticulocyte count
- Examination of the peripheral blood smear for RBC morphology

4. What is the differential diagnosis of childhood microcytic anemia?

The three most common conditions to consider when a child has microcytic anemia include

1. Iron deficiency anemia. This may be nutritional or secondary to blood loss, and the history provides important differentiating clues. The specific studies that may confirm this diagnosis are the serum iron, the total iron binding capacity (TIBC) and the serum ferritin. The transferrin saturation, the serum iron/TIBC, is always low (< 16%) in iron deficiency anemia, as is the serum ferritin.
2. The thalassemia syndromes, α (alpha) and/or β (beta). The diagnosis of homozygous β thalassemia is discussed elsewhere. Heterozygosity β (thalassemia trait) may be differentiated from iron deficiency by using Mentzer's index (MCV/RBC count in millions). An index of >13 indicates iron deficiency, whereas < 12 indicates the trait. Moreover, in thalassemia trait, the iron studies usually produce normal results, and hemoglobin electrophoresis reveals an increase in the amount of Hgb F and Hgb A2 (> 3,5%). α Thalassemia trait is a diagnosis of exclusion, which may be confirmed by genetic analysis of the globin genes.
3. Chronic lead poisoning with associated iron deficiency. A blood lead level is diagnostic.

5. How does one determine the differential diagnosis of normocytic anemia?

A normochromic, normocytic anemia occurs in the following conditions:
- Acute blood loss
- Hemolytic anemias
  - Autoimmune
  - Microangiopathic
  - Disorders of hemoglobin
  - Disorders of red cell membranes
  - Disorders of erythrocyte enzymes

- Marrow failure syndromes that initially are normocytic later may become macrocytic; low reticulocyte count, with other cell lines potentially affected
- Anemia of chronic disease
- Lead poisoning without iron deficiency

6. Describe the diagnostic approach for a child with a hemolytic anemia.

A patient with suspected hemolytic anemia has an elevated reticulocyte count, indicating increased RBC destruction and a compensatory heightened RBC production. The most important diagnostic test is careful review of the peripheral smear, which should provide direction for confirmatory tests that include Coombs' tests, hemoglobin electrophoresis, osmotic fragility and specific enzyme assays.

7. What is anemia of chronic disease, and what are the diagnostic features?

Anemia of chronic disease is the most common cause of anemia in hospitalized patients and those suffering from chronic inflammatory diseases. A common feature is the activation of cellular immunity in conditions as varied as chronic infections, autoimmune disorders and neoplasia. The underlying pathophysiologic mechanisms of this disorder are not clearly understood, though the diagnosis is easily made based on a normocytic or slightly microcytic anemia, low plasma iron, low iron binding capacity (as opposed to high, which occurs in iron deficiency states) and elevated plasma ferritin (low in iron deficiency). Transferrin receptor concentrations in the plasma are normal (increased in iron deficiency).

8. Give the differential diagnosis of macrocytic anemia.

Macrocytosis, defined as an elevated MCV, may result from the following conditions:

- Present in the normal newborn
- Anemia with a massive reticulocytosis, seen following a hemolytic episode in individuals with G6PD deficiency or hereditary spherocytosis
- Liver disease
- Hypothyroidism
- Down's syndrome
- Megaloblastic anemia, which may be nutritional (as in vitamin B12 or folic acid deficiency), may be the result of drugs that interfere with folic acid metabolism such as chemotherapeutic agents, or may be seen with inborn errors of metabolism such as orotic aciduria

9. What is the RBC distribution width (RDW), and what is its significance?

The size of RBCs varies along a narrow distribution curve around the mean, which is the MCV. The RDW gives us an idea of the variability in the size of the erythrocytes about this mean. It is increased in conditions in which there are populations of cells that vary from very small to very large (anisocytosis). It is useful to distinguish the microcytic anemias: thalassemia trait (normal RDW) from iron deficiency (increased RDW), and chronic lead poisoning (markedly increased RDW). The RDW may also be increased in autoimmune hemolytic anemias, in B12-deficient individuals receiving supplements and following a blood transfusion when two distinct populations of cells are present.

10. Define Howell-Jolly bodies and name some of the other inclusions seen in erythrocytes.

These are small, peripheral, darkly stained inclusions in the erythrocyte that represent nuclear remnants. They are seen in asplenic and hyposplenic states, pernicious anemia, dyserythropoeitic anemias and severe iron deficiency. Other inclusions are Cabot's rings, Heinz bodies and basophilic stippling.

11. Describe the significance of target cells and name other red cell morphologic abnormalities on smear.

Target cells, as the name implies, appear to have a central area of hemoglobin surrounded by an area of clearing, which in turn is surrounded by the rest of the cellular hemoglobin. Target cells may be seen on the peripheral smears of individuals with the following conditions:

- Hemoglobinopathies (S, C, D and E) and the thalassemia syndromes
- Hypochromic-microcytic anemias
- Obstructive liver disease
- After splenectomy

Other morphologic abnormalities include spherocytes, poikilocytes, elliptocytes, sickle cells, schistocytes and acanthocytes.

BIBLIOGRAPHY

1. Glader BE: Hemolytic anemia in children. Clin Lab Med 19(1):87–111, 1999.
2. Nathan DG, Orkin SH (eds): Hematology of Infancy and Childhood, 5th Ed. Philadelphia, W.B. Saunders Company, 1998.
3. Hoffbrand AV, Herbert V: Nutritional anemias. Semin Hematol 36(4 suppl 7):13–23, 1999.

2. DEVELOPMENTAL HEMATOLOGY

Sergio Piomelli, M.D.

1. Define fetal erythropoiesis.

In the fetus, at approximately the 4th gestational week, erythropoiesis begins. It is prevalently extravascular in the yolk sac. By the 5th gestational week erythropoiesis starts to appear in the liver. Only in the last trimester the erythropoiesis (and myelopoiesis) takes place in the bone marrow. Simultaneously, major changes occur in the structure of hemoglobin. First, embryonic hemoglobins are formed, then these are replaced by fetal hemoglobin; ultimately, adult hemoglobin predominates.

The first chains to develop are the ϵ chains, similar in structure to the β chains. The ϵ chains initially form symmetrical tetramers (ϵ^4). Next, other embryonic hemoglobins develop: The ζ chains with the ϵ chains form the tetramer $\zeta^2\epsilon^2$. These primitive hemoglobins are called Gower-1.

Slowly the α chain develops. Initially, it pairs with the ϵ chain and forms the complex $\alpha^2\epsilon^2$: the Gower-2 hemoglobin. Finally, the γ chain appears. It first pairs with the ζ chain to form the tetramer $\zeta^2\gamma^2$ (Hgb Portland). Finally, fetal hemoglobin (hemoglobin F = $\alpha^2\gamma^2$) is formed.

In the third trimester, the adult β chain appears, and adult-type hemoglobin (hemoglobin A = $\alpha^2\beta^2$) progressively replaces the hemoglobin F. At birth, approximately 40–60% of the hemoglobin is hemoglobin A. The fetal Hb continues to decline after birth and reaches the very low (1–2%) adult level by 4–5 months of age.

2. Describe erythropoiesis at birth.

At birth, the hemoglobin level is very high (15–18 g/dL) and the red cells are extremely large (120–130μ^3). As the erythropoiesis progressively turns to mostly Hgb A, the red cells decrease in size to <80 μ^3 and the hemoglobin concentration drops to 11–12 g/dL. This low concentration persists throughout infancy and ultimately at puberty starts to slowly rise toward the adult level.

Disorders of Hemoglobin in the Neonatal Period

3. How does occult blood loss before delivery occur?

In most pregnancies, some fetal cells are found in the maternal circulation. In nearly 40% of these pregnancies, up to 40 mL of fetal blood is present in the maternal circulation. Only in a small percentage of cases (<1%), the blood loss is greater and results in fetal anemia. This situation can be usually easily diagnosed by staining the blood film of the mother for fetal cells.

Fetal to fetal transfusion occurs frequently in mozorygotic twins, resulting in one anemic and one polycythemic newborn.

4. Discuss hemoglobinopathies and thalassemias at birth.

Most hemoglobinopathies are not clinically obvious at birth, since fetal hemoglobin synthesis persists and thus obscures the detection of hemoglobins that are abnormal in the β chains.

However, defects of the α chains are clinically obvious in the neonatal period. Normal newborns have four α genes. Newborns with α-thalassemia trait (two or three α genes) show microcytosis and traces of Hgb Bart (γ^4). Newborns with Hgb H disease (one α gene only) show larger concentrations of Hgb Bart and some Hgb H (β^4) and are significantly anemic.

Hydrops fetalis occurs in those fetuses that are homozygous for α-thalassemia (no α genes). As soon as embryonic eythropoiesis stops, these fetuses become profoundly anemic in utero; this leads to congestive heeart failure and diffuse edema (hydropo). When unrecognized, this syndrome is fatal in utero. However, if the diagnosis is made in utero, the fetus may reach gestation with repeated intrauterine transfusions. The newborn will then need chronic transfusion, as the absence of α chains precludes the synthesis of any hemoglobin.

5. Describe other disorders of hemoglobin.

A number of hemoglobin variants have been described. Those that result in a reduction of the red cell life span are of clinical significance. At variance with thalassemia (when hemoglobin synthesis is decreased or absent), in most hemoglobinopathies, the synthesis of hemoglobin is normal, but the hemoglobin function is abnormal.

Hemoglobin defects can result from replacement of one or two amino acids (resulting from a single base substitution in the codon). Depending on the type and the position of the amino acid replacement, the effect on red cell survival may be different. Other hemoglobin defects may be caused by amino acid deletion or to non-homologous crossover, resulting in a fusion hemoglobin, such as Hgb Lepore. In this hemoglobinopathy, the hemoglobin synthesis if impaired, leading to a thalassemia-like syndrome. A different type of abnormality may result from an error in the termination codon. A classic example is hemoglobin Constant Spring, frequent in Southeast Asia; it also leads to a thalassemia-like syndrome.

The most classic example of abnormal hemoglobin resulting from a single base substitution is the replacement of glutamic acid with glycine in the sixth amino-acid position (hemoglobin S). This single change results in a tendency of the hemoglobin molecules to polymerize into filamentous structure when deprived of oxygen, leading to intracellular sickling. When Hgb S is inherited in the homozygous state, this leads to a severe syndrome: Hgb SS, or sickle cell anemia. The effects are profound on all body systems affected by the intravascular sickling and the consequent tissue hypoxia. The replacement of glutamic acid with lysine in the same sixth amino acid position instead results in hemoglobin C, by itself a rather inoffensive alteration. In heterozygous individuals, Hgb C is only manifested by the diffuse presence of target cells, without anemia. In the homozygous individual, it only induces a modest asymptomatic anemia with diffuse targeting. However, when an individual is a compound heterozygote, inheriting both hemoglobins S and C, the resulting clinical manifestation is a mild form of sickle cell anemia.

Individuals who inherit the Hgb S gene and the gene for β-thalassemia are also affected by a clinical syndrome (Hgb S-thalassemia) of a severity comparable to homozygous sickle cell disease. If, however, the gene for thalassemia results in the synthesis of some Hgb A, although at a reduced rate (thalassemia plus), the clinical severity is substantially mitigated.

6. Discuss hemoglobin variants with abnormal function.

Unstable hemoglobins precipitate inside the red cells, leading to the formation of Heinz bodies and to intravascular hemolysis. Iindividuals with these defects are usually heterozygous, as the homozygous state (certainly extremely rare) would be incompatible with life.

Methemoglobins are a group of hemoglobin variants that lead to asymptomatic cyanosis; they have a spectrum similar to that of methemoglobin. Individuals with these hemoglobin abnormalities are heterozygous, have a large concentration of Hgb A and, apart from the cyanosis, are totally asymptomatic. The more common cause of congenital methemoglobinemia, however, reflects a defect in the enzyme methemoglobin reductase, not a hemoglobin defect.

BIBLIOGRAPHY

1. Oski F: The erythrocyte and its disorders. In Nathan D, Oski F (eds): Hematology of Infancy and Childhood, 4th ed. Philadelphia, W.B. Saunders, pp 18–23.

3. SICKLE CELL SYNDROMES

Sujit Sheth, M.D.

1. What are the different disorders described by the term sickle cell disease?

Sickle cell disease encompasses a variety of symptomatic disorders, including homozygous sickle cell disease or HbSS disease; double heterozygotes for HbS; and a host of different genetic mutations, including β thalassemia, Hb C, D, E, O and Lepore. In the United States, 60-70% of individuals with "sickle cell disease" have HbSS disease. Though HbSS and HbS-β^0 thalassemia are considered to be the most clinically severe forms of the disease, there is a great deal of heterogeneity in these disorders, and the severity is variable.

2. Describe the origin of the disease.

Sickle cell disease is believed to have originated in Africa, where it has a high frequency among populations exposed during evolution to the selection pressure of the malarial parasite. Herrick first described the disease in 1910 in a dental student. Individuals of African, Mediterranean, Middle Eastern and Indian ethnicity have the highest prevalence of the disease, though different genotypes occur in different regions. In the United States, HbSS disease affects primarily the African-American population and to a lesser degree, the Hispanic population of immigrants from the Caribbean. It is estimated that one in 8 to 10 African-Americans is a carrier of the trait.

3. What is the underlying pathophysiology of HbSS disease?

The cause of HbSS disease is a mutation in both of the β globin genes, which results in replacement of glutamic acid with valine at position 6 of the β globin chain. This in turn results in an abnormal hemoglobin, hemoglobin S, which polymerizes in its deoxygenated state and causes an alteration in the shape of the erythrocyte. It is this elongated, sickle-shaped cell that gives the disease its name. The abnormal rheology of these cells and the resultant increased viscosity and sludging cause obstruction of blood flow in the smaller venules and capillaries, giving rise to "vaso-occlusion," which is the pathophysiologic basis of most of the clinical manifestations of the disease. In addition, ongoing hemolysis also occurs and gives rise to chronic anemia.

4. What are some of the clinical manifestations of the disease?

Sickle cell disease may affect all of the organs of the body. Important clinical manifestations may be classified as to their etiology and include

Clinical manifestations secondary to hemolysis:

- Anemia: may be exacerbated following hyperhemolytic or aplastic "crises"
- Chronic jaundice: with exacerbations following episodes of hyperhemolysis
- Cholelithiasis
- Retarded growth and sexual maturation secondary to the chronic anemia

Clinical manifestations secondary to vaso-occlusion:

- Recurrent painful "crises" involving the musculoskeleton or abdominal viscera
- Functional asplenia and the resultant susceptibility to bacterial infections
- Stroke
- Splenic sequestration

- Acute chest syndrome
- Avascular necrosis of the femoral or humeral heads
- Chronic organ damage of the kidney, retina and brain
- Leg ulcers, which are particularly prominent in adulthood
- Priapism

5. Define splenic sequestration.

Pooling of blood in the spleen is a frequent occurrence in children with sickle cell disease, particularly in the first few years of life, resulting in what is termed "splenic sequestration crisis." The spectrum of severity in this syndrome is wide, ranging from mild splenomegaly to massive enlargement, circulatory collapse and even death. The diagnosis is usually clinical, based on the enlargement of the spleen with a drop in hemoglobin level by > 2 g/dL. Imaging studies are rarely required to confirm the diagnosis. It is more common in younger children who have HbSS disease and older children and adolescents who have HbSC disease, but it may occur even in adults. Children who have had one episode are far more likely to have a recurrent event, and the morbidity from this complication is significant. Hospitalization and transfusions are almost always required.

6. What is the etiology of the aplastic crisis in patients with sickle cell disease?

In an aplastic crisis, as the name implies, there is a shut down of the bone marrow that is usually limited to the red blood cell precursors. The patient becomes profoundly anemic and may go into high-output cardiac failure. Several viruses are associated with this syndrome in individuals who have a hemolytic disorder. The most common agent is parvovirus B19. This virus has a specific receptor, the P antigen, on the erythroid precursor. The condition is self-limited in most instances, but supportive therapy including transfusion may be necessary.

7. Is it possible to predict or prevent stroke in sickle cell disease?

Yes. Stroke in sickle cell disease results primarily from large vessel disease, with a lesser component of small vessel disease as well. Advances in noninvasive imaging techniques have made it possible to measure flow velocities in the large vessels in the neck and the brain. Flow rates are measured by transcranial doppler (TCD), and if the mean flow velocity is above an arbitrarily chosen 200 cm/sec, the individual is deemed to be at increased risk of stroke. These individuals are enrolled in a chronic transfusion therapy program that has been shown to prevent the first stroke in almost all patients found to be at risk by TCD.

8. What is the "acute chest syndrome"?

The acute chest syndrome is akin to a vaso-occlusive crisis in the lungs and results from occlusion of the microcirculation of the pulmonary bed. The "syndrome" consists of progressive respiratory distress and hypoxia, chest pain, and cough accompanied by infiltrates on a chest x-ray. The etiology is multifactorial and includes stasis, hypoventilation, infection, fat embolization from bone marrow necrosis and microthrombi in the pulmonary circulation, all of which may be involved singly or in combination. There is a massive inflammatory response, a capillary leak may develop, and there is progression to respiratory failure. Management usually includes an exchange transfusion, anti-inflammatory therapy and respiratory support.

9. Are there pharmacologic agents that may modify the clinical course of sickle cell disease?

Yes. Several agents have been used to help ameliorate the clinical severity of the disease. In the past few years, the two agents that have been shown to have some promise are hydroxyurea and butyrate. Both agents cause an induction of fetal hemoglobin synthesis, though the mechanism through which they accomplish this is not clear. Fetal hemoglobin inhibits sickling of the red cells and has been shown to reduce the severity and duration of vaso-occlusive crises.

10. Name the strategies employed for infection prophylaxis.

Functional asplenia develops in almost all individuals with HbSS disease by the age of 3–5 years. Along with stroke and acute chest syndrome, infection is the major cause of morbidity and mortality in children with this disease. Encapsulated organisms such as *Streptococcus pneumoniae, Haemophilus influenzae* and others are the main infectious agents. Penicillin prophylaxis is begun by age 3 months, and continued at least until age 6 years and longer, if possible. Pneumococcal vaccines, including both the new heptavalent conjugate vaccine as well as the older 23-valent polysaccharide vaccine, should be administered. All fevers in patients with sickle cell anemia warrant prompt evaluation, and parenteral broad-spectrum antibiotic coverage must be administered for 48 hours pending blood culture results and resolution of clinical symptoms.

11. Are there curative therapies for sickle cell disease?

Yes, two curative strategies exist for this disease. Bone marrow transplantation from a matched unaffected sibling is curative and has been shown to be safe and effective by several cooperative groups. Results with unrelated donors have been dismal, though the use of stem cells from umbilical cord blood has shown some promise. The other cure is gene therapy. Though vector-mediated transfection of marrow stem cells with the normal β globin gene is an attractive concept, its application to human sickle cell disease has proven to be an enormous challenge.

12. List the indications for chronic transfusion therapy in sickle cell disease.

Children who have already had a stroke must embark on a chronic transfusion program to prevent a second such insult. Following the STOP (stroke prevention) study, children with abnormal TCDs are treated in a similar fashion. Individuals with recurrent acute chest syndrome, severe debilitating pain and chronic organ failure may also be treated with transfusions, but these are usually not as long term. Besides the risks of reactions and the transmission of viral diseases through transfused blood, the major complication is systemic iron loading, which necessitates chelation therapy with deferoxamine.

13. How is HbSC disease clinically different from HbSS disease?

Individuals with HbSC disease tend to have a milder course than those with HBSS disease. They may retain some splenic function into their second decade of life and may thus also have splenic sequestration events later in childhood. In addition, for reasons that are not completely clear, individuals with HbSC disease tend to have more severe retinal disease and must therefore be observed closely.

BIBLIOGRAPHY

1. Embury SH, Hebbel RP, Mohandas: In Steinberg MH (ed): Sickle Cell Disease: Basic principles and clinical practice. New York, Raven Press, 1994.
2. Lane PA: Sickle cell disease. Pediatr Clin North Am 43:639–664, 1996.
3. Steinberg MH: Management of sickle cell disease. N Eng J Med 340:1021–1030, 1999.
4. Walters MC, et al: Bone marrow transplantation in sickle cell disease. N Eng J Med 335:369–376, 1996.

4. THE THALASSEMIAS

Sergio Piomelli, M.D.

1. Define thalassemia.

The thalassemias are congenital disorders of hemoglobin synthesis, when the formation of one of the two chains of hemoglobin (alpha or beta) is reduced or absent. The name *thalassemia* is taken from the Greek word *thalassa*, meaning sea; these syndromes were first described in populations living in the Mediterranean area.

2. What are α- and β-thalassemia?

α-thalassemia occurs when the formation of the α chain is affected. There are four α genes, and α-thalassemia results from the absence of one or more α genes. Individuals with two or three α genes are carriers of α-thalassemia (α-thalassemia trait). The only manifestation is microcytosis. Individual carriers of β-thalassemia (β-thalassemia trait) also have marked microcytosis. Neither trait is clinically significant, but both are genetically relevant. The microcytosis of thalassemia trait needs to be differentiated from the microcytosis of iron deficiency. The easiest differential diagnosis is provided by the measurement of erythrocyte porphyrin levels, which are normal in thalassemia trait (α or β), but elevated in iron deficiency. (Rarely, an individual may have both iron deficiency and thalassemia trait.)

3. Define Hgb H disease.

Individuals who have only one α gene are affected by "Hgb H disease." In their bone marrow, the excess of β chains resulting from the minimal production of α chains leads to the formation of Hgb H. This is β^4 or a tetramer of β chains. Hgb H can carry oxygen but is quite unstablc. In Hgb H disease, the level of Hgb is quite decreased, and splenomegaly is usually present.

4. What is hydrops fetalis?

The total absence of α chains is incompatible with life. When the embrionic hemoglobin synthesis ceases in utero, this results in extreme anemia that leads to congestive heart failure and extreme edema (hydrops fetalis). When the diagnosis is established in utero, the fetus may be salvaged by intrauterine transfusion, but the newborn remains transfusion dependent for life.

5. Define β-thalassemia.

β thalassemia results from the failure of synthesis of the β chain of hemoglobin. The β thalassemias are subdivided into β plus and β minus, depending on the degree of suppression of the β chain synthesis—reduced in the β plus variants, absent in the β minus. In bone marrow normoblasts, the failure of β chain synthesis results in an accumulation of α chains. These precipitate within the cell that is destroyed within the bone marrow. The result is an extreme bone marrow expansion, but since the normoblasts are not viable, there is no production of red cells.

Thalassemia can result from a very large number of different mutations, although in specific regional areas, one mutation is usually predominant.

6. What is Cooley's anemia, or homozygous β-thalassemia?

This is the most severe from of β thalassemia. Children with this defect would, untreated, die by 1 or 2 yr of age. Chronic transfusions are required to sustain life. A regimen of chronic transfusion, maintaining a hemoglobin baseline above 9–10 g/dL results in prevention of all complications and a " normal life."

7. Discuss iron overload in thalassemia major.

The result of chronic transfusion is the accumulation of iron, since each transfusion unit contains approximately 200 mg. The body has no mechanism to eliminate excess iron. Thus, the transfused iron progressively accumulates, leading to death by hemosiderosis by 25–30 yr of age, unless chelation therapy removes the iron and achieves iron balance.

8. What is chelation therapy?

Iron can be eliminated from the body by drugs called chelating agents, that bind the iron and lead to its excretion in urine and/or feces. Deferoxamine B is the standard chelating drug. However, because of its rapid excretion in the urine, it is necessary to administer it by continuous infusion. Usually this is accomplished having a syringe pump 7 or 8 hr per day, usually at night. The treatment with deferoxamine B is cumbersome, expensive and difficult to cope with. However, extensive experience indicates that its use results in the achievement iron balance. Patients who cannot comply with this regimen succumb to the iron overload, usually by cardiomiopathy.

9. Discuss oral chelators.

Because of the difficulty with this regimen, an intensive search for an oral substitute iron chelator has been undertaken. L1 (commercially sold as deferiprone) is an oral iron chelator. Although less efficient than deferoxamine, it is easier to use, resulting in better compliance and thus in comparable iron excretion. However, recent studies have shown that this compound loses efficiency with time and may result in compromising liver function. Although these results are controversial, unless this risk is proven by larger-scale experiments, the use of deferiprone is not advisable.

10. How is bone marrow transplantation used to treat Cooley's anemia?

Cooley's anemia can be cured by bone marrow transplantation. This however, requires a compatible donor. Bone marrow transplantation is very successful in younger patients and does not cause severe liver damage or massive iron overload. In older patients or in patients with liver disease, however, the rate of fatality is prohibitive.

11. Define thalassemia intermedia.

This is a group of syndromes similar to Cooley's anemia. However, in thalassemia intermedia, a Hgb level of 6–7 g/dL can be maintained without transfusion. It may result from a combination of mild β-thalassemia genes, with or without interaction with α-thalassemia. Although these patients do not require transfusion, they have poor function (since most of their hemoglobin is Hgb F, a poor oxygen carrier) and later in life develop "pseudotumors" due to proliferation of their ineffective bone marrow. Therefore, they often must begin chronic transfusion in later life to attempt suppressing their enormously expanded but ineffective erythropoiesis.

BIBLIOGRAPHY

1. McDonagh KW, Nehuis A:. The thalassemias. In Nathan D, Oski F (eds): Hematology of Infancy and Childhood, 4th ed. Philadelphia, W.B. Saunders, pp 783–881.
2. Olivieri NF, Brittenham GM: Iron-chelating therapy and the treatment of thalassemia. Blood 89:739–761, 1997.

5. ANEMIAS SECONDARY TO ENZYME DEFICIENCY

Sergio Piomelli, M.D.

1. Discuss nonspherocytic hemolytic anemias.

With the exception of G6PD (glucose-6 phosphate deydrogenase) deficiency and pyruvate kinase deficiency, the anemias secondary to enzyme deficiency are extremely rare. To contrast them with hereditary spherocytosis (the most common inherited hemolytic anemia), they are often classified as nonspherocytic hemolytic anemias. In these anemias, the red cell morphology is normal, although often there is intense reticulocytosis, easily recognizable since the reticulocytes are red cells of larger size and exhibit a blue tinge on the peripheral smear.

G6PD deficiency is probably the most common genetic defect in the world, observed in millions of individuals in sutropical areas. Because it provides protection against malaria, its frequency increased progressively, reaching the current high levels in most subtropical areas. The protection against malaria is counteracted by the disadvantage resulting from the increased frequency of neonatal hyperbilirubinemia and kernicterus. This results in a "balanced polymorphism." Thus, in most populations involved, the maximum gene frequency is 25%.

G6PD is a sex-linked gene that resides in the X chromosome. Therefore, males may have the complete deficiency, while in most females the defect is only partial. Rarely,·in areas of extreme frequency, female with homozygous inheritance express the full deficiency. Since all female are a genetic mosaic, in some cells one X chromosome is active and the other is inactive. Thus, in female carriers of G6PD deficiency, some cells express the defective gene and some cells express the normal one. The inactivation of one or the other X chromosome (also called "lyonization," after Mary Lyon, who discovered the phenomenon) occurs at random in early development. The majority of heterozygous females have an approximately equal proportion of cell in which the defective or the normal chromosome is inactivated; thus, they exhibit approximately 50% of the normal activity. However, in the enzyme assay, some heterozygous females may appear normal (if in most of their cells the defective X chromosome is inactive) or completely deficient (if in most of their cells the normal X chromosome is inactivated instead).

2. What are the clinical manifestations of G6PD deficiency?

In the steady state, G6PD-deficient individuals only exhibit minimal compensated chronic hemolysis, evidenced by minimal anemia and slight reticulocytosis. However, when challenged by an oxidizing insult (such as naphthalene fumes, sulphonamides or primaquine tablets) the defective red cell cannot counteract the insult with increased production of the reduced form of niccotinamide-adenine dinucleotide phosphate, the normal antidote to oxidative insults. Thus, the defective cells are acutely destroyed within the circulation, resulting in acute anemia with hemoglobinuria, since the hemolysis is intravascular.

The two most common variants of G6PD deficiency are the so-called B^- and A^- (defined by their electrophoretic mobility). The B^- variant is most frequent among Mediterranean individuals. The A^- variant is nearly exclusively found among individuals of African origin. Individuals with the B^- variant, when challenged by an oxidizing insult, experience extreme hemolysis that may lead to death by acute anemia. The A^- variant is less severe, as it results from the production of an unstable enzyme. These individuals have young red cells that are not deficient; however, as the cells age, the deficiency becomes manifest in the older red cells. Thus A- individuals, when challenged by an oxidizing agent, exhibit much less severe anemia and rarely have hemoglobinuria. Once the older, defective cells have been removed, continuation of the oxidizing agent leads to a continuous compensated hemolysis.

Pyruvate kinase deficiency is the most frequent of these disorders. In the glycolytic pathway, this enzyme converts phosphoenolpyruvate to pyruvate, which is then converted by lactic dehydrogenase into lactate. The enzyme defect results in a block in glycolysis at this level, with consequent accumulation of 2-3 dyphosphoglycerate (2-3 DPG) upstream. This is characteristic of this defect and may lead to the diagnosis, even without enzyme assay. Pyruvate kinase deficiency is an extremely severe hemolytic anemia, characterized by intense reticulocytosis and splenomegaly. It induces severe hyperbilirubinemia in the newborn period and may rarely even result in utero in anemia so severe as to lead to cardiac failure and generalized edema (hydrops fetalis).

3. How is pyruvate kinase deficiency treated?

The treatment of choice is splenectomy. This results in stabilization of the Hgb level at a value compatible with normal activity. (The increased 2-3 DPG favors the release of oxygen from the hemoglobin.) There is a paradoxical increase in reticulocytes that may reach as high as 50–70%. Retyculocytes are, in fact, the only cells capable of survival in these patients. Removal of the spleen facilitates their entrance in the circulation; thus, while this ameliorates the anemia, the percentage of reticulocytes is enormously increased.

4. Describe the less-common anemias secondary to enzyme deficieny.

Anemia secondary to defects of all the other enzymes of glucose metabolism have been described, but they are extremely rare. Some defects, such as triose-isomerase-deficiency, have been reported to be associated with hemolysis and mental retardation.

5. What is phospho-fructose-kinase deficiency?

This defect results in markedly decreased concentrations of 2-3 DPG, one of its downstream products. Since this compound modulates the affinity of hemoglobin for oxygen, in the homozygous form of this enxymatic defect, there is paradoxically polycythemia resulting from the cellular relative hypoxia in association with reticulocytosis.

BIBLIOGRAPHY

1. Luzzatto L: G6PD deficiency and hemolytic anemia. In Nathan D, Oski F (eds): Hematology of Infancy and Childhood, 4th ed. Philadelphia, W.B. Saunders, pp 674–695.
2. Mentzer WC: Pyruvate kinase deficiency and disorders of glucolysis. In Nathan D, Oski F (eds): Hematology of Infancy and Childhood, 4th ed. Philadelphia, W.B. Saunders, pp 634–658.

6. ANEMIA SECONDARY TO MEMBRANE DISORDERS

Tamara N. *New,* M.D.

1. What are the different types of red cell membrane disorders?

Hereditary spherocytosis (HS), elliptocytosis, pyropoikilocytosis, stomatocytosis, acanthocytosis, and xerocytosis.

2. What is the pathogenesis of HS?

HS is an autosomal-dominant inherited hemolytic anemia, caused by a deficiency of a red cell skeletal protein. In the majority of cases, there is a defect of spectrin or one of the proteins involved in the attachment of spectrin to the membrane. The degree of spectrin deficiency directly correlates with the severity of the disease. This defect affects the mechanical properties of the red cell. There is a decreased surface/volume ratio, which causes spheroidal, osmotically fragile cells. Due to diminished deformability, cells are sequestered in the spleen.

3. What are the clinical and laboratory manifestations of HS?

Half of the cases present during the neonatal period or early childhood, with a picture consistent with a hemolytic anemia: indirect hyperbilirubinemia, anemia, reticulocytosis, splenomeagly, and a negative Coombs' test. Many times there is a positive family history. Some patients present at a later age with anemia, jaundice, splenomegaly, or with aplastic crisis, usually associated with a viral illness. The anemia may be mild or moderate, depending on the degree of compensation. The peripheral smear is characterized by small, dense, round, spherical red cells. The MCV is usually normal, with an elevated MCHC. Tests for osmotic fragility and acidified glycerol lysis are positive. Complications include erythroblastopenic crisis, causing a sudden and pronounced fall in hemoglobin and reticulocyte count; obstructive jaundice, due to gallstones; accelerated hemolytic crisis, due to pregnancy, severe illness, or exercise.

4. Describe treatment and management options.

Splenectomy eliminates the anemia and therefore reduces the reticulocytosis. Spherocytosis of the red cells continues; however red cell survival improves to near normal. For patients with only mild disease, folic acid supplementation and supportive care are the only requirements.

5. What is hereditary elliptocytosis?

An autosomal-dominant membrane defect, also involving dysfunctional spectrin. Similar to HS, there is a disruption of the surface/volume ratio, which disrupts the mechanical properties of the cell. Most individuals with this disorder are asymptomatic. A small percentage of patients have symptoms similar to those seen in individuals with hereditary spherocytosis. The osmotic fragility test may be normal or abnormal.

6. Discuss the clinical variations of hereditary elliptocytosis.

Mild hereditary elliptocytosis is the most common clinical form of the disease. Patients are symptom free, with normal spleen size and hemoglobin levels. There is often mild, compensated hemolysis with mild reticulocytosis. Individuals with more severe variants can have chronic or sporadic hemolysis. Infants with mild hereditary elliptocytosis are often born with moderately severe hemolytic anemia. These patients present with neonatal jaundice, poikilocytosis, and elliptocytosis. A minority of patients develop dysplastic and ineffective erythropoiesis, with low reticulocyte counts and indirect hyperbilirubinemia. Treatment is the same as for HS.

7. What is hereditary pyropoikilocytosis?

This is an uncommon form of congenital hemolytic anemia. Patients are severely anemic, with hemoglobin levels of 4–8 g/dL. The peripheral smear is contains red cell fragments, spherocytes, triangulocytes, and other bizarre-shaped cells. Patients present early in life with significant anemia, hyperbilirubinemia, and splenomegaly. Osmotic fragility testing is markedly abnormal. Some degree of hemolysis remains following splenectomy, but to a much lesser degree.

8. What is hereditary stomatocytosis?

This disorder is an autosomal-dominant hemolytic anemia in which red cells are characterized as "mouth-shaped." having linear central clearing. Some patients are asymptomatic, while others present with neonatal jaundice, splenomegaly, and anemia. The defect disrupts the cells' water balance, causing cell swelling, cell rigidity, and decreased red cell survival. Splenectomy reduces the rate of hemolysis for more severe patients.

9. What is hereditary acanthocytosis?

This is an autosomal-recessive disorder, characterized by mild hemolytic anemia, fat malabsorption, and a neurologic movement disorder. The distinct appearance of acanthocytes, with irregular projections of various lengths, can be seen in this rare condition or more commonly in acquired conditions: uremia, microangiopathic hemolytic anemia, and cirrhosis.

10. Define xerocytosis.

In this familial disorder, red cells become dehydrated due to altered membrane permeability. Although patients with this condition may have moderate anemia and reticulocytosis, they have relatively few symptoms. Therefore, these patients rarely require treatment.

BIBLIOGRAPHY

1. Lanzkowsky P: Manual of Pediatric Hematology and Oncology, 2nd ed. New York, Churchill Livingstone, 1995, pp 104–111.
2. Nathan DG, Orkin SH: Nathan and Oski's Hematology of Infancy and Childhood, 5th ed. Vol. 1. Philadelphia.W. B. Saunders Company, 1998, pp 544–664.

7. AUTOIMMUNE HEMOLYTIC ANEMIA

Maria Luisa Sulis, M.D.

1. What is the definition of autoimmune hemolytic anemia?

Autoimmune hemolytic anemia (AIHA) occurs secondary to premature destruction of red cells by autoantibodies that bind to antigens on the erythrocyte membrane.

2. Describe the classification of AIHA.

AIHA can be broadly classified as either primary or secondary:

- Primary or idiopathic
  - Warm antibody
  - Paroxysmal cold hemoglobinuria (PCH)
  - Cold antibody
- Secondary
  - Infection: viral, bacterial, *Mycoplasma*
  - Drugs: quinine, aminosalicylic acid, antibiotics, chlorpromazine, insulin
  - Lead
  - Malignancy
  - Systemic autoimmune diseases: systemic lupus erythmatosis, sccleroderma, rheumatoid arthritis
  - Immunodeficiency

3. What are warm and cold antibodies?

Warm antibodies usually consist of immunoglobulin (IG) that bind to erythrocyte membrane antigens more optimally at 37°C; they rarely fix complement. Cold antibodies consist of IgM that optimally bind to erythrocyte membrane antigens at 4°C; cold antibodies usually fix complement. IgG can sometimes behave as cold antibodies and are responsible for PCH.

4. What antigens on the red cells are the targets of the autoantibodies?

Warm antibodies usually bind to the Rh antigens, whereas cold antibodies usually bind to the I/i antigens.

5. What is the most common form of primary AIHA?

Warm IgG–mediated antibodies cause the most common form of AIHA in children. When cold antibodies are responsible for AIHA, they are usually associated with cold agglutinins that occur during infections, specifically during *Mycoplasma* infection and less frequently during infection with cytomegalovirus, Epstein-Barr virus or other viruses. Cold reactive antibodies cause AIHA more frequently in adults.

6. Define PCH.

PCH is a form of autoimmune hemolysis caused by an IgG autoantibody called the Donath-Landsteiner autoantibody. Unlike most IgG, this autoantibody binds to the antigen at cold temperature and can fix complement. The Coombs test may be negative or positive only for complement, so specific diagnostic procedures must be performed to detect this antibody. The degree of hemolysis is usually mild.

7. Is the hemolysis associated with AIHA intravascular or extravascular?

IgM molecules, cold antibodies, are large and can fix complement on the surface of the red blood cell; thus, hemolysis is frequently intravascular. IgG molecules, warm antibodies, are much smaller. They rarely fix complement on the surface of the red blood but instead "coat" the erythrocyte membrane. The coated red cells are then trapped and destroyed in the spleen; thus, hemolysis if frequently extravascular.

8. Discuss the signs and symptoms of AIHA.

The most frequent signs and symptoms in a child with AIHA include fatigue, exercise intolerance, and the passage of dark urine. The physical exam reveals a pale or icteric child; tachycardia and flow murmur may be present as well as hepatosplenomegaly.

9. What are the laboratory findings in AIHA?

The hemoglobin concentration can vary but is usually quite depressed—between 5 and 7 g/dL. The white blood cell count and platelet count are normal. The red blood cell indices are usually within normal limits. The peripheral smear reveals the presence of small spherocytes, schistocytes, and polychromasia secondary to the compensatory reticulocytosis. The indirect bilirubin is elevated, as is the lactic dehydrogenase. The haptoglobin level is low. If the hemolysis is extravascular secondary to warm IgG antibodies, the urine will be normal. The urine will be dark (tea color or Coca-Cola color) if the hemolysis is intravascular secondary to the hemoglobinuria associated with IgM cold antibodies.

10. What is the most helpful laboratory test to establish the diagnosis of AIHA?

The direct Coombs test is the most important laboratory test to confirm the diagnosis of AIHA. The direct Coombs test identifies IgG or complement on the surface of the red blood cell. When only the complement is detected, IgM molecules, cold antibodies, are most likely responsible for the hemolysis. When cold hemolysis is suspected, the Coombs test can be performed at a lower temperature (<37°C) to detect the autoantibodies. Occasionally the Coombs test can be negative in the setting of hemoytic anemia when the titer of autoantibodies is too low to be detected.

11. What is the prognosis of AIHA?

AIHA mediated by cold antibodies is usually self-limiting, although it can be very dramatic. AIHA mediated by warm antibodies can follow a more chronic course.

12. Do patients with AIHA always need to be treated?

No. Only patients with symptoms related to the anemia or in whom the hemoglobin concentration is falling very rapidly require treatment. All patients should be carefully monitored, and good urinary output should be maintained. If the patient has cold-reactive AIHA, keep him or her warm!

13. Describe the treatment options for patients with AIHA.

- Packed red blood cell transfusion: In most cases it is sufficient to transfuse packed red blood cells to reach a hemoglobin level of 6–8 g/dL to avoid cardiopulmonary compromise. At times it may be difficult to find compatible blood secondary to the possibility of hemolytic transfusion reaction.
- Corticosteroids: Corticosteroids may be beneficial especially in patients with IgG mediated warm AIHA; however, i frequently takes 24–48 hr before the effect of steroids may begin to elevate the level of hemoglobin. Recommended dosage is 2 mg/kg of Prednisone for 2–4 weeks, followed by slow tapeering over few months according to the hemoglobin concentration, reticulocyte level, and intensity of Coombs test.

- Intravenous IgG: The use of intravenous IgG may not be a very effective therapeutic option; however, its use is usually more effective in patients with IgM cold-mediated AIHA.
- Exchange transfusion or plasmapheresis may be effective acutely if a simple transfusion of packed red blood cells and corticosteroids fail to raise the level of hemoglobin.
- Splenectomy may be treatment of choice in chronic AIHA; however, it should be reserved to refractory cases of AIHA.

14. What is meant by the term *secondary* AIHA?

Perhaps more than 50% of the cases of the warm-reactive AIHA are secondary to systemic disease and frequently may be the presenting sign or symptom of a new-oneset systemic disease. More benign diseases, such as viral or bacterial infections, can be associated with AIHA that usually resolves once the infection is treated. AIHA is frequently seen in autoimmune diseases, lymphoproliferative disorders, and immunodeficiencies as a reflection of immune dysregulation.

BIBLIOGRAPHY

1. Lanzkowsky P: Manual of Pediatric Hematology and Oncology. 2nd ed. New York, Churchill Livingstone, 1995, pp 104–111.
2. Nathan DG, Orkin SH: Nathan and Oski's Hematology of Infancy and Childhood, 5th ed. Vol. 1. Philadelphia, W. B. Saunders Company, 1998, pp. 544–664.

8. ANEMIA SECONDARY TO IRON DEFICIENCY

Gary M. Brittenham, M.D.

1. What is the most common cause of anemia?

Iron deficiency continues to be the most common cause of anemia, both in the United States and worldwide. In the United States, the prevalence of iron deficiency has been decreased by the amounts of bioavailable iron in the diet, by food fortification, and by the use of iron supplements. However, iron nutrition remains a common problem in some subgroups of the pediatric population, especially toddlers and adolescent girls.

2. Define deficiency and name its stages.

Iron deficiency is a deficit in total body iron that develops when iron requirements exceed iron supply. Three successive stages of increasing severity of iron deficiency may be distinguished:

- Iron depletion: The first stage; consists of a decline in storage iron without a decrease in the level of hemoglobin or other functional iron compounds.
- Iron-deficient erythropoiesis: The second stage; begins when iron stores have been completely exhausted and the production of hemoglobin and other functional iron compounds becomes limited by the lack of iron. In this stage, the effect on hemoglobin production may not be detected by the standards used to differentiate normal from anemic states.
- Iron deficiency anemia: The third and most advanced stage; develops with a further decrease in the total body iron.

3. What signs or symptoms are considered highly specific for iron deficiency?

Pagophagia, koilonychia, and blue sclerae are three manifestations that are very specifically associated with iron deficiency:

- Pagophagia: A form of pica in which ice is the substance obsessively consumed. Pagophagia responds promptly to iron therapy, resolving within a few days to 2 weeks. Iron-deficient changes in the lingual or buccal mucosa have been postulated as an explanation.
- Koilonychia: Occurs when the distal half of the fingernails develop a concave or "spoon" shape resulting from impaired nailbed epithelial growth. Koilonychia are thought to be almost pathognomonic of iron deficiency but occur in only a small proportion of patients.
- Blue sclerae: Sclerae with a definite or striking bluish hue have been reported to be both highly specific and sensitive as an indicator of iron deficiency. The bluish tinge is believed to be the consequence of thinning of the sclera, making the choroid visible. Diminished collagen synthesis, caused by iron deficiency, is postulated as the cause of the thinning of the sclera.

4. Describe the major ill effects of iron deficiency in pediatric populations.

Defective psychomotor development in infants, impaired educational performance in schoolchildren, and diminished physical endurance are the major liabilities of iron deficiency that have been found in controlled studies.

5. What are the causes of iron deficiency?

The causes of iron deficiency are listed below. Any condition producing a sustained increase in iron requirements over iron supply can result in iron deficiency.

- Growth: During infancy, childhood, and adolescence, iron requirements may exceed the supply of iron available from diet and stores. Premature infants, with a lower birth weight and a more rapid postnatal rate of growth, have a high risk of iron deficiency unless given iron supplements. With rapid growth during the first year of life, the body weight normally triples, and iron requirements are at a high level. Iron requirements decline as growth slows during the second year of life and into childhood but rise again during the adolescent growth spurt.
- Blood loss: Loss of blood leads to increased iron requirements that result in iron deficiency. In adolescent females, menstrual blood loss often accounts for increased iron requirements. For adolescents who are blood donors, each donation results in the loss of 200–250 mg of iron. If the source of blood loss is not obvious, then gastrointestinal, genitourinary, and, rarely, respiratory blood loss need to be considered.
- Pregnancy: During gestation, the need for iron increases and without supplemental iron, causes the net loss of the equivalent of about 1,200–1,500 mL of blood. After delivery, if the infant is breast-fed, lactation increases iron requirements by about 0.5–1.0 mg/day.
- Inadequate supply of iron: An insufficient supply of iron may be responsible for the development of iron deficiency. In infants and adolescent females with high iron requirements, diets containing inadequate amounts of bioavailable iron contribute to the development of iron deficiency. The risk of iron deficiency is especially high when iron requirements are increased and the supply of iron is inadequate. For example, infants fed cow's milk often become iron deficient because of the combination of increased iron losses from cow's milk–induced gastrointestinal bleeding and the small amounts of iron of low bioavailability in cow's milk.
- Impaired absorption of iron: Defective absorption is an uncommon cause of iron deficiency. In some patients, intestinal malabsorption of iron is only one aspect of more generalized malabsorption. Gastric surgery, especially partial or total gastric resection, may result in iron deficiency. Iron deficiency due to impaired iron transport is rare.
- Impaired iron transport

6. Discuss the best laboratory methods to establish a diagnosis of iron deficiency.

The combination of the serum ferritin concentration and a new test, the serum transferrin receptor concentration, now make possible the diagnosis of iron deficiency in most clinical circumstances. In cases where both assessment of the iron supply for erythropoiesis and the morphological features of hematopoiesis are needed, bone marrow aspiration and biopsy is the reference method. Staining the marrow with Prussian blue provides information about macrophage iron stores by grading the amounts of marrow hemosiderin and the morphology and proportion of marrow sideroblasts. Sideroblasts are erythroblasts that contain one or more Prussian blue–positive granules, which can be identified by light microscopy.

7. How is the serum ferritin concentration used in the diagnosis of iron deficiency?

In healthy subjects, serum ferritin concentrations generally decrease with depletion of storage iron and increase with storage iron accumulation. If the serum ferritin concentration is decreased to less than about 12 μg/L, the diagnosis of iron deficiency is virtually established. By contrast, serum ferritin concentrations that are normal or elevated do not exclude iron deficiency. Serum ferritin is an acute-phase reactant, with the consequence that production and serum concentrations of ferritin increase with infection, inflammation, acute and chronic liver disease, and malignancy. In some instances, such as liver disease or chemotherapy, ferritin is released from damaged cells and/or the clearance of circulating ferritin is altered. Serum ferritin may also be increased by hemolysis and ineffective erythropoiesis. Thus, the serum ferritin concentration cannot be relied upon to make the diagnosis of iron deficiency in the presence of any of these conditions, all common in hospitalized patients.

8. How is the serum transferrin receptor concentration used in the diagnosis of iron deficiency?

Measurement of serum transferrin receptor concentration is a helpful new laboratory method for the diagnosis of iron deficiency that is especially useful in the presence of inflammation or infection. The transferrin receptor found circulating in plasma is a truncated form of the dimeric cellular transferrin receptor that is shed from cells. The serum concentration reflects the total body mass of tissue transferrin receptor. In normal subjects, about 80% of the cellular transferrin receptors are found on erythroid precursors in the bone marrow, and roughly the same proportion of the circulating soluble transferrin receptors is derived from these erythroid cells. Accordingly, erythroid marrow activity is the principal determinant of the serum transferrin receptor concentration. With erythroid hypoplasia, or aplasia, for example, in patients with aplastic anemia, red cell aplasia, or chronic renal failure, the serum transferrin receptor concentration is decreased. By contrast, with erythroid hyperplasia, the serum transferrin receptor concentration is increased (e.g., in patients with thalassemia major, sickle cell anemia, and other chronic hemolytic disorders). If erythroid hyperplasia can be excluded, an increase in the transferrin receptor concentration is highly specific for tissue iron deficiency. Unlike the serum ferritin concentration, the serum transferrin concentration is not increased with infection, inflammation, or liver disease. Thus, the serum transferrin receptor concentration provides a means of detecting iron deficiency even in the presence of chronic inflammation or infection and for distinguishing the anemia of iron deficiency from the anemia of chronic disease.

9. How is the combination of serum transferrin receptor concentration and serum ferritin best used to make the diagnosis of iron deficiency in the presence of infection or inflammation?

The serum transferrin receptor concentration becomes an even more effective laboratory measure of iron deficiency when used in conjunction with the serum ferritin concentration. The serum transferrin receptor concentration measures the degree of tissue deficiency of iron, whereas the serum ferritin concentration provides an indicator of the amount of storage iron in the body. Calculating the ratio of the serum transferrin receptor concentration to the logarithm of the serum ferritin concentration (TfR/log Ferritin ratio) provides the highest sensitivity and specificity for the diagnosis of iron deficiency. Figures 1–3 compare these measures of iron deficiency in a population of 129 consecutive anemic patients, all of whom had bone marrow examination, the reference method for determining the presence or absence of stainable iron in the marrow. Patients with no stainable iron and no coexistent disorder were diagnosed as uncomplicated iron deficiency anemia. Patients with marrow iron stores present and an infectious disease, a chronic inflammatory disease, or a nonhematological malignancy were considered to have the anemia of chronic disease. Patients with absent iron stores and an infectious disease, a chronic inflammatory disease, or a nonhematological malignancy were classified as having both disorders. As shown in Figures 1 and 2, measurement of the serum ferritin concentration alone or of the serum transferrin receptor concentration alone still left some overlap between the three groups of patients. The TfR/log Ferritin ratio provides an excellent means of detecting iron deficiency; in this population, the sensitivity and specificity were both 1.00. Thus, as shown in Figure 3, the ratio of the serum transferrin receptor concentration to the logarithm of the serum ferritin concentration (TfR/log Ferritin ratio) provides the best available means of diagnosing iron deficiency in the presence of chronic inflammation or infection.

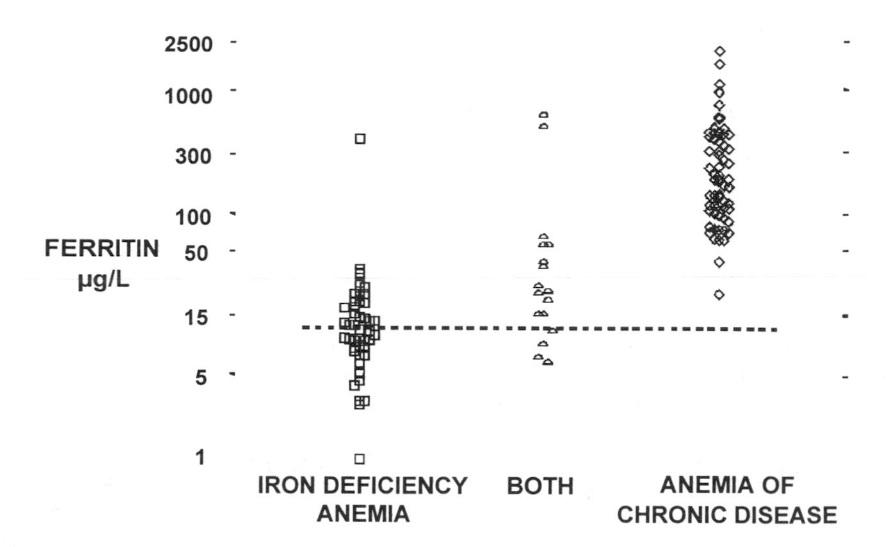

Figure 1. Serum ferritin concentrations in anemic patients with iron deficiency anemia (N = 48), the anemia of chronic disease (N = 64), or both (N = 17; these were patients with absent iron stores on bone marrow examination together with an infectious disease, a chronic inflammatory disease, or a non-hematological malignancy). The *horizontal dashed line* represents a serum ferritin concentration of 12 µg/L. (Redrawn from Punnonen K, Irjala K, Rajamaki A: Serum transferrin receptor and its ratio to serum ferritin in the diagnosis of iron deficiency. Blood 89:1052–1057, 1997, with permission.)

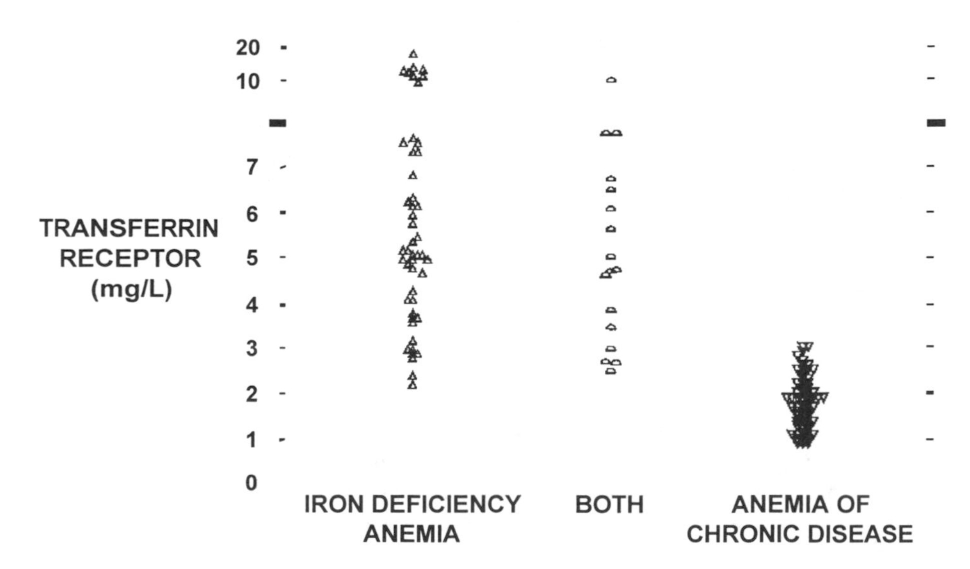

Figure 2. Serum transferrin receptor concentrations in anemic patients with iron deficiency anemia, the anemia of chronic disease, or both. (Redrawn from Punnonen K, Irjala K, Rajamaki A: Serum transferrin receptor and its ratio to serum ferritin in the diagnosis of iron deficiency. Blood 89:1052–1057, 1997, with permission.)

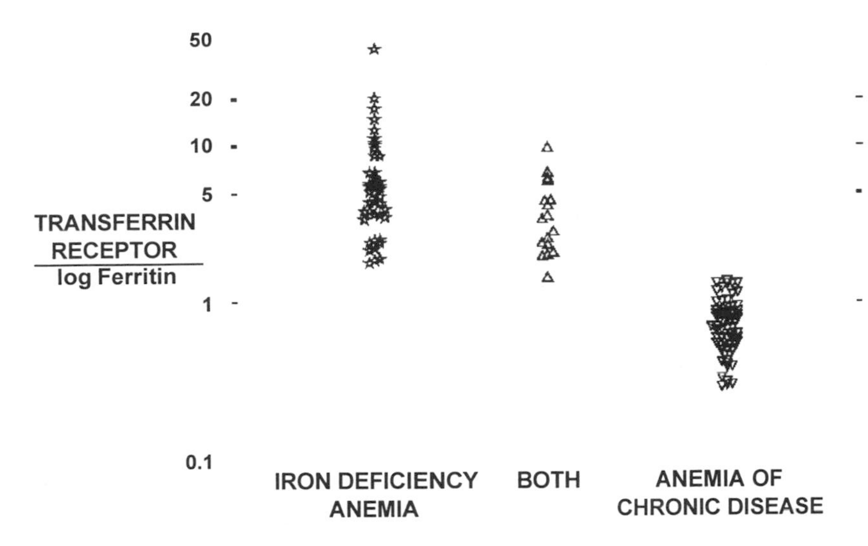

Figure 3. The ratio of the serum transferrin receptor concentration to the log of the serum ferritin concentration in anemic patients with iron deficiency anemia, the anemia of chronic disease, or both. (Redrawn from Punnonen K, Irjala K, Rajamaki A: Serum transferrin receptor and its ratio to serum ferritin in the diagnosis of iron deficiency. Blood 89:1052–1057, 1997, with permission.)

10. What is the best therapy for iron deficiency anemia?

The goal of therapy for iron deficiency anemia is both correction of the deficit in hemoglobin and replenishment of body iron stores. Oral iron is effective, safe, and inexpensive; thus, it is the treatment of choice for almost all patients. Oral and parenteral treatment give similar results. Parenteral iron, with the attendant risks of local and systemic adverse reactions, should be used only in the uncommon patient who cannot absorb or tolerate oral iron or who have iron requirements that cannot be met by oral iron because of a refractory source of chronic blood loss. Rarely, red cell transfusion have to be used with the exceptional patients whose chronic rate of blood loss exceeds the rate of replacement possible even with parenteral iron.

BIBLIOGRAPHY

1. Brittenham GM. Disorders of iron metabolism: iron deficiency and overload. In Hoffman R, Benz EJ, Shattil SJ, et al. (eds): Hematology: Basic Principles and Practice. New York, Churchill Livingstone, 3rd ed, 2000, 397–428.
2. Centers for Disease Control: Recommendations to prevent and control iron deficiency in the United States. MMWR Morbid Mortal Wkly Rep 47:1–29, 1998.
3. Cook JD: Defining optimal body iron. Proc Nutr Soc 58:489–495, 1999.
4. Cook JD, Skikne BS, Baynes RD: Iron deficiency: The global perspective. Adv Exp Med Biol 356:219–228, 1994.
5. Hyman ES: Acquired iron-deficiency anaemia due to impaired iron transport. Lancet 1:91–95, 1983.
6. Kalra L, Hamlyn AN, Jones BJ: Blue sclerae: A common sign of iron deficiency? Lancet 2:1267–1269, 1986.
7. Looker AC, Dallman PR, Carroll MD, et al.: Prevalence of iron deficiency in the United States. JAMA 277:973–976, 1997.
8. Olivares M, Walter T, Cook JD, et al.: Usefulness of serum transferrin receptor and serum ferritin in diagnosis of iron deficiency in infancy. Am J Clin Nutr 72:1191–1195, 2000.
9. Punnonen K, Irjala K, Rajamaki A: Serum transferrin receptor and its ratio to serum ferritin in the diagnosis of iron deficiency. Blood 89:1052–1057, 1997.

9. NEONATAL ANEMIA

Jill S. Menell, M.D.

1. Describe the organs of hematopoiesis during embryogenesis and explain at what gestational age they are important sites of blood cell production.

Early in embryogenesis (~14 days after conception), the blood islands form in the yolk sac. These cells are derived from mesenchyme (embryonic connective tissue) and give rise to the blood vessels and the hematopoietic system. The liver is the next site of blood cell production that begins at 5 to 6 weeks of gestation and is the primary source of blood cells from the third to fifth months of gestation. The spleen contributes to blood cell production during the third to seventh months of gestation. The bone marrow begins to manufacture blood cells around the fourth month of gestation and becomes the primary site by the seventh month.

2. What are normal red blood cell indices for a newborn?

First day postnatal central hemoglobin values are generally 16–20 g/dL from 24 weeks of gestation onward. The MCV averages 135 fL at 24 weeks and gradually decreases to an average value of 119 fL at term. Hemoglobin values can vary by an average of 4 g/dL depending on whether the blood is obtained via capillary (i.e., heel stick) or venous route. The difference may be exaggerated in the sickest infants. It is important to take these factors into account when interpreting the results of blood counts in a newborn.

3. Give the reasons for relative polycythemia in the newborn and the decline in red blood cell production in the first week of life.

Fetuses are exposed to a hypoxic environment in utero. The placenta delivers 35–40 mm Hg of oxygen. The low oxygen tension leads to an increase in red blood cell production analogous to living at high altitudes with lower ambient oxygen levels. As the newborn infant breathes in a normal oxygen environment, red cell production drops dramatically. Within the first few days, production drops two to threefold and drops 10-fold by the end of the first week. Hemoglobin and hematocrit values tend to remain stable in a term infant during the first week and gradually drop to a physiologic nadir over several weeks. Preterm infants have a more rapid drop in their red cell counts, usually within the first week. This is due, in part, to a reduced red blood cell survival in preterm infants.

4. Why are preterm infants at greater risk for development of anemia than those who are full term?

Preterm infants do not have the benefit of longer gestation in the womb. The last trimester of pregnancy is when the most the growth of the fetus occurs. As the body grows, the red cell mass expands and serves as the major iron stores for the infant. Compared to the full term infant, the preterm infant has not had enough time in utero to accumulate sufficient iron stores. Anemia in preterm babies is confounded by a shortened red cell lifespan, iatrogenic blood loss and lack of a normal erythropoietin response.

5. How would you distinguish between acute and chronic blood loss in an anemic newborn?

An infant who experiences acute blood loss at birth exhibits distress—pallor, tachycardia, irregular respirations, weak pulses and hypotension. In general, organomegaly is not a presenting feature. An infant who has had a chronic feto-maternal transfusion is pale and is not in obvious distress unless heart failure has ensued. An infant with acute blood loss may have normal hemoglobin initially and then develop anemia as the blood volume equilibrates. Chronic blood loss presents as anemia in the cord blood. The red cell morphology is normochromic and macrocytic with acute blood loss and hypochromic and microcytic with chronic blood loss. A reticulocyte count is often elevated with acute blood loss but not with chronic loss. Serum iron and iron stores are depleted with chronic blood loss but are normal with acute blood loss. Iron therapy is indicated for both situations; however, the infant with acute blood loss may need resuscitation and transfusions.

6. Describe the approach for treating a newborn with anemia.

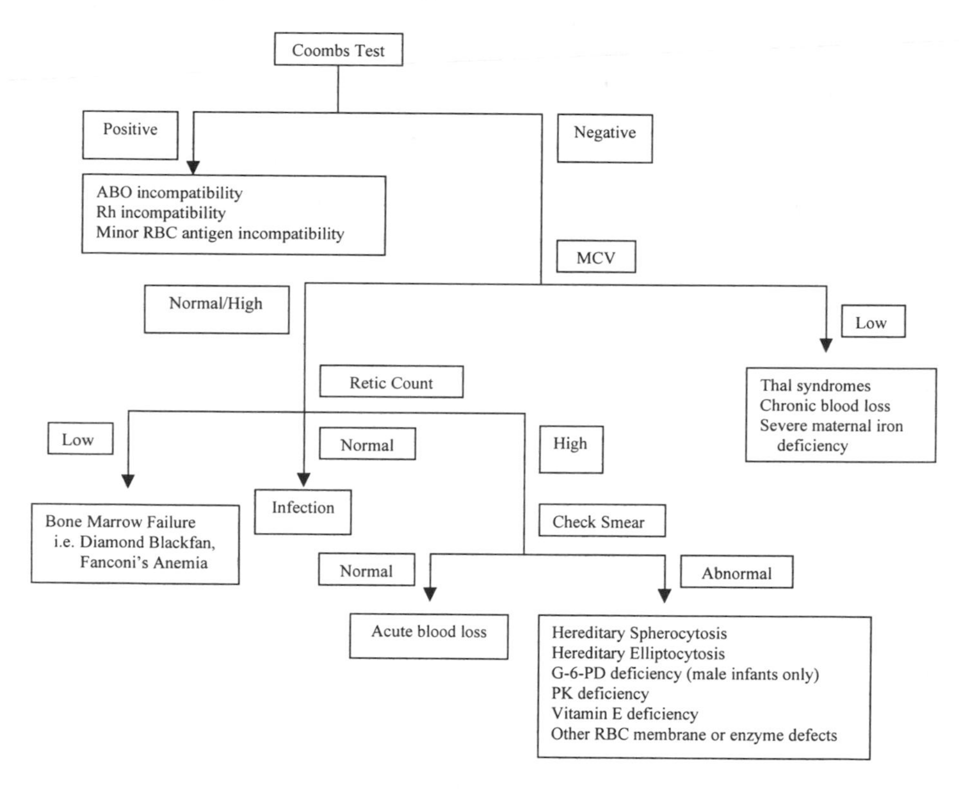

Figure 1. Schematic diagram for the work-up of anemia in the newborn

The initial laboratory studies to evaluate a newborn with anemia are maternal and infant blood types, direct Coombs' test, reticulocyte count, MCV, examination of the peripheral smear and bilirubin level. These studies will guide your further investigative work-up. Hyperbilirubinemia is reviewed below.

7. What are risk factors for feto-maternal hemorrhage and how is the diagnosis established?

Varying degrees of feto-maternal transfusion occur in about half of all pregnancies. Clinically significant bleeding occurs in less than 1% of births. The episode may be preceded by traumatic amniocentesis or external cephalic version. The infant's condition at birth depends on whether this is an acute event. Serum bilirubin levels tend to be low as the red cell volume is reduced.

The diagnosis is established by demonstration of fetal cells in the maternal circulation. The most common method is the Kleihauer-Betke technique of acid elution. The fetal hemoglobin is resistant to elution in an acid environment, whereas adult hemoglobin is not. The fetal cells stain pink and the adult cells do not. The volume of blood lost by the infant can be calculated from the percentage of fetal cells detected in the maternal blood. This method can result in false-positive or exaggerated findings in instances where the mother may have an elevated fetal hemoglobin, as in β-Thalassemia trait, sickle cell disease, or hereditary persistence of fetal hemoglobin. The Kleihauer-Betke technique is not useful if there is an "ABO set up," as the fetal cells will be rapidly cleared from the maternal circulation.

8. Describe the causes of a microcytic anemia in the newborn.

The differential diagnosis for a microcytic anemia in a newborn includes thalassemia syndromes, chronic blood loss or iron deficiency anemia. Iron deficiency anemia is an extremely rare event in the newborn unless the mother is severely iron deficient. The placenta is very efficient at extracting iron from the maternal circulation. Iron deficiency may occur with chronic feto-maternal transfusion or in the anemic twin in a twin-to-twin transfusion.

As fetal hemoglobin contains alpha-globin chains, a person with deletions of two or more alpha-globin genes will have microcytic red cells. The anemia is mild with two deletions (α-thal trait), more severe with three deletions (hemoglobin H disease) and profound with four deletions (hydrops fetalis). Newborn screening will often detect a fast-moving hemoglobin (Bart's hemoglobin, γ_4) when alpha gene deletions are present. More rarely, abnormalities of the gamma globin gene may cause a microcytic anemia in the newborn.

9. What is the risk for development of Rh immunization in an Rh-negative woman?

Half of pregnancies have some degree of feto-maternal transfusion. RhD immunization is not always predictable based on the volume of fetal cells. The prevalence of Rh immunization in ABO-compatible pregnancies is 16%. When ABO incompatibility is present, the risk is 1.5–2%. Spontaneous abortion confers a risk of 1.5–2% and the risk after a therapeutic abortion is 4–5%. The risk in any one pregnancy depends upon the blood group of the fetus. If the father is heterozygous for RhD, then there is a 50% chance that the fetus will be Rh negative. All offspring of a homozygous father will be obligate carriers and all pregnancies will be at risk.

Rh immunization can be reduced by 96% when prophylaxis with Rh immunoglobulins (RhIG) is employed. RhIG is administered to all Rh-negative pregnant women on performance of invasive procedures (i.e., chorionic villous sampling [CVS], amniocentesis, etc.), or spontaneous or therapeutic abortion, at 28 weeks of gestation and after delivery of an Rh-positive fetus. Since the inception of immune prophylaxis, the incidence of hemolytic disease of the newborn has been reduced dramatically.

10. Describe the optimal management of the fetus with Rh hemolytic disease.

The mother is screened at the first antenatal visit for alloreactive antibodies with an indirect Coombs' test. If antibodies are present or the mother has had a previously affected fetus, then the blood type of the fetus is determined. If the father is Rh negative, no further investigation is necessary. If the father is known to be homozygous for RhD then the fetus is an obligate carrier and is at risk. If the father's blood type is unknown or he is heterozygous, then the polymerase chain reaction can be used with CVS, amniocentesis or maternal blood (new technique) to detect the presence of the D allele. If the fetus is Rh negative, then no further invasive procedures are indicated.

A mother who has had a previous severely affected infant should be followed by percutaneous umbilical blood sampling (PUBS) at 20-22 weeks with determination of the fetal hematocrit. Intrauterine intravenous transfusion (IUIVT) should be given for a hematocrit <30%. A

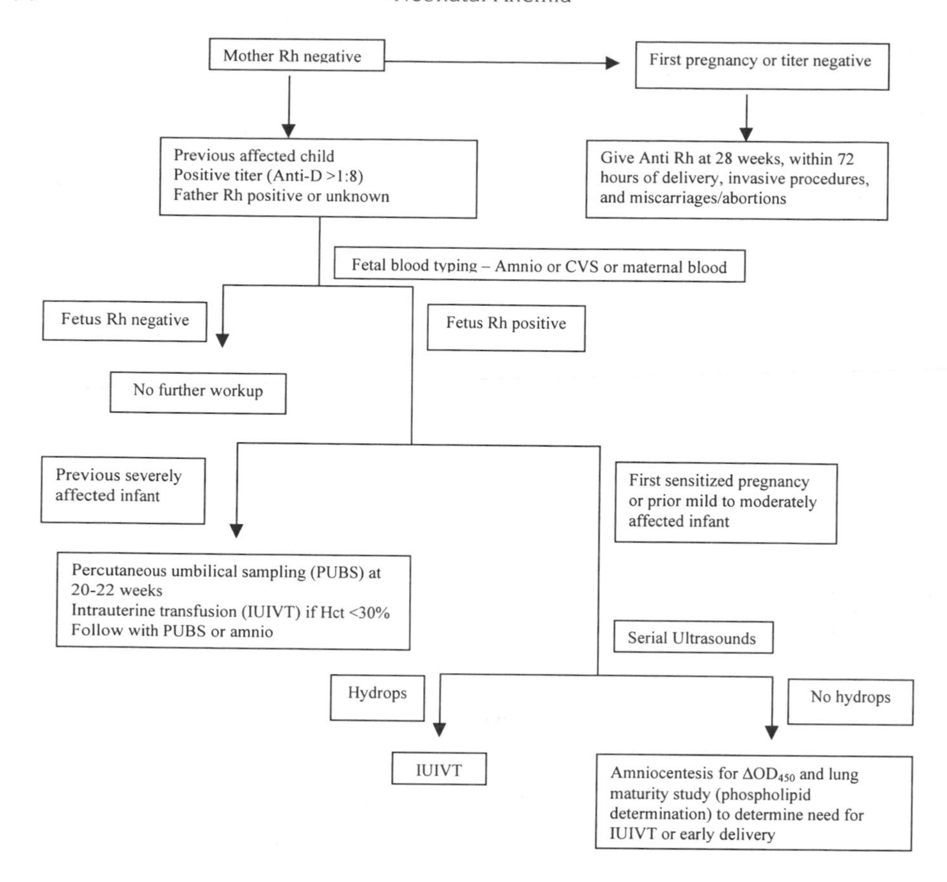

Figure 2. Algorithm for the care of an Rh-negative pregnancy

sensitized mother with no prior history or a mildly to moderately affected previous child should be followed by serial ultrasounds. Presence of fetal hydrops is an indication for IUIVT.

If hydrops is not detected, then an amniocentesis is performed to determine the optical density difference at 450 μm (ΔOD450) and the lipid profile. The ΔOD_{450} gives a prediction of the fetal outcome based on the methods of Freda and of Liley (Figure 3). The lipid profile measures lung maturity to determine if the baby may be delivered safely. If the ΔOD_{450} indicates that the fetus is severely affected and the lungs are mature, then the infant should be delivered. If the lungs are immature and the fetus is severely affected, then IUIVT is indicated. Transfused red cells should be Rh negative, CMV negative and irradiated.

11. Discuss the optimal management of the newborn with Rh hemolytic disease.

Transfusions in utero do not preclude a problem in the newborn period. Hyperbilirubinemia is generally more of a concern after delivery as the antibody and hemolysis persist. Hydropic infants will need ventilator support and immediate exchange. A partial exchange may be done initially to correct the anemia. In stable infants, phototherapy should be instituted immediately. The bilirubin should be followed carefully. If there is a rise of 1 mg/hr or the level is approaching 20 mg/dL in full-term (or 10–15 mg/dL in pre-term infants) within the first few days of life, then a double-volume exchange transfusion with Rh negative whole blood should be performed. This removes Rh-positive cells, bilirubin and the offending antibody. Bilirubin

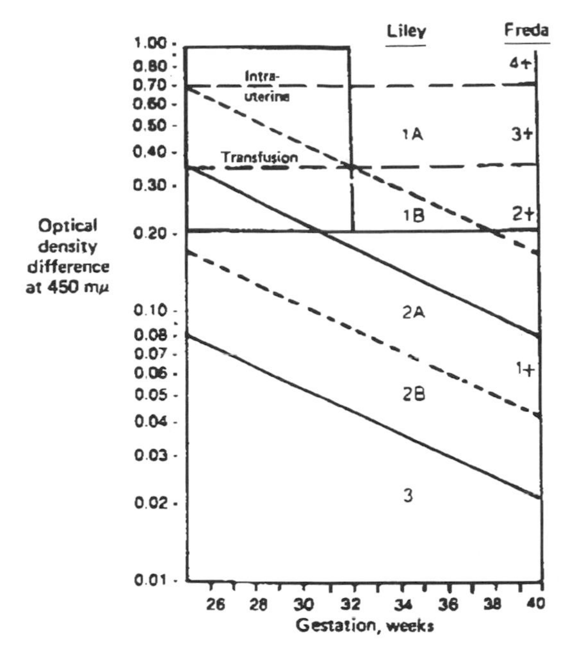

Figure 3. Assessment of fetal prognosis by the methods of Liley and of Freda. L iley's method of prediction. *Zone 1A*: Condition desperate, immediate delivery or intrauterine transfusion required, depending on gestational age. *Zone 1B*: Hemoglobin less than 8 g/dl, delivery or intrauterine transfusion urgent, depending on gestational age. *Zone 2A*: Hemoglobin 8–10 g/dl, delivery at 36–37 weeks. *Zone 2B*: Hemoglobin 11.0–13.9 g/dl, delivery at 37–39 weeks. *Zone 3*: Not anemic, deliver at term. Freda's method of prediction: *Zone 4+*: Fetal death imminent, immediate delivery or intrauterine transfusion, depending on gestational age. *Zone 3+*: Fetus in jeopardy, death within 3 weeks, delivery or intrauterine transfusion as soon as possible, depending on gestational age. *Zone 2+*: Fetal survival for at least 7–10 days, repeat amniocentesis indicated, possible indication for intrauterine transfusion, depending on gestational age. *Zone 1+*: Fetus in no immediate danger. (From Robertson JG: Evaluation of the reported methods of interpreting spectrophotometric tracings of amniotic fluid analysis in Rhesus isoimmunization. Am J Obstet Gynecol 95:120, 1966, with permission.)

and the anti-D antibody are not completely removed as they are in the interstitial tissues as well. The infant should continue phototherapy and be monitored frequently for continued hemolysis. A repeat exchange transfusion may be required for increased bilirubin. Infants who undergo exchange in the newborn period are more likely to develop early iron deficiency and should be followed for several months to ensure that they do not develop late anemia.

12. What is the diagnostic approach to jaundice in the newborn?

The following algorithm is a schematic approach to treating the neonate with jaundice (Figure 4). It is beyond the scope of this chapter to exhaustively review the work-up for each of these disorders.

Unless there is clearly hemolysis present, every newborn with jaundice should have one direct bilirubin determination to avoid missing a potentially devastating disorder such as biliary atresia.

13. Describe the reasons for "physiologic jaundice."

Jaundice in a newborn is usually present when the serum bilirubin is above 3 mg/dL.

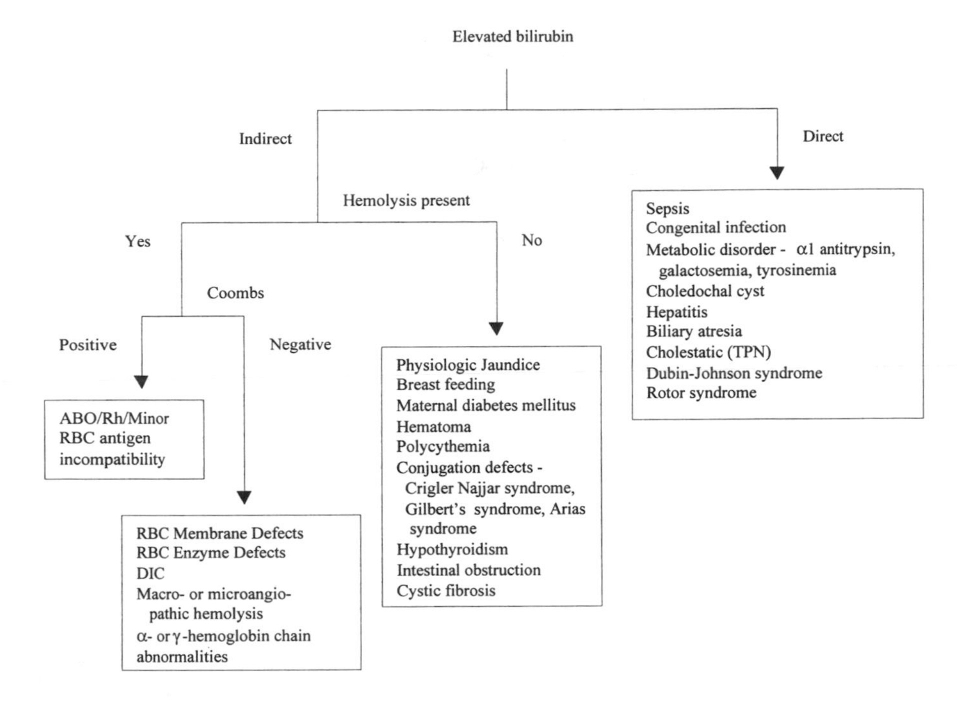

Figure 4. The approach to the jaundiced newborn

Physiologic jaundice results from an increased bilirubin load to an immature liver. Newborn red blood cells have a shortened life span as compared with adult red blood cells. The majority of bilirubin is produced from the breakdown of heme in senescent red blood cells. A shortened red cell life span leads to an increased bilirubin load.

The liver converts unconjugated bilirubin to a water-soluble (conjugated) form by a process called glucuronidation. The newborn's liver has a decreased capacity for bilirubin conjugation. Jaundice in the newborn is confounded by increased enterohepatic circulation of bilirubin. Abundant β-glucuronidase in the newborn intestinal mucosa hydrolyzes conjugated bilirubin. Newly formed unconjugated bilirubin is then reabsorbed into the portal circulation. Breastfeeding can increase enterohepatic circulation of bilirubin and prolong or exaggerate jaundice.

In a full-term infant, physiologic jaundice peaks at the fourth day of life at a level of approximately 12 g/dL. If the indirect bilirubin is greater than 7 mg/dL at 36 hr, then hemolysis is likely. Infants who are jaundiced beyond 7 days of life should be suspected of having a congenital disorder of bilirubin metabolism.

14. How does phototherapy work?

Bilirubin absorbs blue light in the range of 420–470 nm. Unconjugated bilirubin is highly water insoluble. When light photons pass through the skin of the newborn, the energy causes a conformational change in the bilirubin molecule. The newly formed substance is water-soluble and is excreted in the bile and urine without the need for conjugation. Increasing the body surface area exposed to the light maximizes phototherapy. The infant should be monitored carefully for hyperthermia and dehydration. In addition, the eyes should be shielded to prevent damage by ultraviolet light.

15. What are the indications for phototherapy and exchange transfusion?

The primary reason for intervention for unconjugated hyperbilirubinemia is the prevention of bilirubin neurotoxicity or kernicterus. This is due to direct damage to certain areas of the brain, including the basal ganglia, hippocampus, cerebellum and subthalamic nuclei by bilirubin. The physical signs of kernicterus include lethargy, poor suck, rigidity, impaired Moro reflex, opisthotonos, high-pitched cry and seizures.

The factors predisposing to kernicterus are not completely understood. Albumin binding of unconjugated bilirubin and the maturity of the blood-brain barrier are thought to be the two most important factors. Indications for phototherapy depend on the age of the patient, the gestational age and the general condition of the infant.

Current American Academy of Pediatrics guidelines recommend the following for a healthy term infant (> 37 weeks gestation):

Table 1. Guidelines for Phototherapy in the Healthy Term Infant

	TOTAL SERUM BILIRUBIN, mg/dL (pmol/L)			
AGE, hr	CONSIDER PHOTOTHERAPY	PHOTOTHERAPY	EXCHANGE TRANSFUSION IF PHOTOTHERAPY FAILS	EXCHANGE TRANSFUSION AND PHOTOTHERAPY
< 24	—	—	—	—
25-48	≥12 (170)	≥15 (260)	≥20 (340)	≥25 (430)
49-72	≥15 (260)	≥18 (310)	≥25 (430)	≥30 (510)
> 72	≥17 (290)	≥20 (340)	≥25 (430)	≥ 30 (510)

This table is useful only for those infants older than 24 hrs and those who are healthy. In infants younger than 24 hr, clinical jaundice is considered pathologic and should be worked up further. Early jaundice is likely related to hemolysis.

Phototherapy should lower the serum bilirubin 1–2 mg/dL within 4–6 hr and should maintain it at a level below the exchange transfusion level. If this is not the case, then exchange is indicated. Phototherapy is usually discontinued when the serum bilirubin drops below 10 mg/dL.

Infants younger than 37 weeks' gestation are at risk at lower bilirubin levels. Aside from gestational age, other factors affecting the integrity of the blood brain barrier and bilirubin binding to albumin include perinatal asphyxia, hypoxia, acidosis, sepsis, hypothermia and hypoglycemia. For premature infants or those who have had complications at birth, phototherapy and exchange transfusion should be considered at lower levels than those designated for the healthy term infant. For the infant with very low birth weight, phototherapy should begin at birth, and exchange transfusion should be considered when the bilirubin approaches 10 mg/dL.

16. Discuss the clinical features of ABO incompatibility.

As compared with Rh hemolytic disease of the newborn, ABO hemolytic disease is a much milder disorder in the majority of cases. There are several reasons for this. First, most anti-A and anti-B antibodies are IgM and do not cross the placenta. Usually only a small amount of IgG antibodies are present. Second, newborn red cells have fewer antigenic sites for A and B as compared with adult red blood cells. Antibodies work more efficiently when the antigens are in close proximity. Third, A and B antigens are expressed on many tissues within the body so that fewer "free" antibodies are available for binding to the red cells.

In ABO hemolytic disease, the mother is typically type O and the infant is type A or B. ABO incompatibility occurs in approximately 20% of pregnancies. Only 25–30% of pregnancies at risk will show a positive result on Coombs' testing. In general, fewer than 2% have severe enough hemolysis to require exchange transfusion. Jaundice is more prominent in ABO hemolysis than is severe anemia. Infants with positive Coombs' test results may be at risk for late anemia due to the persistence of the antibody. They should be monitored during the first months for an exaggerated physiologic anemia.

17. Describe the causes of non-immune hemolysis in the newborn.

Infants with hemolytic disease typically present with jaundice and splenomegaly. Causes of non-immune hemolysis include red cell membrane defects, red cell enzyme defects, disseminated intravascular coagulopathy, macro- or microangiopathic hemolysis, hemoglobinopathies (α- or γ-hemoglobin abnormalities).

Red cell membrane defects often present with hemolysis or hyperbilirubinemia in the newborn period. These include hereditary spherocytosis, elliptocytosis, stomatocytosis, xerocytosis and pyropoikilocytosis. As newborn red cells often have abnormal shapes, the exact diagnosis may not be apparent based on the peripheral smear. Hereditary spherocytosis will usually be obvious, whereas, the other disorders may not. A family history is important, as these are often autosomal dominant disorders. Osmotic fragility testing is not accurate in the newborn due to the nature of the fetal red cell.

Disorders of red cell enzymes may manifest with jaundice in the first few days of life. The most common is glucose-6-phosphate dehydrogenase deficiency. This should be suspected in male infants of African American or Mediterranean descent with jaundice. Measuring levels of the enzyme are not reliable when the reticulocyte count is elevated. Checking the maternal levels or specific DNA testing will establish the diagnosis. Pyruvate kinase deficiency is the next most common enzymatic defect. Other enzymes in the glucose metabolism pathways are much less common but should be considered after more common diagnoses have been excluded.

Infections leading to disseminated intravascular coagulopathy may be a cause of non-immune hemolysis. The infant often appears quite sick and has other abnormalities including a bleeding diathesis with thrombocytopenia. Prompt work-up and treatment of the underlying condition are imperative.

Macro- or microangiopathic hemolysis should be considered in infants with thrombocytopenia and hemolytic anemia not due to sepsis. The disorders associated with this include cavernous hemangiomas or hemangioendotheliomas, large thrombi, renal artery stenosis and severe aortic coarctation.

Defects in hemoglobin synthesis or structure are generally confined to the alpha and gamma chains, as they make up fetal hemoglobin. Beta chain defects, such as sickle cell disease and β-thalassemia do not present in the newborn period. Alpha- and gamma-chain structural defects generally are mild disorders as they only affect one gene. An exception is Hb Hasharon, which is a single amino acid substitution in the α-chain (14 Asp$\rightarrow$His) that produces an unstable hemoglobin more pronounced in fetal than adult hemoglobin. The hemolytic anemia usually lessens within the first few months of life with the switch to adult hemoglobin. Gamma-chain structural defects are often noted incidentally on newborn screening. HbF-Poole is a gamma-chain defect that presents as Heinz body hemolytic disease in the newborn period and resolves after a few weeks of life.

BIBLIOGRAPHY

1. American Academy of Pediatrics Provisional Committee for Quality Improvement and Subcommittee on Hyperbilirubinemia: Practice guidelines: Management on hyperbilirubinemia in the healthy term newborn. Pediatrics 94(4), 1994.
2. Bowman JM: Immune Hemolytic Disease. In Nathan DG, Orkin SH (eds.). Nathan and Oski's Hematology of Infancy and Childhood, 5th ed. Philadelphia, W.B. Saunders, 1998, pp. 53–78.
3. Brugnara C, Platt OS: The neonatal erythrocyte and its disorders. In Nathan DG, Orkin SH (eds.). Nathan and Oski's Hematology of Infancy and Childhood, 5th ed. Philadelphia, W.B. Saunders, 1998, pp. 19–52.
4. Jackson M, Branch DW: Isoimmunization in pregnancy. In Gabbe SG, Niebyl JR, Simpson JL (eds.).

Gabbe: Obstetrics—Normal and Abnormal Pregnancies, 3rd ed. Philadelphia, Churchill Livingstone, Inc., 1996, pp. 899–932.
5. Lanzkowski P: Anemia during the neonatal period. In Lanzkowski P (ed.). Manual of Pediatric Hematology and Oncology, 3rd ed. San Diego, Academic Press, 1999, pp. 13–32.
6. Robertson, JG: Evaluation of the reported methods of interpreting spectrophotometric Tracings of amniotic fuid analysis in rhesus immunization. Am J Obstet Gynecol 95:120–126, 1966.
7. Valencia GB: Neonatal jaundice. In Finberg L (ed.). Saunders Manual of Pediatric Practice. Philadelphia, W. B. Saunders, 1998, pp. 55–58.
8. Whitington PF, Alonso EM: Disorders of bilirubin metabolism. In Nathan DG, Orkin SH (eds.). Nathan and Oski's Hematology of Infancy and Childhood, 5th ed. Philadelphia, W.B. Saunders, 1998, pp. 79–113.

10. NORMAL HEMOSTASIS

Margaret T. *Lee*, M. D.

1. Discuss the mechanisms involved in hemostasis.

Hemostasis involves the interplay of the blood vessel, the platelets and the coagulation system to arrest or control bleeding from a site of vascular injury. When a blood vessel is damaged, the following events occur:

- Vasoconstriction
- Platelet adhesion and aggregation mediated by von Willebrand factor and fibrinogen forming a platelet plug
- Exposure of collagen and tissue factor from the damaged endothelium causes initiation of coagulation by the activation of factor VII and subsequent activation of a series of clotting factors leading to the formation of fibrin clot
- Regulation of extension of the blood clot by the natural anticoagulants
- Activation of the fibrinolytic system causing lysis of the clot
- Remodeling and healing of the injury site after control of bleeding

2. Describe the events that lead to the formation of a fibrin clot.

Coagulation is initiated by two mechanisms: the extrinsic and the intrinsic pathways. It is believed that the extrinsic pathway is the critical mechanism triggered in vivo in response to trauma, whereas the intrinsic pathway plays a role in the continued formation of fibrin. The extrinsic pathway is initiated when during an injury, tissue factor found in the cells surrounding the vascular bed comes in contact with and activates factor VII and forms a complex in the presence of calcium ions. The factor VIIa–tissue factor complex then converts factor X to Xa (as well as IX to IXa). Factor Xa binds to factor Va in the presence of calcium and phospholipid and forms the prothrombinase complex that rapidly converts prothrombin to thrombin. In the intrinsic pathway, factor Xa is formed by a series of enzymatic conversion of factor XII, factor XI, prekallikrein, high-molecular-weight kininogen and factor IX. The activated factor IX, along with factor VIIIa as a cofactor in the presence of calcium and phospholipid, then forms the tenase complex, which converts factor X to Xa. Thrombin generated from these pathways is a key effector enzyme that converts fibrinogen to fibrin. It also causes feedback amplification of coagulation by activation of factors V, VIII, XI and XIII. Fibrin is then covalently crosslinked by factor XIIIa to form a stabilized clot.

3. Discuss the regulation of blood coagulation by the anticoagulant or inhibitor pathway.

Blood coagulation is regulated by several natural anticoagulants to limit and localize thrombus formation at the site of injury. This occurs at each level of the pathway either by enzyme inhibition or by modulation of its cofactors. The tissue factor pathway inhibitor (TFPI) inactivates the factor VIIa–tissue factor complex. Antithrombin III inactivates thrombin and other serine proteases (XIIa, XIa, Xa and IXa). Its action is enhanced in the presence of heparin or heparan sulfate in the vessel wall. The protein C system inactivates factors Va and VIIIa. This is initiated by thrombin, which binds to thrombomodulin (an endothelial cell membrane protein) and forms activated protein C (APC). APC acts most efficiently in the presence of its cofactor protein S, which exists in the plasma as either a free protein or bound to the complement component C4b–binding protein.

4. Describe the fibrinolytic system.

The fibrinolytic system is responsible for lysis of fibrin clot. It is composed of plasminogen and its activators and inhibitors. Plasminogen is converted to plasmin through activation by tissue plasminogen activator (tPA) which is synthesized and released from vascular endothelium, or by urokinase which is produced in the kidney. The fibrinolytic process is regulated by specific protease inhibitors: 1) PAI-1 (plasminogen activator inhibitor), which inhibits the plasminogen activators (tPA and urokinase), and 2) α2-antiplasmin, which inhibits plasmin. Plasmin acts on both fibrinogen and fibrin, forming the fibrinogen-fibrin degradation products (FDPs). Cross-linked fibrin lysed by plasmin leads to the production of fragments such as D-dimer.

5. Where are the coagulation proteins synthesized?

All the coagulation proteins are synthesized in the liver, except for factor VIII, which, although synthesized mainly by the hepatocytes, is also made elsewhere (e.g., the endothelium).

6. Which are the vitamin K–dependent factors and proteins?

Vitamin K is important for the synthesis of the procoagulant factors II, VII, IX and X and the anticoagulants proteins C and S. Vitamin K promotes the post-translational modification of specific glutamic acid residues to g-carboxyglutamic acid that is essential in their calcium binding to negatively charged phospholipid surfaces.

7. Which clotting factors are "acute phase reactants"?

Factor VIII, fibrinogen and von Willebrand factor are often elevated during infection and the inflammatory processes.

8. Discuss the historical data that are essential in making a diagnosis of a bleeding disorder.

Obtaining a good and reliable history is important in making an accurate diagnosis of a bleeding disorder. The type of bleeding (e.g., skin, mucous membrane, joint or deep muscle bleeds), its severity and the duration of symptoms must be evaluated. History of any bleeding from surgery (such as circumcision, tonsillectomy, biopsy or dental procedure) or trauma is a good indicator of bleeding risks. A careful family history must be obtained, as many common bleeding disorders are familial or inherited, such as von Willebrand's disease and the hemophilias. Acquired causes must also be sought, such as intake of drugs that are known to affect hemostasis (e.g., aspirin, warfarin, certain anticonvulsants and antibiotics), as well as medical conditions known to be associated with bleeding (e.g., liver or kidney disease, lupus and other autoimmune disorders).

9. What laboratory tests are used for the screening of hemostasis?

- Platelet count
- Prothrombin time (PT): measures the "extrinsic pathway"
- Activated partial thromboplastin time (aPTT): measures the "intrinsic pathway"
- Thrombin time (TT): the time required for plasma to clot after the addition of thrombin. It measures the quality and amount of fibrinogen and the rate of conversion of fibrinogen to fibrin. It is prolonged in hypofibrinogenemia and dysfibrinogenemia and by substances that interfere with the thrombin-induced fibrinogen conversion to fibrin, such as heparin and FDPs.
- Fibrinogen concentration. Fibrinogen is not prolonged in the other commonly used screening tests (PT, APTT, TT) until the level is well below the normal (< 100 mg/dL).
- Bleeding time: used to assess the vascular and platelet phase of hemostasis. It measures the time required for a skin incision to stop bleeding. The test is standardized by

using a template that regulates the length and depth of the skin incision and maintaining a certain amount of pressure with a blood pressure cuff.

10. What is the "mixing study"?

A mixing study is done when the APTT is prolonged to differentiate factor deficiency and the presence of an inhibitor. Normal plasma is added to the patient's plasma (in equal volume), and the APTT assay is performed on the mixture. If the APTT of the mixture corrects or becomes normal, factor deficiency is present (factors VIII, IX, XI, XII, PK or HMWK). If, however, the APTT remains prolonged, this indicates the presence of an inhibitor (lupus anticoagulant or inhibitor specific to factor VIII, IX or XI).

11. What are some of the artifacts in sample collection and processing of coagulation testing that affect interpretation of the test?

A properly collected and processed sample is crucial in the interpretation of coagulation tests. Some of the causes of errors include:

- Traumatic and repeated punctures and slow blood flow contaminate the sample with procoagulant materials in the tissue juice (tissue factor or thrombin), causing shortening of the APTT and positive D-dimer or FDPs.
- High hematocrit: This results in less amount of plasma in proportion to the citrate anticoagulant, thereby causing extra citrate to bind calcium and thus prolong the clotting time.
- Incomplete filling of collection tube ("short" draw): If the amount of blood drawn is reduced in proportion to the citrate anticoagulant, the excess citrate depletes the calcium in the plasma and leads to prolongation of PT/PTT.
- Heparin contamination may occur when specimens are drawn from arterial or venous catheters flushed with heparin. To obtain an accurate coagulation test 3 to 5 millimeters of blood must be discarded prior to collecting the sample to get rid of the heparin.

12. Are there any screening tests for the natural inhibitors or anticoagulants?

No. Reduced amounts of the natural anticoagulants or inhibitors do not cause "shortening" of the PT or APTT. Specific assays for measuring the activity and concentration of the anticoagulants antithrombin III, protein C and protein S are available for testing.

REFERENCES

1. Dahlback B: Blood coagulation. Lancet 355:1627–1632, 2000.
2. Lusher JM: Approach to the bleeding patient. In Nathan DG and Orkin SH (eds): Hematology of Infancy and Childhood. Philadelphia, W.B. Saunders, 1998, pp 1574–1584.

11. NEONATAL HEMOSTASIS

Margaret T. Lee, M.D.

1. How is the coagulation system in the newborn period different from that in the adult?

The coagulation system in the newborn is considered to be immature, with many of the coagulation proteins reduced at birth. In the procoagulant system, the contact factors (high-molecular-weight kininogen, prekallikrein, factors XII and XI); and the vitamin K–dependent factors (II, VII, IX and X), are reduced to about 30–50% of the adult range in the term newborn infant and are further reduced in the preterm infant. On the other hand, factors V and VIII, and fibrinogen are present in the normal adult range even in the premature neonate. Except for modest elevation of α2-macroglobulin, the coagulation inhibitors (antithrombin, protein C and protein S) are also reduced to $\leq$ 50% of normal. Moreover, there are a few clotting factors in the neonate that exhibit unique structural and functional differences from the adult proteins. For instance, "fetal" fibrinogen has increased sialic acid content associated with a prolonged thrombin time and reptilase time. The functional significance of this is unknown. Newborns also have increased von Willebrand factor, which has an altered multimeric structure with increased high-molecular-weight forms producing increased reactivity with ristocetin.

2. Describe how this difference in the coagulation system between newborns and adults affect the commonly used coagulation screening tests.

The reduced level of most of the coagulation proteins is reflected as prolongation of the coagulation screening tests. The prothrombin time (PT) is only minimally prolonged in the normal term infant, whereas the activated partial thromboplastin time (APTT) is markedly prolonged due to the reduced levels of the contact factors disproportionately affecting the APTT. In the premature infant, these test results are even more prolonged. Because of this, results for these tests must be interpreted based on established reference range for neonates according to their gestational as well as postnatal age, and in consideration of the interlaboratory variation in relation to the adult normal range for that laboratory.

3. When do these coagulation proteins reach the adult values?

The procoagulant proteins that are decreased at birth gradually increase postnatally and reach the adult values by about 6 months of age. However, although the values fall within the adult normal range, the mean levels remain reduced throughout infancy when compared with the mean levels of adults. The inhibitors also increase during the first 3–6 months of life, except for protein C, which remain significantly reduced until the early teenage years.

4. What is the normal platelet count in the newborn?

The platelet count at birth for both term and preterm infants is the same as that of the adult normal range (150–450 $\times$ 10^9/L). Data from fetal blood sampling show that the fetal platelet count is within the adult normal range as early as 15–18 weeks of gestation.

5. How do bleeding disorders present in the neonate?

The clinical presentation of bleeding disorder in the neonate tends to differ from that seen in older children and adults. Neonates can present with bleeding from the scalp, large cephalhematomas, intracranial hemorrhage, bleeding from the umbilicus, bleeding following circumcision, oozing from venipuncture sites or heelsticks and sometimes gastrointestinal bleeding. Hemarthrosis and deep muscle bleeding are rather unusual.

6a. A two-day-old, healthy full-term male infant developed bleeding following circumcision. What laboratory evaluation is indicated in this patient?

In a healthy full-term infant who presents with bleeding manifestation, severe thrombocytopenia from immune causes, congenital or inherited factor deficiences as well as vitamin K deficiency should be considered. Initial screening tests include a platelet count and coagulation studies including PT, APTT, thrombin time and fibrinogen. Bleeding time is usually not performed because it is difficult to interpret in the newborn. Specific factor assays are indicated if the PT or APTT is prolonged and if hemophilia is suspected.

6b. The laboratory work-up reveals an isolated prolongation of APTT of 95 seconds. What are the possible diagnoses?

Factor VIII (hemophilia A) and factor IX (hemophilia B) are the two most common congenital factor deficiencies that can cause isolated prolongation of the APTT. These are both x-linked recessive and therefore manifest in males. The severe forms (factor levels $< 1\%$) can present in newborns. Factor XI deficiency can also prolong the APTT. It is autosomally inherited, the homozygous forms are relatively rare and consanguinity is often present.

6c. How would you treat this patient to control the bleeding?

Replacement therapy with the appropriate factor concentrate is indicated to control the bleeding. However, when the diagnosis of a specific factor deficiency is pending, fresh frozen plasma (FFP), which contains all the clotting factors, is the blood product of choice. Cryoprecipitate contains factor VIII but does not have factors IX or XI.

7. A 5-day-old full-term female infant presents with prolonged bleeding from the umbilical cord. Initial laboratory evaluation showed normal platelet count and normal results for coagulation studies (PT, APTT, fibrinogen). What further work-up is needed, and what could be the diagnosis?

The coagulation screening tests do not include factor XIII, therefore if this is suspected, a specific assay must be performed. Homozygous deficiency of this factor classically presents with delayed umbilical cord bleeding. The urea solubility test is a useful screening test for homozygous deficiency. A bleeding time may also be performed to evaluate possible platelet dysfunction, although this will be difficult to interpret in the newborn. Data should also be obtained from the parents for inherited bleeding disorders.

8. What are the three forms of hemorrhagic disease of the newborn (HDN) secondary to vitamin K deficiency?

Hemorrhagic disease of the newborn, which can present with various hemorrhagic manifestations such as gastrointestinal, postcircumcisional, umbilical or intracranial bleeding occurs in three forms:

- Early: The early form occurs within the first 24 hours after birth and is due to maternal ingestion of medications that pass through the placental circulation and affect the neonatal production of vitamin K. These drugs include warfarin, carbamazepine, barbiturates, phenytoin, rifampin, isoniazid and certain cephalosporins.
- Classic: The classic form manifests between days 2 and 7 of life and is caused by inadequate intake of vitamin K seen in breast-fed babies with marginal intake of breast milk.

Commercial infant formulas contain higher amounts of vitamin K compared with breast milk. The classic form of HDN is prevented by the routine practice of prophylactic administration of vitamin K at birth.

- Late: The late form of HDN presents 2 weeks to 6 months after birth because of inadequate intake (low vitamin K content in breast milk) or inadequate absorption in hepatobiliary disease. This form occurs more frequently in boys and has a high incidence of intracranial bleeding. Intramuscular injection of vitamin K at birth provides improved protection against late-onset HDN compared with oral vitamin K.

9. Why are neonates and young infants prone to thrombosis?

Within the pediatric age group, the peak incidence of thrombotic disorders occurs in neonates and infants younger than 1 year. Although the immature coagulation system in the newborn is "physiologic" the balance is perturbed in favor of thrombin formation rather than clot inhibition, especially in sick infants. In vitro studies on thrombin regulation in neonates and cord blood indicate that their blood exhibits a deficiency of thrombin inhibition and reduced plasmin generation.

10. What are some of the commonly associated conditions that predispose to neonatal thrombosis?

The majority of neonatal thromboses occur in association with indwelling vascular catheters. Other associated conditions include polycythemia, hypoxia, infection, maternal diabetes, and maternal lupus anticoagulant. Neonatal thromboses most frequently involve the large major vessels, such as the inferior vena cava, renal veins, aorta and middle cerebral artery.

11. Describe the treatment for thromboses in the neonate.

The optimal treatment for neonatal thrombosis remains undefined. Depending on the clot extent and symptoms, treatment options include supportive therapy; anticoagulation with heparin; thrombolytic therapy with streptokinase, urokinase or tPA; and surgery. Anticoagulants are usually given in the short term (10–14 days), with either unfractionated heparin or low-molecular-weight heparin (LMWH). Oral anticoagulation or LMWH is sometimes given for long-term anticoagulation of extensive thrombosis.

12. Why is it difficult to treat neonates with heparin?

Newborns require higher doses of heparin compared with older children and adults for anticoagulation. This reflects the physiologic variation in neonatal hemostasis and pharmacokinetics. Heparin works by accelerating the inactivation of thrombin and other activated clotting factors by antithrombin, which is physiologically reduced in the neonate, thereby causing "heparin resistance." Furthermore, heparin has a faster clearance in the newborn because of an increased volume of distribution.

13. Discuss the mechanisms and causes of thrombocytopenia in the newborn.

The underlying mechanisms of thrombocytopenia in the newborn can be broadly categorized as either decreased bone marrow production or increased peripheral destruction or consumption. In many conditions, it is not easy to delineate the exact mechanism, and a combination of both occurs. The best approach to identify the etiology is to look for the most common causes in the particular setting, whether the infant is well or sick, and searching for any relevant maternal factors and significant family history. The table below enumerates the many possible causes of neonatal thrombocytopenia.

Causes of Neonatal Thrombocytopenia

- Increased platelet destruction
  - a) Immune-mediated
    - Neonatal alloimmune thrombocytopenia
    - Maternal immune thrombocytopenic purpura
    - Maternal autoimmune diseases
    - Maternal drug ingestion
  - b) Non-immune mediated
    - Birth asphyxia
    - Disseminated intravascular coagulation
    - Necrotizing enterocolitis
    - Giant hemangiomas (Kasabach-Merritt syndrome)
    - Thrombosis
    - Cardiac anomalies
    - Hypersplenism
- Decreased platelet production
  - a) Bone marrow aplasia
    - Thrombocytopenia with absent radii
    - Amegakaryocytic thrombocytopenia
    - Fanconi's anemia
    - Trisomy syndromes and other chromosomal abnormalities
  - b) Bone marrow replacement
    - Congenital leukemia
    - Neuroblastoma
    - Osteopetrosis
    - Histiocytosis
- Mixed or uncertain etiology
  - a) Congenital intrauterine infections
  - b) Maternal pre-eclampsia
  - c) Phototherapy
  - d) Rh hemolytic disease
  - e) Polycythemia
  - f) Genetic disorders (Alport's, metabolic disorders)
  - g) Other hereditary thrombocytopenias (Bernard-Soulier syndrome, May-Hegglin anomaly and Wiskott-Aldrich syndromes)

14. What is the treatment for neonatal thrombocytopenia?

Except in cases of maternal autoimmune thrombocytopenia, platelet transfusion with cytomegalovirus-negative, white blood cell–depleted platelet concentrate remains the treatment of choice for severe thrombocytopenia in the neonate. The primary aim for platelet transfusion is to maintain a platelet count that will prevent the risk of significant hemorrhage, particularly intracranial bleeding. A dose of 10 mL/kg of platelet concentrate should raise the platelet count 75–100 $\times$ 10^9/L. In the future, perhaps the megakaryocytopoietic cytokines such as thrombopoietin and IL-11 may be used in the prevention and treatment of thrombocytopenia in the neonate.

15. What is the platelet count "trigger" for treatment in the newborn?

There is no general consensus as to a "safe" platelet count in the neonate. In general, treatment guidelines vary according to the gestational and postnatal age, with a higher trigger for premature babies in the immediate postnatal period when the risk for intraventricular hemorrhage is greatest and the presence of other interconcurrent conditions such as sepsis and disseminated intravascular coagulation is most prevalent. Many sick neonates also have significant platelet dysfunction associated with the thrombocytopenia. Therefore, despite the lack of objective evidence, most generally consider treatment at a level of 50×10^9/L for premature infants—especially in the first week of life—as well as for surgery and "sick" clinically unstable neonates. The threshold is lowered to 20–30 $\times 10^9$/L in stable term infants when the count has been stable or increasing.

16. Define neonatal alloimmune thrombocytopenia (NAIT).

Thrombocytopenia in the neonate resulting from immune-mediated platelet destruction caused by alloantobodies produced and transferred by the mother against a specific fetal platelet antigen that the baby inherited from the father and that is absent in the mother. This is the platelet equivalent of Rh hemolytic disease of the newborn. Typically, this is suspected in an otherwise healthy full-term newborn with no other obvious causes for thrombocytopenia who presents with petechiae, gastrointestinal bleeding, or, in as many as 20% of cases, intracranial hemorrhage. Clinical diagnosis is supported by poor response to random donor platelet transfusion and response to washed maternal platelets. The diagnosis is confirmed by determination of platelet alloantigen phenotype of the parents and detection of maternal antibody with specificity for paternal or fetal platelet antigen. The most common platelet antigen involved is the human platelet antigen HPA-1a (previous nomenclature, PIA-1). Unlike Rh hemolytic disease of the newborn, in which the first-born baby is not affected, NAIT can occur in about 50% of cases during the first pregnancy.

17. Discuss the management of NAIT.

NAIT is a self-limiting condition with eventual recovery of the platelet count in 2–4 weeks. However, until the platelet count recovers, the neonate is at an increased risk for life-threatening hemorrhage because of severe thrombocytopenia in the immediate newborn period. The mainstay of treatment is transfusion of compatible, antigen-negative platelets, usually most easily obtained from the mother, as donors for antigen-negative platelets often are not readily available. High-dose intravenous immunoglobulin (IVIG) also may be given as an adjunct treatment, although its effect is usually delayed and less predictable. Optimal antenatal management to prevent risk of recurrence in future pregnancies remains controversial. Options include maternal infusion of IVIG with or without corticosteroids once thrombocytopenia in the fetus is identified. Early elective delivery by caesarian section is generally advocated.

18. Differentiate neonatal autoimmune thrombocytopenia (NITP) from NAIT.

In NITP, IgG autoantibodies from the mother who has an underlying immune thrombocytopenia or other autoimmune diseases, such as systemic lupus erythematosus, are passively transferred to the baby who may subsequently develop thrombocytopenia secondary to immune destruction of platelets. The antibodies are directed against antigens common to both mother and baby, unlike in NAIT, in which the antibodies are only directed against the baby's platelets. Therefore, in NITP, the mother has a low platelet count, whereas in NAIT, maternal platelet count is normal. The platelet count in NITP can be normal at birth, with nadir at 2–5 days after delivery. Bleeding problems in utero or during delivery are rare. This is also a self-limiting condition, with platelet recovery in 2–3 months. Treatment options in cases of severe thrombocytopenia ($< 50 \times 109$/L) include IVIG and corticosteroids.

BIBLIOGRAPHY

1. Chalmers EA, Gibson BE: Hemostatic problems in the neonate. In Lilleyman J, Hann I, Blanchette V (eds): Pediatric Hematology. London, Churchill Livingstone, 1999, pp 651–678.
2. Edstrom CS, Christensen RD, Andrew M: Developmental aspects of blood hemostasis and disorders of coagulation and fibrinolysis in the neonatal period. In Christensen RD (ed): Hematologic problems of the neonate. Philadelphia, W.B. Saunders, 2000, pp 239–271.
3. Roberts I: Management of thrombocytopenia in neonates. Br Jf Haematol 105:864–870, 1999.
4. Sola MC, Christensen RD: Developmental aspects of platelets and disorders of platelets in the neonatal period. In Christensen RD (ed): Hematologic problems of the neonate. Philadelphia, W.B. Saunders, 2000, pp 273–309.

12. DISORDERS OF COAGULATION

Margaret T. Lee, M.D.

1. Classify hemophilia A and B according to the degree of severity.

The severity of the clinical manifestation of hemophilias A and B (deficiency of factor VIII and IX, respectively), correlates with the level or activity of the factor in the plasma. Thus, the disease is best classified according to these levels:

- Mild: 0.05–0.30 U/ml
- Moderate: 0.01–0.05 U/ml
- Severe: < 0.01 U/ml

2. Can hemophilias A and B be distinguished based on their clinical presentation?

No. Both factors VIII and IX are part of the same coagulation sequence in the intrinsic pathway leading to the formation of the fibrin clot. Individuals affected by either type of coagulation factor deficiency have the same type of bleeding commonly characterized by joint and soft tissue hemorrhages. Both hemophilia A (factor VIII deficiency) and hemophilia B (factor IX deficiency) are x-linked recessive and are therefore seen in male patients. The only way to differentiate hemophilias A and B is by performing specific plasma factor assays.

3. Does a negative family history exclude the diagnosis of hemophilia?

No. About 20–30% of newly diagnosed individuals with hemophilia have disease caused by spontaneous mutations and thus do not have previously identifiable affected family member.

4. Are there female hemophiliacs?

Hemophilias A and B are x-linked recessive genetic diseases and therefore occur in male subjects almost exclusively. However, there are a few reported cases of hemophilia in female patients, presumably due to extreme lyonization, homozygosity (inheritance of the hemophilia gene from each parent) or coinheritance of type 2N von Willebrand's disease (qualitative variant with reduced binding of factor VIII).

5. List the principles of replacement therapy in hemophilia.

- Bleeding must be treated promptly and appropriately.
- The dose of factor replacement is determined by its volume of distribution, the half-life, and the hemostatic requirement of the type of bleeding.
- Factor VIII: 1 U/kg of factor concentrate raises the factor level by 2%. The dose is calculated by multiplying the weight in kilograms by the desired percentage increment, divided by 2. The half-life of factor VIII is 8–12 hours.
- Factor IX: 1 U/kg of factor concentrate raises the factor level by 1% The dose is calculated by multiplying the weight in kilograms by the desired percentage increment. The half-life of factor IX is 24 hours.
- Therapeutic level desired for the specific type or site of bleeding. In general, routine hemarthroses and soft tissue bleeds require 30–40% correction while life-threatening hemorrhages require 80–100%.
- Recommended dosage for specific hemorrhages:

Site of bleeding	*Hemophilia A*	*Hemophilia B*
Joint	20 U/kg, then QD as needed	30 U/kg, then QOD as needed
Muscle, subcutaneous	20 U/kg, then QD as needed	30 U/kg, then QOD as needed
Oral mucosa	20 U/kg (+ anti-fibrinolytic agent*)	30 U/kg (+ anti-fibrinolytic agent*)
Epistaxis	20 U/kg + anti-fibrinolytic agent* + pressure)	30 U/kg (+ anti-fibrinolytic agent* + pressure
Life-threatening bleed (Central nervous system, airway, massive gastro-intestinal); Major trauma and surgery	50 U/kg stat, then 25 U/kg Q 12 hours for 10–14 days, or continuous infusion at 4U/kg/hour to maintain 100% for 24 hours, then 2–3 U/kg/hour to maintain > 50% for 5–7 days, then > 30% for 5–7 days	80 U/kg stat, then 20–40 U/kg Q 24 hours to maintain > 40% for 5–7 days, then > 30% for 5–7 days
Genitourinary	20 U/kg + bed rest + fluid hydration + prednisone if bleeding persists	30 U/kg + bed rest + fluid hydration + prednisone if bleeding persists

Q = every, QD = every day; QOD = every other day.
*Anti-fibrinolytic agents: epsilon aminocaproic acid (Amicar), tranexamic acid (Cyklokapron).

6. What is a "target joint?"

In individuals with severe hemophilia, frequent recurrent bleeding into a particular joint ("target" joint) can occur without trauma. This occurs because repeated joint bleeding leads to synovial inflammation and thickening, which establishes a subsequent vicious cycle of rebleeding into the joint.

7. What are factor inhibitors?

Inhibitors are antibodies that block the function of a specific coagulation protein. Inhibitors develop most commonly in individuals with congenital factor deficiencies, such as hemophilia, after exposure to factor concentrates. They develop in 25–30% of children with severe hemophila A and less often (1–3%) in children with hemophilia B. There are certain factor concentrate replacement products that are thought to be particularly immunogenic and promote antibody production. In addition, certain abnormalities in the factor VIII or factor IX gene are associated with a higher predisposition to inhibitor development. Inhibitors may be detected either on routine screening or when the patient fails to respond to appropriate replacement therapy during a bleeding episode. The amount of inhibitor is measured by the Bethesda assay, in which one Bethesda unit (BU) is defined as the quantity of the inhibitor that results in the loss of 50% factor activity in 2 hours at 37°C. Inhibitors may also occur in patients with no history of a factor deficiency, but this is very rare in children.

8. Discuss treatment options for hemophiliacs who develop inhibitors.

Individuals with low-titer inhibitors (< 5 BU) often can be treated with higher doses of factor concentrates that would overcome the antibodies and control the bleeding. However, patients who have high titers are refractory to this therapeutic option. Alternative treatment options that are available for hemophilia A patients with inhibitors include porcine factor VIII concentrate (factor VIII derived from pigs), standard or activated prothrombin complex concentrate (PCC or APCC) and recombinant factor VIIa. Some individuals with inhibitors have cross-reacting antibodies to the porcine product and therefore, their use is limited to those with little or no known cross-reacting antibodies. The PCC and APCC (containing factors II, VII, IX and X) are proven effective and useful in controlling hemorrhages in patients with inhibitors, although it is not entirely clear how they work in "bypassing" the need for factor VIII. These agents are thrombogenic and have caused acute myocardial infarction after repeated infusions. Recombinant VIIa recently has been licensed for use in the United States and appears to be safe and effective. An attempt to suppress or eradicate inhibitors also can be done by immune tolerance induction, in which large doses of factor VIII are given daily for several months. In addition, some have also used intravenous immunoglobulin and cyclophosphamide as immunosuppresive agents.

For patients with hemophilia B with inhibitors, the treatment options also include PCC or APCC and the recombinant factor VIIa. Immune tolerance regimens are less effective in these patients.

9. Name the two major functions or physiologic roles of von Willebrand factor (VWF).

Von Willebrand factor plays an important role in the initial stages of hemostasis by enhancing platelet adhesion and aggregation. First, it mediates the adhesion of platelets to the endothelium by binding with the platelet receptor glycoprotein (Gp)Ib and then subsequently facilitating platelet aggregation by its interaction with the platelet receptor GPIIb-IIIa complex. Secondly, VWF acts as a carrier protein for the coagulation factor VIII, such that reduced level of VWF results in low level of factor VIII by the increased degradation of factor VIII by activated protein C.

10. Describe the classification or types of von Willebrand disease (VWD).

- Type 1 VWD: most common type, found in 80% of patients with VWD disease; patients with type 1 disease have a mild or partial quantitative deficiency of VWF.
- Type 2 VWD: represents 15–20% of cases; patients with type 2 disease have qualitative defects of VWF, which may be further subclassified into the following:
  - a) Type 2A: qualitative variant with decreased platelet-dependent function associated with absence of high and intermediate-molecular-weight multimers
  - b) Type 2B: qualitative variant with increased affinity for binding gylcoprotein Ib.
  - c) Type 2M: qualitative variant with decreased platelet-dependent function associated with normal multimers
  - d) Type 2N: qualitative variant with reduced binding of Factor VIII
- Type 3: severe type, with virtual complete absence of VWF.

11. What are the clinical manifestations of VWD?

Patients with VWD mostly have the type 1 variant with only partial deficiency of VWF. Clinically they present with skin or mucous membrane bleeding that often requires medical attention or can lead to anemia. Examples include recurrent nose-bleeds requiring nasal packing or cautery, prolonged bleeding after dental extraction or oral surgery, menorrhagia, bleeding from skin lacerations that last for hours and spontaneous gastrointestinal bleeding unexplained by other local causes. Patients with the type 2 variants have similar presentations, except for type 2B, which also has accompanying thrombocytopenia. Type 3 patients manifest a more severe phenotype: They do not only present with the same mucocutaneous hemorrhages seen in type 1 patients, they also have joint and soft tissue bleeds similar to those seen in hemophila A patients because of their low levels of factor VIII. Given that VWD is an inherited bleeding condition, patients commonly have a strong family history of similar bleeding manifestations. Most cases of types 1, 2A and 2B disease are autosomal dominant conditions with variable penetrance and expressions. Types 2N and 3 are believed to be autosomal recessive, with patients being either homozygotes or compound heterozygotes for the VWF gene defects.

12. How does desmopressin (DDAVP) work for the treatment of VWD?

Desmopressin is a synthetic analog of the antidiuretic hormone vasopressin. It increases the plasma VWF and factor VIII by 2- to 8-fold within an hour of administration by releasing VWF from its endothelial cell storage, with secondary stabilization of additional factor VIII. It can be given intravenously (0.3 μg/kg) or through the intranasal route (150–300 μg), with peak response at 30–90 minutes after administration. It is safe and effective, with mild side effects such as facial flushing, headache, mild changes in blood pressure and an increase in the pulse rate. Its most serious side effects are hyponatremia and seizures secondary to water retention, especially in infants. This can be avoided by water restriction for several hours after infusion. After repeated administration, patients can develop tachyphylaxis (diminished response), presumably from exhaustion of the endothelial cell stores of the VWF. Most patients with type 1 VWD will respond to DDAVP, while those with the severe type 3 will not respond and need transfusion with either cryoprecipitate or plasma-derived intermediate-purity Factor VIII, such as Humate-P. The therapeutic effect of DDAVP in type 2 VWD is variable and is contraindicated in the type 2B variant.

13. What is hemophilia C?

Factor XI deficiency has been termed hemophilia C, although it does not share the same clinical manifestations as hemophilias A and B or share a similar mode of inheritance. Unlike hemophilias A and B, hemophilia C is an autosomal recessive disorder most commonly seen in Ashkenazi Jews. The clinical presentation is variable, and there is no good correlation between the factor level and the bleeding tendency. It is generally a mild bleeding disorder, and most significant bleeds occur only in association with surgery or trauma. Patients can present with easy bruising, epistaxis and menorrhagia but no joint or deep muscle bleeds. There is isolated prolongation of activated partial thromboplastin time (APTT), and specific factor assay is needed to confirm the diagnosis. Because clinically significant bleeding is not common, replacement therapy with plasma infusions is usually only indicated for high-risk surgical procedures like neurosurgical, cardiac, urologic and ear, nose and throat procedures. Mucous membrane and dental bleeding usually respond well to adjunctive treatment with antifibrinolytic agents like epsilon aminocaproic acid or tranexamic acid.

14. Name three acquired causes of combined prolongation of prothrombin time (PT) and APTT and describe the coagulation factor abnormalities associated with each.

- Vitamin K deficiency—Vitamin K–dependent factors (II, VII, IX and X) are low, while the rest are normal.
- Liver disease—All clotting factors are low except the acute phase reactants factor VIII (and VWF) and fibrinogen, which are elevated or normal until the late or severe stage of hepatic injury.
- Disseminated intravascular coagulation (DIC)—Except in the early or mild stage, all clotting factors are diminished.

15. Why do patients with mild vitamin K deficiency or early liver disease present initially with only an isolated prolonged PT with normal APTT?

Factor VII is a key enzyme in the extrinsic pathway and is measured in vitro by the PT. Among all the procoagulant proteins and the vitamin K–dependent factors, factor VII has the shortest half-life (4–6 hours) and is therefore easily depleted in both vitamin K deficiency and liver disease compared with the other factors, resulting in isolated prolongation of the PT.

16. List some common causes of vitamin K deficiency that result in diminished function of the vitamin K–dependent factors.

Vitamin K is a fat-soluble compound that occurs naturally in the diet (fruits and vegetables) as well as synthesized by the bacterial flora in the gut. Deficiency states can be seen in malnutrition or starvation, prolonged antibiotic therapy and warfarin ingestion, as well as conditions that cause fat malabsorption, such as biliary obstruction, pancreatic insufficiency, short-bowel syndrome, cystic fibrosis and diarrhea.

17. What is DIC?

Disseminated intravascular coagulation is an acquired disorder characterized by generalized activation of the coagulation system, causing widespread fibrin formation that results in thrombosis of small and mid-size vessels, compromising blood supply to organs. Subsequently, consumption of platelets and clotting factors also occurs, which can cause bleeding. This is always a secondary event associated with a number of disease processes, such as infection (commonly bacterial), trauma or injury, malignancy and giant hemangiomas. Laboratory evaluation reveals evidence of coagulation activation and depletion of all clotting factors (procoagulants and anticoagulants) as well as platelets causing prolonged PT and APTT, low fibrinogen, low platelet count and elevated fibrin split products, or D-dimers.

18. Describe the lupus anticoagulant.

The lupus anticoagulant (LA) is a heterogeneous group of antiphospholipid antibodies that cause laboratory artifact of prolonging clot-based coagulation tests. The name is a misnomer. The term *lupus* was used because the abnormality was first described in patients with systemic lupus erythematosus (SLE); the term *anticoagulant* was used because of the prolonged coagulation assays, particularly the APTT. Paradoxically, many patients with LA do not have bleeding, despite the elevated APTT, unless associated with other coagulation abnormalities such as a low prothrombin level. Instead, these patients tend to develop thrombosis. In addition, many patients who have LA do not have SLE. Indeed, LA is commonly found in children on routine coagulation screening (e.g., prior to surgery) associated with previous viral illness or antibiotic therapy and is usually transient and does not cause any hemostatic problems.

19. Define thrombophilia.

The term *thrombophilia* was first used to describe several members of a family with increased prevalence of venous thromboembolism associated with deficiency of antithrombin III, a physiologic anticoagulant. Now the term refers to a group of hereditary abnormalities of the hemostatic system that predispose to thromboembolism, such as deficiency in protein C, protein S and antithrombin; dysfibrinogenemias; and defects in the fibrinolytic system.

20. What is factor V Leiden?

Factor V Leiden is a point mutation in the factor V protein with replacement of arginine by glycine at position 506 (R506Q), making it resistant to degradation by activated protein C. It appears to be the most common form of congenital thrombophilia. It can be diagnosed by screening with APTT-based assay for activated protein C resistance or directly by DNA analysis.

21. Discuss the clinical presentation of thromboembolic disorders in children.

Thromboembolic disorders are less common in children than in adults. In the pediatric population, the age groups found to be at greatest risk are neonates, infants younger than 1 year and teenagers. In the majority of the cases (> 95%), these disorders are acquired or secondary to other risk factors for thrombosis such as central venous catheters and other underlying medical conditions such as prematurity, congenital heart disease, cancer, surgery, systemic lupus erythematosus and others. The congenital prothrombotic disorder with single-gene defect (heterozygous) usually presents after puberty and rarely during childhood. When thrombosis occurs during childhood, a secondary risk factor such as a central venous catheter is usually present. Those with homozygous congenital prothrombotic disorders usually present during childhood, often within the first hours of life, depending on the specific defect and the severity. Examples are newborns with homozygous protein C or S deficiency who present with purpura fulminans (hemorrhagic necrosis of the skin) or cerebral or ophthalmic thrombosis. Thromboembolic complications can be either venous or arterial. Deep venous thrombosis usually occurs in the extremities and presents with pain, swelling and discoloration of the affected limb. Other possible sites of venous thrombosis are the inferior vena cava, renal vein, right atrium, portal vein and cerebral sinus. Arterial thrombosis usually is related to catheters, such as umbilical artery catheterization in neonates, and cardiac catheterization through the femoral artery, but can also occur spontaneously, as in ischemic stroke.

BIBLIOGRAPHY

1. Andrew M, Michelson A, Bovill E: Guidelines for antithrombotic therapy in pediatric patients. J Pediatr 132:575–588, 1998.
2. DiMichele D: Hemophilia 1996: New approach to an old disease. Pediatr Clin North Am 43:709–736, 1996.
3. Levi M, Cate HT: Disseminated intravascular coagulation. N Engl J Med 341:586–592, 1999.
4. Schneppenheim R, Thomas K, Sutor A: Von Willebrand disease in childhood. Semin Thrombosis Hemostasis 21:261–271, 1995.

13. DISORDERS OF PLATELETS

Margaret T. Lee, M.D.

1. What is pseudothrombocytopenia?

Pseudothrombocytopenia, or spurious thrombocytopenia, is an erroneously low platelet count obtained from an automated blood counter that is secondary to platelet clumping, observed on peripheral smear. This can be caused by a poorly collected specimen that is clotted, the presence of EDTA-dependent platelet agglutination, platelet cold agglutinins or platelet satellitism (platelets around neutrophils or monocytes). An accurate platelet count can be obtained by doing a manual count on a freshly collected sample from a finger stick.

2. Differentiate the signs and symptoms of bleeding secondary to a platelet disorder from that of a coagulation disorder.

Bleeding due to platelet disorders typically consists of skin and mucous membrane bleeds such as petechiae, small ecchymoses, gum bleeding epistaxis, gastrointestinal bleeding, and menorrhagia, whereas deep subcutaneous, muscle and joint bleeds are characteristic of coagulation disorders.

3. Define idiopathic (immune) thrombocytopenia purpura (ITP).

Thrombocytopenia secondary to increased destruction of platelets by the macrophages in the reticuloendothelial system, particularly the spleen, consequent to antibodies formed against platelets in response to a viral illness or underlying defects of immune regulation. It is one of the most common acquired bleeding disorders in children.

4. How does one make a diagnosis of ITP?

The diagnosis of ITP is highly clinical. A good and thorough history and physical examination, along with a complete blood count (CBC) and review of the peripheral smear, are all that is essential. In acute ITP, the history is typically brief and the physical examination unremarkable, except for the bleeding signs and symptoms that are related to the degree of thrombocytopenia. The CBC shows a low platelet count, usually severe, with normal white blood cell count (WBC) and hemoglobin/hematocrit. On the peripheral smear, the platelets are reduced and many appear large, indicating an active bone marrow trying to compensate for the increased peripheral destruction. A bone marrow examination is not routinely necessary unless the patient has an atypical presentation. Antiplatelet antibody assays are not crucial in making the diagnosis, as these tests lack sufficient sensitivity and specificity.

5. Differentiate acute from chronic ITP.

Features of Acute and Chronic ITP

FEATURES	ACUTE	CHRONIC
Presentation	Abrupt	Insiduous
Age	Usually young (2–10 years)	Adolescents and adults
Sex	Equal in boys and girls	More common in female patients
Associated conditions	Antecedent viral infections	Autoimmune disorders
Duration of thrombocytopenia	< 6 months	>6 months

6. Discuss the treatment of ITP in children.

ITP in children is usually acute and self-limited. Therapy is only palliative and not curative. The goal of treatment is to obtain a rapid increase in the platelet count to prevent a life-threatening bleed from severe thrombocytopenia, such as an intracranial hemorrhage. The decision to treat is based on the platelet count, severity of bleeding symptoms, lifestyle and activity of the patient and other comorbid conditions that may increase the risk of bleeding. In general, when the platelet count is > 30,000 and the patient is asymptomatic, no treatment is required except for restriction of activity and avoidance of drugs that can affect platelet function, such as aspirin and nonsteroidal anti-inflammatory agents. Treatment is given when the platelet count is < 10,000, even with only minor purpura, and in patients with a platelet count between 10,000 and 30,000 who have significant bleeding. The currently available treatment options are intravenous immunoglobulin (IVIG), corticosteroids and anti-Rh(D) antibody.

7. Describe the mechanism of action of IVIG in the treatment of ITP.

IVIG works by blocking the Fc receptors on the macrophages, thereby sparing destruction of the IgG-coated platelets and allowing them to remain in the circulation. It also contains anti-idiotypic antibodies that can bind to circulating antibodies, thereby rendering them ineffective in binding to platelets.

8. How does anti-Rh(D) antibody work in the treatment of ITP?

Anti-Rh(D) antibody given intravenously can be used to treat ITP in patients who are Rh(D) positive. The patient's Rh(D)-positive red blood cells (RBCs) are coated by the anti-Rh(D) antibodies. These antibody-coated RBCs are then destroyed by the reticuloendothelial system occupying the Fc receptor in these macrophages, thereby sparing the destruction of the antibody-coated platelets.

9. What are the indications for splenectomy in childhood ITP?

In childhood ITP, splenectomy is indicated in chronic cases that are not responsive to the conventional agents and when it becomes difficult to sustain a safe platelet count without causing undesirable side effects from the medications. It is also done in emergency situations of life-threatening hemorrhage when a rapid rise in platelet count is necessary. Because of the high risk for sepsis after splenectomy in younger children and the greater chances for remission in childhood ITP, splenectomy is usually postponed until the patient reaches 6 years of age. Before splenectomy, the patient should receive the pneumococcal vaccine; post-operatively, prophylactic penicillin is indicated to prevent infection with *Streptococcus pneumoniae* and other encapsulated organisms.

10. Name some of the hereditary thrombocytopenias, their mode of inheritance and pertinent clinical features.

Features of Hereditary Thrombocytopenias

DISORDER	INHERITANCE	PLATELET SIZE	FEATURES
Thrombocytopenia with absent radii (TAR) syndrome	Autosomal recessive	Normal	Present at birth, absent radii, but normal thumbs, ↓ megakaryocytes, ↓ platelet aggregation to epinephrine and collagen
Chédiak-Higashi syndrome	Autosomal recessive	Normal	Oculocutaneous albinism, recurrent infections, large granules in white cells, ↓ platelet aggregation to epinephrine and collagen

Bernard-Soulier syndrome	Autosomal recessive	Large	Abnormal platelet function with ↓ aggregation to ristocetin secondary to reduced membrane GPIb-V-IX complex, prolonged bleeding time
Montreal platelet syndrome	Autosomal dominant	Large	Abnormal platelet function with ↓ aggregation to thrombin
Gray platelet syndrome	Autosomal recessive	Large	Agranular megakaryocytes, pale staining platelets secondary to ↓ alpha granules
May-Hegglin anomaly	Autosomal dominant	Large	Dohle bodies in granulocytes
Alport's syndrome	Autosomal dominant	Large	Nephritis, sensorineural deafness, white blood cell inclusions
Wiskott-Aldrich syndrome	X-linked	Small	Thrombocytopenia, eczema, immunodeficiency, recurrent infections

11. List some of the drugs that can cause immune-mediated thrombocytopenia.

- Heparin
- Valproic acid
- Digoxin
- Quinine
- Penicillins
- Cimetidine
- Quinidine

12. Name some of the hereditary platelet function disorders, their mode of inheritance, and platelet aggregation defects.

Features of Hereditary Platelet Function Disorders

DISORDER	INHERITANCE	PLATELET AGGREGATION DEFECT
Glanzmann's thrombasthenia	Autosomal recessive	Deficiency in GP IIb-IIIa, ↓ to all agonists except normal ristocetin aggregation
Bernard-Soulier syndrome	Autosomal recessive	Deficiency of GP Ib-V-IX complex, normal to all agonists except ↓ ristocetin aggregation
Pseudo von Willebrand disease	Autosomal dominant	Defect of GP Ib, increased binding of von Willebrand factor (VWF), ↑ ristocetin aggregation
Storage pool defects:		Abnormal aggregation to several agonists
Dense body deficiency	Autosomal recessive	Decreased thrombin release of ADP and serotonin, decreased dense bodies
Alpha granule deciciency (Gray platelet syndrome)	Autosomal recessive	Decreased alpha granules
Scott syndrome	Autosomal recessive	Normal aggregation platelet factor 3 deficiency

13. List some diseases or conditions that are associated with platelet function defects.

- Uremia
- Liver disease
- Leukemia: especially myeloid, myelodysplasia, myeloproliferative disorders

- Glycogen storage diseases, chronic hypoglycemia
- Valvular heart defects
- Cardiopulmonary bypass
- Nephrotic syndrome
- Hemolytic uremic syndrome, thrombotic thrombocytopenic purpura
- Infections: HIV, infectious mononucleosis

14. Name some of the drugs that are known to cause platelet dysfunction.

- Nonsteroidal anti-inflammatory agents
  Aspirin: causes irreversible effect on platelet function
  Indomethacin, ibuprofen, phenylbutazone, sulfinpyrazone: reversible effect
- Beta-lactam antibiotics: penicillins, cephalosporins
- Valproic acid
- Dextran
- Heparin
- Other drugs that can cause in vitro platelet dysfunction
  Antihistamines
  Phenothiazines
  Tricyclic antidepressants
  Anesthetics: halothane
  Beta-blocker: propranolol

15. What are the options for treatment of platelet function disorders?

Bleeding episodes in patients with known hereditary platelet function disorders without severe thrombocytopenia can be managed with desmopressin (DDAVP) infusions, except in Glanzmann's thrombasthenia and Scott syndrome. The potential role of DDAVP is to stimulate the release of VWF, enhancing platelet adhesion and aggregation. In severe forms or in those that are associated with significant thrombocytopenia, platelet transfusions can be given. Adjunctive treatment with antifibrinolytic agents like epsilon-amino-caproic acid is also helpful. The treatment for the acquired platelet function disorders is generally management of the primary disease. DDAVP infusions and cryoprecipitate transfusions to raise VWF concentration, as well as red cell transfusions and erythropoietin to correct the anemia, are used to treat platelet dysfunction in uremic patients.

16. Discuss thrombocytosis and its classification.

Thrombocytosis is defined as platelet count above the normal value (150,000–450,000). It can be either primary or secondary. Primary or essential thrombocytosis results from a stem cell defect and is seen in myeloproliferative disorders such as idiopathic thrombocythemia, polycythemia vera, chronic myelogenous leukemia and idiopathic myelofibrosis. This is very rare in children. Secondary or reactive thrombocytosis arises as a "reaction" to a predisposing condition such as hypoxia, infections, shift of platelet pool or platelet loss. This is common in children, particularly in young infants.

17. Name the conditions or illnesses associated with reactive or secondary thrombocytosis in children.

- Infections: pneumonia, meningitis, chronic osteomyelitis
- Hypoxia: pulmonary diseases, cardiac disorders, anemia
- After surgery or trauma
- After splenectomy
- Autoimmune disorders: Kawasaki syndrome, juvenile rheumatoid arthritis, collagen vascular disorders

- Inflammatory diseases: Crohn's disease, ulcerative colitis, rheumatic fever
- Hematologic disorders: iron deficiency anemia, chronic hemolytic anemias,hemoglobinopathies, rebound after thrombocytopenia
- Malignancy: neuroblastoma, lymphoma, hepatoblastoma
- Renal: nephrotic syndrome
- Drugs: epinephrine, corticosteroids, vinca alkaloids
- Following stress

18. What are the indications for treatment of thrombocytosis?

Primary thrombocytosis is associated with thrombosis as well as bleeding complications from disturbed platelet function. Treatment options include myelosuppressive agents, such as hydroxyurea, busulfan and interferon; platelet pheresis; and platelet aggregation inhibitors like aspirin and dypiridamole. In contrast, in secondary thrombocytosis, complications are extremely rare and the increased platelet count is generally transient, lasting only a few days or weeks. Except in Kawasaki syndrome, in which there is a known risk for thrombotic complications, reactive thrombocytosis generally does not require treatment. At times, antithrombotic prophylaxis like aspirin is advised when there are other existing risk factors for thrombosis, such as immobilization, vessel damage or hyperviscosity.

BIBLIOGRAPHY

1. Blanchette V, Carcao M: Approach to the investigation and management of immune thrombocytopenic pur pura in children. Semin Hematol 37:299–314, 2000.
2. Hathaway WE, Goodnight SH: Hereditary function defects. In Disorders of Hemostasis and Thrombosis: A Clinical Guide. Columbus, McGraw-Hill, Inc., 1993, pp 94-102.
3. Hathaway WE, Goodnight SH: Acquired platelet function disorders. In Disorders of Hemostasis and-Thrombosis: a Clinical Guide. Columbus, McGraw-Hill, Inc., 1993, pp 103–108.
4. Smith OP: Inherited and congenital thrombocytopenia. In Lilleyman J, Hann I, Blanchette V (eds): Pediatric Hematology. London, Churchill Livingstone, 1999, pp 419–435.
5. Sutor AH: Thrombocytosis in childhood. Semin Thrombosis Hemostasis 21:330–339, 1995.

14. CHILDHOOD IMMUNOLOGICAL DISORDERS

Kiery A. Braithwaite, M.D., and Mitchell S. Cairo, M.D.

1. What are the signs and symptoms that leads one to suspect an immune deficiency in a child?

Infections with unusual organisms, unusual sites of infection, poor and/or unusual response to specific infections and multiple organisms causing infection.

2. Name the most common congenital disorder of the immune system.

IgA deficiency, which occurs in an estimated 1/200 to 1/1000 people, is the most common congenital disorder of the immune system. Excluding IgA deficiency, the incidence of a primary immunodeficiency is approximately 1 in 10,000. This translates into approximately 400 new cases per year in the United States, with an estimated 5000–10,000 total cases. For comparison, the overall incidence is one-fourth that of cystic fibrosis (1 in 2500), and slightly more frequent than phenylketonuria (1 in 14,000). More specifically, both DiGeorge's syndrome and severe combined immunodeficiency (SCID) occur in 1 in 66,000 people, while chronic granulomatous disease (CGD) has a frequency of 1 in 181,000.

3. Describe the clinical manifestations of patients with selective IgA deficiency. What other disorders are associated with this disorder?

Although most patients with IgA deficiency are asymptomatic and unaware of the underlying disorder, it is associated with a large number of conditions such as allergic disorders, gastrointestinal disorders, neurological disease and autoimmune phenomenon. Despite secretory IgA's role in maintaining mucosal integrity, these patients' susceptibility to infections and illnesses is considered normal. The reason behind this is unclear, although most attribute it to compensatory mechanisms by the immune system. For the few patients who are symptomatic, recurrent sinopulmonary infection is the most frequent illness associated with selective IgA deficiency.

4. What is the most common malignancy in children with immunodeficiencies?

Non-Hodgkin's lymphoma (NHL) is the most common malignancy seen in pediatric patients who are immunocompromised. This includes patients with inherited immunodeficiencies, including Wiskott-Aldrich syndrome (WAS), SCID, and ataxia-telangiectasia, as well as children with acquired diseases such as HIV/AIDS. Furthermore, patients who receive immunosuppressive medications for organ, bone marrow and/or stem cell transplants have an increased risk of developing B cell lymphomas.

5. Which malignancies have an increased incidence in children with HIV/AIDS?

Malignancy in children with HIV/AIDS is less frequent than in the adult AIDS population. NHL is the leading AIDS-associated pediatric malignancy; thus, all children diagnosed with NHL should be tested for HIV. NHL in the pediatric AIDS patient is typically Burkitt's lymphoma, and the typical chromosomal translocation t(8;14)(q24;q32) that is associated with Burkitt's lymphoma is frequently appreciated. Fortunately, these patients respond favorably to standard NHL chemotherapy regimens.

Leiomyomas and leiomyosarcomas are the second leading cancers in pediatric AIDS patients. They may be associated with Epstein-Barr virus infection. Unfortunately, treatments have not proven as successful as those for NHL and recurrences are frequent.

Kaposi's sarcoma (KS) and leukemia are the third and fourth occurring malignancies arising in pediatric AIDS patients. KS, however, is much less common in children than in adults with AIDS.

6. The clinical triad of eczema, thrombocytopenia and immunodeficiency characterizes what genetic disorder?

Wiskott-Aldrich syndrome is a rare x-linked recessive disease characterized by immunological defects involving B and T cells, thrombocytopenia and eczema. The genetic defect has been localized to the p11 region of the X chromosome, which codes for the WAS protein (WASP). WASP is expressed on lymphocytes, megakaryocytes and their progenitors, and splenic and thymic cells. Immunologically, patients have defective T cell function, poor antibody response to polysaccharide antigens, as well as a characteristic serum immunoglobulin pattern with elevated levels of IgA and IgE but depressed levels of IgM. Hematologically, patients have thrombocytopenia, which is characterized by small platelets and decreased peripheral survival. A child with WAS has an increased susceptibility to developing autoimmune diseases and malignancies such as NHL. Overwhelming infection and severe hemorrhage may be life threatening and without successful allogeneic stem cell transplantation, the overall prognosis is poor.

7. How is the thrombocytopenia in WAS typically managed?

While awaiting allogeneic stem cell transplantation, children with WAS are constantly threatened by recurrent infections and bleeding episodes, which may range from minor to life-threatening. While infections are usually managed with antibiotics, the thrombocytopenia has traditionally been treated with platelet transfusions and, at times, splenectomy. Splenectomy effectively boosts platelet counts but subsequently predisposes the already immunodeficient WAS patient to increased susceptibility to infection. Frequent platelet transfusions, on the other hand, predispose the patient to alloimmunization and future allogeneic graft failure. Recently, the thromobopoietic growth factor, IL-11, was used to effectively elevate platelet counts and decrease the need for platelet transfusions in two WAS children prior to allogeneic stem cell transplant.

8. What congenital immunodeficiency is considered the most severe?

Severe combined immunodeficiency comprises a heterogeneous group of disorders caused by a variety of genetic mutations leading to profound defects in both cellular and humoral immunity. Within a few months of age, infants with SCID present with recurrent bacterial, viral and opportunistic infections such as persistent thrush, extensive diaper rash, intractable diarrhea, failure to thrive and a persistent cough. Untreated, most children die within the first 2 years of life. Patients demonstrate dramatic susceptibility to infection, very low levels of T cells, and hypogammaglobulinemia. Physical examination reveals hypoplastic peripheral lymph nodes and tonsils, as well as an absent thymus.

The most common form of SCID is x-linked, accounting for 50–60% of all SCID diagnoses. It is associated with a gamma chain mutation of the IL-2 receptor. This particular gamma chain is an essential element of several interleukin receptors that participate in the development of normal lymphocytes. Other variants of SCID include adenosine deaminase deficiency, Nezelof syndrome, Omenn's syndrome, reticular dysgenesis and SCID with defective expression of human leukocyte antigen (HLA).

9. Which variant of SCID did the "bubble boy" have?

Adenosine deaminase (ADA) deficiency. ADA is an enzyme of the purine metabolic pathway that catalyzes the irreversible deamination of adenosine and deoxyadenosine into inosine and 2'deoxyinosine, respectively. Although ADA is present in all cells, immature lymphocytes are especially sensitive to the toxic effects of excessive adenosine and deoxyadenosine. Children with ADA deficiency (15% of SCID patients) generally have more profound lymphopenia than in other types as well as unique skeletal abnormalities. There are four clinical phenotypes in ADA deficiency; unfortunately, 80–90% of patients present with the overwhelming immunodeficiency of the "bubble boy" due to undetectable levels of ADA. A very small percentage of patients have partial immunity, as only 1–5% of the normal levels of ADA are necessary for competent immune function.

10. Name the classic radiographic abnormality seen in children with ADA deficiency.

Approximately 50% of patients with ADA deficiency have flared costochondral junctions noted on routine chest x-ray. Although this finding is characteristic and may occasionally precipitate the diagnosis of ADA deficiency, it is not necessarily specific and is seen in other disorders. The absence of a thymic shadow on chest x-ray is also observed in patients with SCID.

11. Discuss the role of enzyme replacement in ADA deficiency.

Patients with ADA deficiency can be treated with weekly or biweekly injections of polyethylene glycol-modified bovine ADA (PEG-ADA). The immune system's response is variable, and approximately 20% of children do not respond to enzyme replacement. However, the majority of patients have significant clinical improvement, which correlates with a rise in their B and T cell counts within a few months of therapy. Patients with chronic infections as well as failure to thrive stabilize within a few months; respiratory infections and diarrhea diminish in frequency and severity, and opportunistic infections become rare. Not surprisingly, children with milder forms of ADA deficiency tend to respond more favorably to enzyme replacement therapy.

HLA-matched allogeneic stem cell transplantation (SCT), as well as gene therapy, which is currently under investigation, may provide a potential cure for ADA-deficient patients. However, PEG-ADA's ability to stabilize severe symptoms by partially reconstituting immune function benefits patients awaiting a suitable donor. Enzyme replacement is additionally important in ADA-deficient children undergoing gene therapy. By boosting peripheral T cell counts, PEG-ADA provides a source of autologous T cells, which may then be collected and reintroduced with the new gene. Continuing enzyme replacement during these early gene therapy trials also maintains an established regimen of treatment while simultaneously testing a novel therapy.

12. Discuss the role of gene therapy in SCID.

Severe combined immunodeficiency associated with ADA deficiency was the first congenital disease to be treated with gene therapy. In 1990, a clinical trial was initiated using a retroviral vector to transfer the ADA gene into autologous T cells of two children with ADA deficiency. PEG-ADA replacement therapy was continued during the trial, thus avoiding the ethical dilemma of withholding a known life-sustaining treatment. Moreover, because peripheral T cells were utilized to transfer the gene, multiple transfusions of autologous T cells with the ADA gene were necessary. Both children demonstrated a normalization of their peripheral T cell counts, an increase in ADA enzyme activity and an improvement in antibody response to vaccines; furthermore, both children were able to attend school and had a similar number of sick days, as compared with other children. More recently, efforts have been made to direct gene therapy at earlier bone marrow stem cells, thus avoiding the need for multiple transfusions of autologous T cells. Two children with x-linked SCID were recently treated using a retroviral vector to transfer complementary DNA into CD34 positive cells. Thus far, initial follow-up studies in both children demonstrate clinical benefits with successful correction of their disease manifestations.

13. Which congenital immunodeficiency is associated with a partial or complete absence of the thymus?

The DiGeorge syndrome is a congenital disorder associated with developmental anomalies in the third and fourth pharyngeal pouches during embryogenesis. This results in either hypoplasia or aplasia of the thymus and parathyroid glands, causing partial or complete DiGeorge syndrome, respectively. Other structures developing simultaneously are also frequently affected, often leading to both congenital heart disease and dysmorphic facies. Patients typically present with hypocalcemic seizures during the neonatal period. The degree of T cell deficiency varies from minor to severe corresponding to the degree of thymic hypoplasia. For children with partial DiGeorge, the T cell function can often improve spontaneously. However, in complete DiGeorge, T cell function is severely impaired, and only a few treatment options exist. HLA-identical bone marrow transplant has successfully restored T cell function due to the adoptive transfer of mature T cells present in the donor bone marrow. Recently, transplant of allogeneic fetal and/or neonatal thymus tissue during the neonatal period has also resulted in immune reconstitution. It is also important to note that it is not the degree of immunodeficiency that determines the prognosis in these children, but rather the severity of congenital heart disease.

14. Recurrent pyogenic infections and partial oculocutaneous albinism is found in what genetic disorder?

Chédiak-Higashi Syndrome (CHS) is a rare autosomal recessive disease characterized by complex immunological defects, partial oculocutanous albinism, and the presence of giant cytoplasmic granules in all granule-forming cells. These giant inclusion bodies in peripheral leukocytes and their bone marrow precursors are the diagnostic hallmark of CHS. The pathogenesis of this disease is poorly understood but results in several immunological defects including impaired activity of neutrophils and natural killer cells, abnormal chemotaxis, neutropenia and decreased antibody-dependent cellular cytotoxicity. Patients suffer from severe, recurrent infections that are treated with antibiotics.

15. What is the "accelerated phase" in CHS?

Most patients with CHS die within the first two decades of life secondary to the development of an "accelerated phase." This phase is characterized by jaundice, hepatosplenomegaly, lymphadenopathy, pancytopenia and extensive tissue infiltration by lymphoid cells. Once patients enter this phase, the outcome is usually fatal, although the combination of steroids and cytotoxic agents can sometimes prolong life. Allogeneic bone marrow transplantation has been shown to be the only curative treatment for CHS and should be considered prior to the onset of the accelerated phase.

16. What are the clinical manifestations associated with complement deficiencies?

Congenital complement deficiencies, while rare, have been described for all components of the pathway. Interestingly, depending on the particular deficiency, there are two classic clinical manifestations. Patients with C1q, C1r, C1rs, C2 and C4 deficiencies are usually associated with collagen-vascular diseases, such as systemic lupus, chronic glomerulonephritis, dermatomyositis and cutaneous vasculitis. On the other hand, patients with C3 and C5-C9 deficiencies typically have predisposition to recurrent bacterial infections; particularly, they have increased susceptibility to disseminated neisserial infections, resulting in recurrent gonococcal arthritis and meningococcal meningitis.

C2 is the most common complement deficiency. It usually manifests itself with the development of a collagen-vascular disease and less frequently with increased vulnerability to infection. However, an increased susceptibility to pneumococcal bacteremia is reported in a small subset of patients with C2 deficiency and should be considered in any child older than 2 years presenting with pneumococcal bacteremia who has no known risk factors.

17. Describe x-linked agammaglobulinemia (XLA).

XLA is the prototypical syndrome of pure B cell deficiency. Characterized by a developmental defect of maturing B cells, there are normal levels of pre-B cells within the bone marrow but an absence of B cells in the peripheral blood and lymphoid tissue. This is additionally associated with an absence of plasma cells and immunoglobulins. XLA is inherited in an x-linked recessive manner and results from a tyrosine kinase mutation (Btk, Bruton's tyrosine kinase). Cell-mediated immunity is intact. Affected male infants typically present with recurrent respiratory and/or gastrointestinal bacterial infections between 4 and 12 months of age. Prior to this, newborns are protected by placenta-derived maternal IgG. On physical examination, patients have hypoplastic tonsils, lymph nodes and adenoids, tissues that are all normally rich in B cells. The thymus is normal, in contrast to its absence in SCID. Serum studies in XLA will reveal profoundly depressed levels of all immunoglobulin classes.

18. Children with XLA are most susceptible to infection with what organisms?

Affected males are usually healthy until approximately 9–12 months of age and then develop recurrent pyogenic infections. *Haemophilus influenzae, Streptococcus pneumoniae, Staphylococcus aureus*, and *Pseudomonas* are the most prevalent organisms isolated from patients with XLA. Infections frequently localize to the respiratory tract, causing repeated bouts of otitis media, sinusitis, bronchitis and pneumonia. Septic arthritis involving the large joints is another common finding in these children.

Because cellular immunity is intact in XLA, resistance to viruses is normal, with one notable exception: enteroviruses. An increased susceptibility to the enterovirus family, including echovirus, coxsackie virus and poliovirus, occurs in XLA, as antibody helps neutralize these viruses from invasion. These virures usually infect the gastrointestinal tract, thus, frequent diarrhea is common. Enteroviruses may secondarily spread to the blood and central nervous system resulting in chronic meningoencephalitis, as well as a syndrome resembling dermatomyositis. Other manifestations of XLA less commonly reported include growth hormone deficiency, neutropenia, alopecia, glomerulonephritis, amyloidosis and malabsorption. Isolated studies have also described an increased prevalence of lymphoreticular malignancies and colorectal cancer in XLA.

19. Describe the conventional treatment method used for XLA.

Prophylactic therapy with intravenous immunoglobulin (IVIG) is the most effective treatment for XLA. Children who receive high doses of IVIG to sustain IgG levels near normal (> 500 mg/dL) have significantly fewer infections and hospitalizations. Although many infections respond to antibiotics, without IVIG, recurrent infection leads to anatomical destruction such as chronic pulmonary insufficiency. The combination of early diagnosis, aggressive initiation of prophylactic IVIG, and the judicious use of antibiotics allow many patients to reach adulthood when previously they rarely survived early childhood. It is important to note though that while IVIG does substantially improve prognosis, it has its limitations; namely, it only replaces IgG and not the other immunoglobulins, and it doesn't prevent all infections.

20. What is the pathophysiology of CGD?

The neutrophils in CGD patients are incapable of killing intracellular bacteria. Phagocytosis of bacteria by the CGD neutrophil is normal; however, the neutrophil is subsequently unable to kill the ingested microorganisms due to the failure of the NADPH oxidase system to generate superoxide and other reactive oxygen species. Thus, patients with CGD can manifest a normal reaction to infection with fever, an appropriate local inflammatory response and leukocytosis. However, the failure to kill the ingested microorganisms leads to their persistence within the neutrophils, forming a nidus for chronic inflammation and granuloma formation. CGD is inherited either as an x-linked or recessive disorder and is associated with different genetic mutations that can be differentiated by Western blot analysis. The nitroblue tetrazolium (NBT) test is both sensitive and specific for CGD and is useful for establishing diagnosis. In normal patients, a positive result occurs when neutrophil-generated superoxide reduces the soluble yellow NBT dye to an insoluble deep blue dye. However, in CGD, the dye remains yellow, yielding a negative test.

21. Patients with CGD are most susceptible to infection with what microbes?

CGD patients are especially susceptible to infections with catalase-positive microorganisms, including *Staphylococci, Serratia marcescens, Nocardia, E. coli, Pseudomonas* and *Aspergillosis*, as well as opportunistic fungi such as *Candida*. On the other hand, catalase-negative microbes, such as *Streptococcus pneumoniae* and *Haemophilus influenzae* do not pose problems for CGD patients, because these microbes generate enough hydrogen peroxide themselves within the phagocytic vacuoles to contribute to their own demise.

22. What test should be performed in any CGD patient prior to blood transfusion?

There is an association between CGD and the rare Kell blood phenotype, Ko. Although there is no defect in the development and function of erythrocytes in CGD, anemia may be a common secondary manifestation due to severe recurrent infections, as well as gastrointestinal pathology, such as persistent diarrhea, steatorrhea and vitamin B12 malabsorption. Thus, Kell phenotyping is routinely recommended in CGD patients to avoid potential risk of sensitization. If the patient is Ko positive, transfusions should be avoided. If necessary, Ko-positive erythrocytes should be used.

23. Discuss the use of stem cell transplants in patients with primary immunodeficiencies.

Allogeneic SCT offers a cure for the majority of patients with severe genetic immunodeficiencies, including SCID, WAS, CHS and CGD. HLA-identical bone marrow transplants have even been utilized in DiGeorge's syndrome to successfully restore cell-mediated immunity by the adoptive transfer of mature T cells from the donor bone marrow. HLA-identical related SCT is frequently associated with the best outcome, but closely matched unrelated SCT has also proven efficacious in these diseases. Furthermore, matched and mismatched umbilical cord blood donors recently have proven to be an additional adequate source of transplantable hematopoietic cells.

In utero SCT additionally has been successfully performed in patients diagnosed prenatally with SCID. This technique is potentially advantageous because it allows for immunologic reconstitution prior to the onset of a life-threatening infection. However, whether this outweighs the risks associated with chorionic villus sampling and intraperitoneal transfusions should be carefully considered.

BIBLIOGRAPHY

1. Blaese RM, Culver KW, Miller AD, et al. T lymphocyte-directed gene therapy for ADA-SCID: Initial trial results after 4 years. Science 270:475–480, 1995.
2. Braithwaite K, Abu-Ghosh A, Anderson L, Cairo MS. Effect of interleukin-11 in decreasing the need for platelet transfusions and bleeding symptoms in children with severe thrombocytopenia (TCP) secondary to Wiskott-Aldrich Syndrome (WAS) prior to allogeneic stem cell transplantation (ALLO SCT) [abstract]. Pediatr Res 47:247a, 1999.
3. Buckley RH, Schiff SE, Schiff RI, et al. Hematopoietic stem-cell transplantation for the treatment of severe combined immunodeficiency [see comments]. N Engl J Med 340:508–516, 1999.
4. Cavazzana-Calvo M, Hacein-Bey S, de Saint Basile G, et al. Gene therapy of human severe combined immunodeficiency (SCID)-X1 disease [see comments]. Science 288:669–672, 2000.
5. Haddad E, Le Deist F, Blanche S, et al. Treatment of Chédiak-Higashi syndrome by allogenic bone marrow transplantation: Report of 10 cases. Blood 85:3328–3333, 1995.

6. Hershfield MS. PEG-ADA replacement therapy for adenosine deaminase deficiency: An update after 8.5 years. Clin Immunol Immunopathol 76:S228–232, 1995.
7. Markert ML, Boeck A, Hale LP, et al. Transplantation of thymus tissue in complete DiGeorge syndrome [see comments]. N Engl J Med 341:1180–1189, 1999.
8. Ochs HD, Smith CI. X-linked agammaglobulinemia. A clinical and molecular analysis. Medicine (Baltimore) 75:287–299, 1996.
9. Rosen FS, Cooper MD, Wedgwood RJ. The primary immunodeficiencies. N Engl J Med 333:431–440, 1995.
10. Wagner JE, Rosenthal J, Sweetman R, et al. Successful transplantation of HLA-matched and HLA-mismatched umbilical cord blood from unrelated donors: analysis of engraftment and acute graft-versus-host disease. Blood 88:795–802, 1996.

15. DISORDERS OF GRANULOCYTE FUNCTION AND GRANULOPOIESIS

Jill S. Menell, M.D.

1. Describe the signs and symptoms suggestive of a defect in white blood cell number or function.

The skin and mucous membranes are the first line of defense. Once these barriers are broken, the white blood cells, specifically neutrophils, come into play. When neutrophils are defective or the count is low the most common abnormalities are skin and mucous membrane infections. Common presentations include cutaneous cellulitis, superficial or deep abscesses, furunculosis, pneumonia and septicemia. Also common are gingivitis, aphthous ulcers, perirectal inflammation and otitis media. Recurrent respiratory infections, such as pneumonia or sinusitis, also raise suspicion of a white cell disorder. Neutrophils elaborate cytokines and recruit other cells to mediate an inflammatory response. With profound neutropenia, patients may present with high fevers and no obvious focus of infection. The usual inflammatory signs may be absent. Infants who have frequent infections should be evaluated for an underlying defect in their white cells or other branch of the immune system.

2. What are the common pathogens noted in patients with neutrophil disorders?

The most common organisms are skin and gut flora. Patients with other underlying immune defects (such as those involving lymphocytes as well as neutrophils) or those who are neutropenic secondary to chemotherapeutic agents are further at risk for viral, fungal and parasitic pathogens due to a more global immunodeficiency. Individuals with chronic granulomatous disease are unable to mount a respiratory burst to destroy the organisms. They are commonly infected with *Staphylococcus aureus* or more unusual pathogens, such as *Pseudomonas cepacia*, *Serratia marcescens*, *Candida* species, and *Aspergillus fumigatus*.

3. Give the normal values for white blood cell and neutrophil counts.

White blood cell (WBC) and neutrophil counts vary with age and race. Newborns have high WBC counts of 10-30,000/μL, predominantly neutrophils. These numbers drop sharply after the first few days of life. An infant's WBC count after the first month of life runs slightly higher than that of older children and adults (6–17,000/μL) and the differential is predominantly lymphocytes, 60–70%, with 20–30% neutrophils. Toddlers and preschool-age children have approximately equal numbers of lymphocytes and neutrophils. Older children and adolescents have mostly neutrophils, with WBC counts similar to those of adults (5–11,000/μL).

Neutropenia is defined as an absolute neutrophil count (ANC) less than 1,000/μL for infants younger than 1 yr and 1,500/μl for individuals older than 1 yr. The ANC is calculated by multiplying the total WBC count by the percentage of neutrophils. African Americans have 200–600 neutrophils/μL fewer, compared with caucasians. An ANC of 1000-1500/μL is considered mild neutropenia, 500–1000/μL is moderate, and <500/μL is severe neutropenia. These definitions are useful, in that severe neutropenia is associated with the more severe infections.

4. What are the clinical features of isoimmune and autoimmune neutropenia?

Isoimmune neutropenia is analogous to Rh hemolytic disease or alloimmune thrombocytopenia of the newborn. Maternal antibodies directed against fetal neutrophil antigens cross the placenta and mediate immune destruction of the neutrophils. The mother lacks the fetal WBC antigens that are inherited from the father. The most common antigens are NA1 and NA2, which are isotypes of the FcγRIIIB receptor. These infants may be quite ill with infections secondary to profound neutropenia, or they may be asymptomatic. Omphalitis, skin infections, pneumonia, sepsis and meningitis are the most common infections. Neutropenia is a common feature of neonatal sepsis in general. The diagnosis of isoimmune neutropenia is established by detecting antineutrophil antibodies in the maternal and infant sera. Paternal blood is helpful to establish that the mother's serum reacts with *his* cells.

Autoimmune neutropenia of infancy is generally a benign disorder. Affected individuals are often found incidentally with a routine blood count or when diagnosed with a minor infection. Despite ANCs of <500/μL, 80–90% of patients do not have severe infectious complications. The total WBC count is normal. Some patients exhibit increased numbers of monocytes and eosinophils. The median age at diagnosis is 8 months, with a range of 3–30 months. There is a female-to-male predominance of 3:2. Other signs of autoimmune disease are absent. The disease is self-limited, often resolving by the age of 4 yr. Most infections are managed with oral antibiotics. Patients with recurrent infections may benefit from prophylaxis with co-trimoxazole 5 mg/kg, split into two doses per day. Granulocyte colony-stimulating factor (G-CSF) appears to be useful for severe infections.

Autoimmune neutropenia may be associated with systemic disease such as systemic lupus erythematosis, common variable immunodeficiency and immunoglobulin (IgA) deficiency.

5. Describe the approach to treating a patient with neutropenia.

The history should include previous neutrophil measurements, recent viral infections, current and past infections, growth and development, congenital anomalies, medication history or toxic exposures and a family history of infections or unexplained infant deaths.

The physical exam should focus on signs of underlying disease; i.e., growth and development, phenotypic abnormalities, lymphadenopathy, organomegaly, pallor bruising and petechiae. Sites of infection should be evaluated carefully, including mucous membranes, gingiva, skin, ears, lungs and the perianal area.

The laboratory work-up should be determined based on the history and physical exam. If the child appears otherwise well and the past medical history is unremarkable, then the likely diagnosis is an intercurrent viral illness responsible for the neutropenia. In this case, a complete blood count (CBC) and a peripheral smear may be the only tests indicated. If there are no suspicious cells on the smear and the other cell lines are normal, then it is reasonable to repeat the count in 3 or 4 weeks to document recovery of normal counts. Persistent neutropenia warrants antineutrophil antibody testing, especially in infancy. Serum B_{12} and folate levels may be indicated based upon dietary history and the presence of a high mean corpuscular volume (MCV) or other changes in the CBC. A bone marrow aspirate is not indicated in the child who is not having frequent infections.

Children with a significant infectious history associated with chronic neutropenia require more extensive evaluation. CBCs should be obtained two times per week for 6 weeks to document whether cycling of the blood cells is occurring. This would distinguish cyclic neutropenia from severe congenital neutropenia. Children with a malabsorption history should be assessed for pancreatic exocrine function and skeletal survey to evaluate for metaphyseal chondrodysplasia.

Bone marrow aspirate and biopsy are indicated for any child with more than isolated neutropenia (i.e. anemia, high MCV with normal B_{12} and folate levels or thrombocytopenia). The bone marrow should be sent for cytogenetic testing, special stains and flow studies as indicated.

A steroid mobilization test may prove useful in predicting those patients who may have a less severe clinical course.

6. Distinguish between the different forms of congenital neutropenia.

Severe congenital neutropenia or Kostmann's syndrome is an autosomal recessive disorder of neutrophil maturation. The bone marrow shows arrest of myeloid maturation at the promyelocyte stage. Patients have profound neutropenia from birth (commonly <200 cells/μL) and develop fever, skin infections (omphalitis), stomatitis and perirectal abscesses. They often succumb to overwhelming infections. This is a premalignant condition with progression to myelodysplastic syndrome or acute myelogenous leukemia. Monosomy 7 is a common cytogenetic abnormality in the development of malignancy.

Cyclic neutropenia is a rare autosomal dominant disorder of neutrophil production, in which the neutrophils and other cells oscillate in number every 21 ± 3 days. The neutropenic nadir is usually <200 cells/μL and generally persists for 3–5 days. Some individuals have longer or shorter cycles, with a range of 15–36 days. Infections are frequent during the neutropenic phase. They may be minor with aphthous ulcerations, gingivitis, periodontitis, or pharyngitis associated with cervical lymphadenopathy. More serious infections include pneumonia, mastoiditis, and vaginal or rectal ulcerations. Ten percent of individuals succumb to overwhelming infections. The severity of the illness tends to lessen in older individuals.

Chronic benign neutropenia may be familial or sporadic. These individuals have severe neutropenia without recurrent infections. They often have increased numbers of monocytes and eosinophils. The bone marrow shows maturation through the band stage. Response to a steroid challenge is noted. Infections are usually mild.

Reticular dysgenesis is a failure of the stem cells to form both myeloid and lymphoid precursors. Severe neutropenia and moderate to severe lymphopenia is present with agammaglobulinemia. The red cells and platelets are unaffected. Patients often develop fatal bacterial or viral infections.

X-linked hyper IgM immunodeficiency is often associated with cyclic or persistent neutropenia. Neutropenia may be secondary to an autoimmune phenomenon.

Abnormal physical findings will help to distinguish some of the forms of congenital neutropenia. The Shwachman-Diamond syndrome is associated with metaphyseal chondrodysplasia, dwarfism, pancreatic exocrine dysfunction and neutropenia. Common features are chronic diarrhea secondary to malabsorption, failure to thrive and recurrent infections (pneumonia, otitis media).

Cartilage-hair hypoplasia is found in individuals of Amish decent and is characterized by short-limbed dwarfism, fine hair and neutropenia. These individuals may have associated immune dysfunction that leads to severe infections.

Dyskeratosis congenita is an X-linked recessive disorder characterized by nail dystrophy, leukoplakia, and reticulated hyperpigmentation of the skin. Most of these individuals survive to adulthood. Dyskeratosis congenita is thought to be secondary to a defect in DNA repair. Bone marrow transplantation is curative; however, these individuals are at higher risk for complications.

Fanconi's anemia is an autosomal recessive disorder associated with a long list of congenital anomalies. The more common are skin disorders (60%—hyperpigmentation, café au lait spots, hypopigmented areas), short stature (57%), upper limbs (48%—thumb abnormalities with or without radial anomalies, clinodactyly, polydactyly, ulnar abnormalities), hypogonads in male patients (37%), head or face abnormalities (27%—microcephaly, hydrocephalus, micrognathia, peculiar face, bird facies, flat head, frontal bossing), eye disorders (26%—small eyes, strabismus, epicanthal folds, hypertelorism), and renal problems (23%—ectopic or pelvic kidney, horseshoe kidney, hypoplastic or dysplastic kidney, absent kidney, hydronephrosis, hydroureter). There are many other anomalies with a frequency of <20%. Fanconi's anemia may present as an isolated cytopenia, or the other cell lines may be affected as well. The underlying defect is a problem with DNA repair. The diagnosis is established by demonstrating an increase in spontaneous chromatid strand breaks and enhanced sensitivity to clastogenic agents such as diepoxybutane.

Chédiak-Higashi syndrome is a rare autosomal recessive disorder with partial oculocutaneous albinism and giant cytoplasmic inclusions in the neutrophils, monocytes and lymphocytes. Cells containing granules are affected (melanosomes in the skin, white cells and platelets). Ineffective myelopoiesis leads to neutropenia. Impaired neutrophil function and neutropenia lead to recurrent infections. Platelet dysfunction leads to increased bleeding symptoms. The peripheral smear is diagnostic with the abnormal inclusions in the white cells. Patients may develop an accelerated phase with massive proliferation of T lymphocytes in the liver, spleen and bone marrow, resulting in worsened cytopenias.

Several inborn errors of metabolism are associated with neutropenia and other cytopenias. These include glycogen storage disease type IB, methylmalonic acidemia, isovaleric acidemia and prioponic acidemia.

7. Describe acquired causes of neutropenia.

Infection is probably the most common cause of an acquired neutropenia, with viruses being the most common. There may be a history of a nonspecific viral illness in the preceding days to weeks prior to presentation. Viral causes of neutropenia include: cytomegalovirus, Epstein-Barr virus, hepatitis, herpes simplex, human immunodeficiency virus, influenza A and B, measles, mumps, parvovirus, respiratory syncitial virus, roseola, varicella and others. Bacterial causes of neutropenia include gram-negative sepsis, paratyphoid and typhoid fever, brucellosis, tuberculosis and tularemia. Other rare infectious causes of neutropenia include fungal (histoplasmosis), protozoan (leishmaniasis, malaria), rickettsial (rickettsial pox, Rocky Mountain spotted fever, typhus fever).

Many medications can either affect bone marrow production or cause an immune-mediated destruction of the neutrophil. The broad categories of medications that may cause neutropenia include chemotherapy, heavy metals, analgesic/anti-inflammatory, antipsychotic/antidepressant, anticonvulsant, antithyroid, cardiovascular, antihistamine, antimicrobial, antiretroviral and other miscellaneous medications. It is important to review a medication history and determine if a medication may be responsible for the neutropenia prior to an extensive work-up.

Immune mechanisms, either isoimmune or autoimmune, may be a cause of an acquired neutropenia, as discussed earlier. Nutritional causes of neutropenia include severe generalized deficiencies (such as starvation, anorexia nervosa or marasmus), megaloblastic disorders (vitamin B_{12} or folic acid) or copper deficiency. Splenomegaly may cause neutropenia due to sequestration of WBCs in the enlarged organ. Infiltration of the bone marrow by leukemic or extrinsic tumor cells (neuroblastoma or other metastatic solid tumor) may be associated with neutropenia as well. Nutritional deficiencies, splenomegaly and bone marrow infiltration are often associated with involvement of more than one cell line (i.e., thrombocytopenia, anemia). Bone marrow failure syndromes and myelodysplastic syndrome may begin as an isolated cytopenias involving the leukocytes.

8. What are the clinical features of leukocyte adhesion disorder?

Leukocyte adhesion disorder presents in early infancy with frequent infections. A classic feature is omphalitis and delayed separation of the umbilical stump. The neutrophils are deficient in or missing the CD11/CD18 family of receptors. These molecules are responsible for adhesion of the neutrophils to sites of inflammation. The WBC and neutrophil counts are high, since the cells are unable to exit the circulation due to the lack of these surface receptors. Patients also exhibit impaired wound healing. Individuals with severe disease die in early childhood.

9. Describe the clinical features of a patient with chronic granulomatous disease. How is the diagnosis established?

Chronic granulomatous disease (CGD) is a qualitative disorder of the neutrophil. The neutrophils have normal chemotactic and phagocytic function but are unable to kill catalase positive organisms. The disease is caused by mutations in the genes involved in the NADPH oxidase system that is responsible for generating reactive oxygen species in the lysosomes. Approximately two-thirds of cases are inherited in an X-linked recessive mode involving the membrane protein, cytochrome oxidase b_{558} (91 kDa protein). The others are inherited in an autosomal recessive pattern with involvement of cytosolic proteins 22, 47 or 67 kDa.

The clinical presentation is severe recurrent bacterial or fungal purulent disease. The common sites of infection are lungs, skin, gastrointestinal tract, liver and lymph nodes. Generalized lymphadenopathy and hepatosplenomegaly are common physical findings. The infections are often with organisms not ordinarily considered pathogens. The common offending pathogens are catalase positive and include *S. aureus*, *P. cepacia*, *S. marcescens*, *Candida* species, and *A. fumigatus*.

The diagnosis is established with the nitroblue tetrazolium test. Normal neutrophils generate superoxide radicals that change the dye from yellow to blue. CGD neutrophils are unable to produce the blue color change.

10. What are some general guidelines for the treatment of patients with disorders of neutrophil number and function?

Individuals with neutropenia without recurrent infections should be monitored periodically, but no specific therapy is indicated. Parents and caretakers should be advised of some general precautions which include a heightened awareness of the danger of fevers with prompt evaluation by a physician, good oral hygiene and avoiding rectal temperatures. Patients with fever and severe neutropenia (ANC <500 cell/μL) should be treated as bacterial sepsis until proven otherwise. The incidence of bacterial sepsis is approximately 20% with fever and severe neutropenia. Broad-spectrum antibiotics to cover skin and gastrointestinal flora are indicated until bacterial cultures are negative. Patients in septic shock should receive a beta-lactamase resistant antibiotic and an aminoglycoside for gram-negative organisms. A rapid response time is imperative.

G-CSF has been proven to reduce the rate of infections in a number of inherited and acquired disorders of neutropenia. These include severe congenital neutropenia (Kostmann's syndrome), cyclic neutropenia, Shwachman-Diamond syndrome and dyskeratosis congenita. G-CSF is useful in immune neutropenia when associated with a severe infection.

Prophylaxis with co-trimoxazole (5–10 mg/kg divided into two doses per day) has been shown to dramatically reduce infections in patients with chronic neutropenia and CGD. This should be considered in the infant with autoimmune neutropenia and recurrent infections.

Gamma interferon (50 mcg/m^2/dose three times per week) should be used long term in patients with CGD. Aggressive surgical drainage of abscesses is also warranted in these patients.

Stem cell transplantation is the only cure for the severe congenital neutropenias and bone marrow failure states.

11. Name the disorders associated with atypical lymphocytes.

Atypical lymphocytes are T cells that are generally large with foamy, vacuolated cytoplasm. The borders of the cell are indented by surrounding red blood cells. Some may appear immature with nucleoli. These cells are most commonly seen in viral infections. Epstein-Barr virus and cytomegalovirus are the two most common viruses to consider when the atypical lymphocyte count exceeds 20% of the peripheral WBC count. Other causes of marked atypical lymphocytosis include infectious hepatitis, posttransfusion syndrome and drug hypersensitivity (p-amino salicylic acid, phenytoin, mephenytoin and organic arsenicals).

Less dramatic atypical lymphocyte counts (<20%) are associated with many viruses, such as mumps, varicella, measles, rubella, herpes simplex, herpes zoster, and roseola. Other infectious agents include brucellosis, tuberculosis, toxoplasmosis, rickettsialpox and syphilis. Hematologic causes of atypical lymphocytes include Langerhans' cell histiocytosis, leukemia, lymphoma and agranulocytosis. Lead poisoning and stress are other miscellaneous causes of atypical lymphocytosis.

12. What are the causes of eosinophilia?

Allergy is the most common cause of eosinophilia in children in the United States. Acute allergic reactions can be associated with counts exceeding 20,000/μL. Chronic allergies are associated with more modest increases in eosinophils (2,000/μL). Allergic entities associated with increased eosinophils include asthma, hay fever, drug reaction and allergic bronchopulmonary aspergillosis. Dermatologic disorders associated with eosinophilia include atopic dermatitis, eczema, scabies, acute urticaria, pemphigus and toxic epidermal necrolysis. Gastrointestinal disorders, such as Crohn's disease, ulcerative colitis, eosinophilic gastritis and milk precipitin disease are associated with increased eosinophils. One third of patients with chronic hepatitis will exhibit an increased eosinophil count. Abdominal radiation is associated with increased eosinophils. Malignant diseases, such as brain tumors, Hodgkin's and non-hodgkin's lymphoma and myeloproliferative disorders may have an associated eosinophilia. Eosinophilia may be seen in a variety of other disorders, including immunodeficiency disorders (particularly Wiskott-Aldrich syndrome), autoimmune disorders, chronic peritoneal dialysis or hemodialysis, congenital heart disease and TAR syndrome (thrombocytopenia with absent radii).

Outside of the United States, the most common cause of eosinophilia is parasitic infestation. Helminthic organisms include *Ascaris lumbricoides*, trichinosis, echinococcus, visceral larva migrans, hookworm, strongyloides and filariasis. Protozoan parasites include malaria, toxoplasmosis and pneumocystis.

The hypereosinophilic syndrome is rare in children. It is a spectrum of disease that includes Löffler's pulmonary syndrome (self-limited) to severe chronic conditions that are eventually fatal. These conditions are defined as persistent eosinophilia of >1500/μL for longer than 6 months, no evidence of malignancy or other cause of the increased count and signs and symptoms of organ involvement with infiltration of eosinophils. The bone marrow shows increased numbers of eosinophils but no immature forms to suggest leukemia. Nonspecific symptoms include fever, weight loss and fatigue. Cardiac damage by the eosinophils and their byproducts is the usual cause of death.

BIBLIOGRAPHY

1. Alter BA, Young NS: The bone marrow failure syndromes. In Nathan DG, Orkin SH (eds): Nathan and Oski's Hematology of Infancy and Childhood, 5th ed. Philadelphia, W.B. Saunders, 1998, pp 237–335.
2. Boxer LA, Blackwood RA: Leukocyte disorders: Quantitative and qualitative disorders of the neutrophil, part I. Pediatr Rev 17:19–28, 1996.
3. Boxer LA, Blackwood RA: Leukocyte disorders: Quantitative and qualitative disorders of the neutrophil, part II. Pediatr Rev 17:47–50, 1996.
4. Bux J, Behrens G, Jaeger G, Welte K: Diagnosis and clinical course of autoimmune neutropenia in infancy: Analysis of 240 cases. Blood 91:181–186, 1998.
5. Dinauer MC: The phagocyte system and disorders of granulopoiesis and granulocye function. In Nathan DG, Orkin SH (eds): Nathan and Oski's Hematology of Infancy and Childhood, 5th ed. Philadelphia, W.B. Saunders, 1998, pp 19–52.
6. Lekstrom-Hines JA, Gallin JI: Immunodeficiency diseases caused by defects in phagocytes. N Engl J Med 343:1703–1714, 2000.

16. STORAGE DISORDERS

James H. Garvin, Jr,. M.D., Ph.D.

1. How common are storage disorders?

Storage disorders are the group of inherited metabolic diseases ("inborn errors of metabolism") in which a particular metabolic pathway is blocked due to an absent or defective enzyme or transport protein. Accumulation of toxic levels of substrate (or intermediate metabolites from an alternate pathway) leads to symptomatic disease. Although each individual condition is rare, the collective incidence of these disorders is about 1 in 5000 live births. Inheritance is usually autosomal recessive, with both parents being asymptomatic carriers. The risk will be increased if there is parental consanguinity.

2. Although inheritance of most storage disorders is autosomal recessive, which of these disorders shows x-linked inheritance?

Hunter's syndrome and adrenoleukodystrophy are transmitted as x-linked recessive traits. This has practical implications for genetic counseling.

3. When do these disorders typically present?

Disorders of protein and carboydrate metabolism and mitochondrial disorders usually present acutely in the neonatal period. Less-severe variants may be diagnosed later in childhood. Glycogen storage disorders, lysosomal storage disorders, fatty acid oxidation defects and disturbances of purine and pyrimidine synthesis usually present more insidiously in infancy or childhood. Sphingolipidoses may be diagnosed throughout childhood. Sphingolipidoses with onset between 3 and 6 months of age include type II Gaucher's disease, type A Niemann-Pick disease, Tay-Sachs disease, Farber's disease and globoid-cell leukodystrophy (Krabbe's disease). Disorders with later onset include infantile metachromatic leukodystrophy (age 6 months to 2 years) and types I and III Gaucher's disease, types B and C Nemann-Pick disease, juvenile metachromatic leukodystrophy and Fabry's disease (age 2 years to adolescence).

4. Name the principal types of storage disorders and give examples of each.

The principal types of storage disorders are listed in Table 1. Related conditions include skeletal dysplasias (osteogenesis imperfecta, osteopetrosis), cystinosis, hyperlipoproteinemias and the porphyrias.

Classification of Storage Diseases

METABOLIC DEFECT	TYPES OF DEFECT	EXAMPLES
Disorders of Protein Metabolism	Aminoacidopathies	• Phenylketonuria • Tyrosinemia • Maple syrup urine disease (branched-chain ketoaciduria)
	Organic acidemias	• Methylmalonic acidemia • Isovaleric acidemia • Lactic acidemia
	Urea cycle enzyme defects	• Citrullinemia • Carbamyl phosphate synthetase deficiency • Ornithine transcarbamylase deficiency

Continued on next page

Classification of Storage Diseases (continued)

METABOLIC DEFECT	TYPES OF DEFECT	EXAMPLES
Disorders of carbohydrate metabolism	Carbohydrate intolerance	• Galactosemia • Hereditary fructose intolerance
	Glycogen storage disorders	Liver glycogenoses • von Gierke's disease (glucose-6-phosphatase deficiency) Muscle glycogenoses • Pompe's disease (acid maltase deficiency) • McArdle's disease (phosphorylase deficiency)
Lysosomal storage disorders	Sphingolipidoses	• Tay-Sachs disease (hexosaminidase A deficiency) • Gaucher's disease (glucocerebrosidase deficiency) • Niemann-Pick disease (sphingomyelinase deficiency) • Generalized gangliosidosis (β-galactosidase deficiency) • Sandhoff disease (hexosaminidase A deficiency) • Farber disease (ceramidase deficiency) • Fabry's disease (ceramide trihexosidase deficiency) • Wolman disease (acid lipase deficiency)
	Leukodystrophies	• Metachromatic leukodystrophy (arylsulfatase A deficiency) • Globoid cell leukodystrophy (Krabbe's disease) (galactocerebosidase deficiency)
	Mucopolysaccharidoses	• Hurler syndrome, Scheie's syndrome, Hurler-Scheie compound (α-L-iduronidase deficiency) • Hunter's syndrome (iduronate sulfatase deficiency) • Sanfilippo's syndrome types A, B, C, D (heparan *N*-sulfatase deficiency, α-*N*-acetyltransferase deficiency, α-acetyltranserase deficiency, α-acetylglucosamine-6-sulfatase deficiency) • Maroteaux-Lamy syndrome (galactosamine-4-sulfatase deficiency) • Sly syndrome (β-glucuronidase deficiency) • Morquio syndrome (galactose-6-sulfatase deficiency)
	Mucolipidoses	• Sialidosis (glycoprotein sialidase deficiency) • I-Cell disease (lysosomal hydrolase deficiency) • Mannosidosis (α-mannosidase deficiency)
	Glycogenoses	• Acid maltase deficiency (see above)
Fatty acid oxidation defects		• Carnitine deficiency (medium chain acyl CoA dehydrogenase deficiency)

Classification of Storage Diseases (continued)

METABOLIC DEFECT	TYPES OF DEFECT	EXAMPLES
Disorders of purine and pyrimidine metabolism		• Lesch-Nyhan syndrome (HGPRT deficiency) • Adenosine deaminase deficiency • Nucleoside phosphorylase deficiency • Orotic aciduria
Mitochondrial disorders		• Leigh's disease (pyruvate dehydrogenase deficiency) • Kearns-Sayre syndrome • Mitochondrial encephalomyopathy—lactic acidosis—and stoke-like symptoms
Peroxisomal disorders		• Zellweger syndrome • Adrenoleukodystrophy • Refsum disease (phytanic oxidase deficiency)

5. Which storage disorders are included in neonatal screening?

Most states require screening for phenylketonuria (United States incidence 1/14,000) and galactosemia (1/60,000). Some states also mandate screening for biotinidase deficiency (1/70,000), maple syrup urine disease (1/100,000) and homocystinuria (1/100,000).

6. Compare and contrast the clinical features of storage disorders presenting in newborns versus older infants and children.

Disorders Presenting in Newborns and Young Infants

- Acute onset of vomiting, failure to feed, hypotonia or hypertonia, respiratory distress, seizures, lethargy, coma (carbohydrate intolerance, organic acidemias, urea cycle enzyme defects)
- Abnormal hair or skin (organic acidemias, urea cycle enzyme defects)
- Abnormal odor (organic acidemias)
- Hepatomegaly and liver dysfunction (galactosemia, fatty acid oxidation defects, carnitine deficiency)
- History of sudden infant death in a sibling

Disorders Presenting in Older Infants and Children

- Dysmorphic or coarse features and skeletal abnormalities (lysosomal disorders, especially mucopolysaccharidoses)
- Developmental delay
- Recurrent vomiting and failure to thrive, with symptoms appearing after dietary change (urea cycle enzyme defects, carbohydrate intolerance)
- Hepatosplenomegaly and liver dysfunction
- Slowly progressive encephalopathy (sphingolipidoses, mucopolysaccharidoses)
- Seizures (urea cycle enzyme defects, lysosomal or peroxisomal disorders)
- Ataxia and hypotonia or hypertonia
- Mental retardation and unexplained neuropsychiatric symptoms in an older child or adolescent

7. What are some typical laboratory findings in storage disorders?

- Metabolic acidosis (organic acidemias, maple syrup urine disease, urea cycle enzyme defects, carbohydrate intolerance, fatty acid oxidation defects)
- Hypoglycemia (carbohydrate intolerance, glycogen storage diseases, primary lactic acidosis)
- Mellituria (carbohydrate intolerance)

- Hyperammonemia (urea cycle enzyme defects, organic acidemias)
- Anemia, neutropenia, thrombocytopenia (organic acidemias)
- Abnormal liver function tests (carbohydrate intolerance, fatty acid oxidation defects)
- Abnormal serum amino acid or carnitine or urine organic acid quantitation
- Abnormal enzyme level or DNA analysis in leukocytes, skin fibroblasts or liver tissue
- Histologic abnormalities in skin, liver and skeletal muscle

8. Bone marrow infiltration is a manifestation of which storage disorders?

"Foam cells" are seen in the bone marrow in all types of Gaucher's disease and Niemann-Pick disease. They have also been described in generalized (G_{M1}) gangliosidosis, G_{M2} gangliosidosis (Sandhoff variant), sialidosis, several types of mucolipidosis, Farber disease and Wolman disease. Cystine crystals may be found in the bone marrow of patients with cystinosis. Pancytopenia, bone marrow hypoplasia and extramedullary hematopoiesis are features of infantile malignant osteopetrosis.

9. A term infant appears well at birth, but shortly after starting formula feeding becomes acutely ill with vomiting, lethargy and episodes of apnea. Sepsis work-up is negative, and the possibility of a storage disorder is considered. Describe the initial approach to management, including emergency measures.

- Discontinuation of oral intake and restriction of protein and carbohydrates.
- Correction of hypoglycemia and metabolic acidosis, if present.
- Evaluate for organic acidemia. If mellituria present, evaluate for galactosemia.
- Treatment of hyperammonemia (sodium phenylacetate, sodium benzoate, hemodialysis).
- Evaluate for urea cycle enzyme defect. Arginine may be effective.
- Levocarnitine in primary carnitine deficiency, and empirically in hyperammonemic states.
- Pyridoxine for refractory seizures in infants.
- Specific dietary regimens depending on disorder.
- Supplemental vitamins (thiamine, biotin, riboflavin, cobalamine).

10. Definitive treatment for storage disorders includes enzyme replacement therapy (as in Gaucher's disease), bone marrow or liver transplant (to restore normal enzyme production) and ultimately, gene therapy. For which storage disorders is bone marrow transplant currently recommended?

Allogeneic bone marrow transplant is currently recommended for Hurler syndrome, Maroteaux-Lamy syndrome, Sly syndrome, childhood-onset adrenoleukodystrophy, globoid cell leukodystrophy, metachromatic leukodystrophy, mannosidosis and aspartylglucosaminuria. Early timing of transplant is critical, to circumvent otherwise progressive neurologic deterioration. For example, the late infantile form of metachromatic leukodystrophy is generally too advanced at the time of diagnosis for bone transplant to have an impact. Results have also been unsatisfactory in Hunter's syndrome, Sanfilippo's syndrome (all types) and Morquio syndrome.

BIBLIOGRAPHY

1. Clarke JTR: A Clinical Guide to Inherited Metabolic Diseases. New York, Cambridge University Press, 1996.
2. Scriver CR: The Metabolic and Molecular Bases of Inherited Diseases, 7th ed. New York, Mc-Graw Hill, 1995.

17. HEMATOLOGICAL MANIFESTATIONS OF SYSTEMIC DISEASE

Maria Luisa Sulis, M.D., *and Tamara New*, M.D.

1. Describe the systemic diseases that have hematological manifestations.

Diseases of the cardiac, pulmonary endocrine, gastrointestinal, metabolic, and nervous systems frequently have hematologic manifestations. Renal and/or liver failure, collagen vascular disease, and infection also often have hematologic manifestations.

2. What are the hematological disorders seen in cardiac disease?

Polycythemia is a well-known consequence of cyanotic heart disease, as a compensatory mechanism to increase oxygen-carrying capacity. Coagulation abnormalities appear to be associated with the degree of polycythemia. The exact cause is not clear; however, it has been postulated that the tissue hypoxia that results from the hyperviscosity may cause a consumptive process. Thrombocytopenia is also related to cyanotic heart disease. The degree of thrombocytopenia correlates with the severity of the polycythemia and with ongoing hypoxia. Platelet production in the bone marrow has been demonstrated to be normal; however, platelet survival is diminished. These patients may additionally have platelet aggregation defects. Individuals who have prosthetic heart valves generally have some hemolysis of red blood cells due to direct mechanical injury. The degree of hemolysis may or may not be severe enough to cause anemia.

3. Discuss the hematological disorders seen in renal disease.

Renal disease is most commonly associated with anemia. This anemia is classified as normocytic, normochromic anemia. The anemia is caused by a deficiency of erythropoietin, which is primarily produced in the kidney. Red cell survival also may be decreased due to uremia when renal disease is severe. Uremia also has an affect on the clotting factor levels, specifically factors V, VII, IX, and X. Platelet survival and platelet function also may be diminished in renal disease. Patients on dialysis will become deficient in folic acid, and can have transient sequestration of granulocytes, resulting in granulocytopenia. Patients should be on three-times-a-week erythropoietin replacement, plus daily folate and iron supplementation.

4. What hematological disorders are seen in liver disease?

Liver disease has most commonly been associated with coagulation abnormalities; however, it can be associated with anemia as well. The liver is involved in the synthesis of many of the clotting factors; therefore, when there is liver dysfunction, factor levels are diminished. The vitamin K–dependent factors are the factors that are primarily affected: factors II, VII, IX, and X. Factor VII, is the most severely and acutely affected factor because its synthesis takes place almost entirely in the liver. Factor VII also has the shortest half-life of all the factors. Factor VIII is generally unaffected in liver disease or is elevated. When the liver damage is caused by obstruction, fibrinogen may be elevated, as may be factors XI and XII and antithrombin III. In severe hepatocellular disease, which significantly affects synthetic liver function, the coagulation profile is often consistent with disseminated intravascular coagulation. The anemia associated with liver disease is multifactorial. The anemia, unlike most anemias due to systemic diseases, is macrocytic, which is due to folate deficiency. There is decreased red cell survival, which is probably due to dysfunction of the antioxidant system.

Patients who develop portal hypertension may develop hypersplenism and subsequent splenic sequestration. If patients are folate deficient, they should be on daily supplementation. Vitamin K supplementation may help to transiently correct the coagulation defects.

5. What pulmonary diseases are associated with abnormal hematologic findings?

Hypoxia leads to polycythemia and in severe instances, thrombocytopenia. Pulmonary hemosiderosis is a condition that results in recurrent hemorrhage into the lungs. This condition may be secondary to collagen vascular disease, glomerulonephritis, or systemic lupus, or it may be idiopathic. It is associated with an anemia of iron deficiency.

6. Which endocrine disorders are associated with hematologic abnormalities?

Hyperthyroidism causes increased red cell mass. Although it affects some of the metabolic functions of the red cell, this does not adversely affect the cell's lifespan. Occasionally associated neutropenia and thrombocytopenia are present. Hypothyroidism, on the other hand, does cause a normocytic normochromic anemia. Some patients with hypothyroidism also have low levels of factors VIII, VII, IX, and XI and diminished platelet function. Anemia is also associated with both hypopituitarism and adrenal insufficiency. The later is probably due to overall reduction in basal metabolism .

7. What is the "anemia of chronic disorders"?

This form of anemia is common in several diseases, from collagen diseases to cancer to infections. The etiology is multifactorial. Shortened red cell survival is likely to be due to extracorpuscolar, environmental factors; the bone marrow response to the degree of anemia is inadequate and the absorption or the utilization of iron from the reticuloendothelial system (RES) is impaired. Occasionally, iron deficiency anemia coexists. In some cases, there is defective production of erythropoietin.

8. Describe the laboratory findings typical of the "anemia of chronic disease."

The anemia is usually normochromic and normocytic; it is occasionally hypochromic and microcytic, in which case the differential diagnosis with iron deficiency anemia can be difficult. Plasma iron, total iron binding capacity, and transferrin saturation are usually diminished, whereas the ferritin can be normal or increased.

9. What other hematological findings are typical of collagen vascular diseases?

Iron deficiency anemia is frequently seen in rheumatoid arthritis, in part due to decreased iron absorption and in part because of microscopic gastrointestinal bleeding secondary to nonsteroidal anti-inflammatory drug intake. Hemolytic anemia can be seen in systemic lupus erythematosus and aplastic anemia in scleroderma. Leukocytosis or leukopenia can be present as a result of inflammation, immune destruction, or bone marrow depression. Thrombocytopenia is frequent in all collagen disorders, usually due to autoimmune destruction. Patients with systemic lupus erythematosus can present with prolonged partial thromboplastin time (PTT) due to the presence of an anticoagulant (lupus anticoagulant), probably an antibody directed against a still unknown target. It carries a risk of thrombosis that is not yet defined in children.

10. Name the hematological abnormalities are associated with diabetes mellitus.

The most common finding is the Hgb A_{1c}, which is a glycohemoglobin (fusion between Hgb and an aldehyde or a ketone) also present in the normal population but markedly increased in diabetics; it is an important marker of diabetic control. Diabetic control is also important for red cell survival, while acidosis influences oxygen delivery and 2,3-diphosphoglycerate levels (they both increase). Frequently, anemia of chronic disease occurs. The function of the neutrophils is usually impaired. Diabetic patients also have increased risk of thrombosis. This is multifactorial in origin: There is increased platelet aggregation, increased factor VIII, XI, XII and decreased angiotensin III and fibrinolysis. The increased risk of thrombosis is also well described in infants of diabetic mothers.

11. What are the hematological manifestations of common infections?

Commonly, pediatric infections cause abnormalities in all of the three cell lines, sometimes in the form of complication of infectious process, other times as natural, necessary response of the immune system against the infectious pathogen.

- Red cells: Anemia due to inflammation is very common in young children, being second only to iron deficiency anemia. The etiology is multifactorial, as seen in the anemia of chronic disease, but hemolytic anemia seems to be the most common etiology. The degree of hemolysis is dependent on the pathogen and the severity of the infection. Severe hemolytic anemia is seen in bacterial sepsis (especially from *Clostridium, Pneumococcus, Meningococcus,* and *Hemophilus*), whereas mild anemia is seen in common viral infections. Even common, mild infections can cause anemia, so it's wise to wait until complete resolution of infection before starting a full work-up. Parvovirus infection is a very well-known cause of anemia, mostly from bone marrow suppression and especially in patients with congenital hemolytic anemia (sickle cell, thalassemia, G6PD deficiency), in whom it can cause "aplastic crises."
- White cells: Neutrophilia is an "healthy" response of the organism to infections, particularly bacterial infections and usually the degree of neutrophilia, as well as the degree of bandemia, correlates with the severity of the infections. Neutropenia in the setting of a bacterial infection is an ominous sign, indicating overwhelming sepsis or inability to mount an adequate response, as in newborns or preemies. Lymphocytosis is common in viral infections, particularly infectious mononucleosis and pertussis. Eosinophilia is frequent in parasitic infections.
- Platelets: Both thrombocytopenia and thrombocytosis are common findings during infectious episodes. Thrombocytosis is more frequently seen during viral infections, especially congenital, or in severe sepsis, particularly in neonates. It usually resolves once the infection is under control, but it may take few weeks. It is mandatory to check the coagulation profile in the setting of a severe infectious process, particularly when thrombocytopenia is present, because of the possibility of associated disseminated intravascular coagulation (DIC).

12. Define DIC.

DIC is a serious clinical disorder secondary to severe underlying diseases, more often sepsis, major trauma with major tissue injury, malignancy (in particular APML), thrombotic thrombocytopenic purpura (TTP), hemolytic-uremic syndrome. It is due to abnormally increased and uncontrolled generation of thrombin and plasmin, formation of microthrombi, and consumption of platelets and coagulation factors. The most common symptom is hemorrhage. There is no specific test to diagnose DIC, but it is usually the combination of the clinical picture and the findings of thrombocytopenia, prolonged prothrombin time and PTT, decreased fibrinogen, and increased D-dimers that lead to the diagnosis.

13. When is treatment indicated for patients with hematologic manifestations of infection warranted?

In general the most effective treatment of the hematological abnormalities associated with infections is the treatment of the infection itself. Transfusion of packed red blood cells is indicated only when the child is symptomatic from the anemia; this will more likely happen in children who have underlying hemolytic disorders. The majority of the time, the anemia is mild and resolves once the infection is over. Platelet transfusion is indicated when the degree of thrombocytopenia represents a significant risk of hemorrhage. Thrombocytosis due to infections is not associated with increased thrombotic risk; therefore, it does not require any intervention. Treatment for DIC is indicated only in the presence of bleeding or when the laboratory parameters are significantly abnormal in coexistence of other risk factors for bleeding. The treatment is supportive and requires replacement of platelets, fresh frozen plasma, and cryoprecipitate.

REFERENCES

1. Abshire TC: The anemia of inflammation: a common cause of childhood anemia. Pediatr Clin North Am. 43:623-637, 1996.
2. Lanzkowsky P: Manual of Pediatric Hematology and Oncology, 2nd ed. New York, Churchill Livingstone, 1995, pp 104–111.
3. Nathan DG, Orkin SH: Nathan and Oski's Hematology of Infancy and Childhood, 5th ed. Vol. 1. Philadelphia, W. B. Saunders Company, 1998, pp 544–664.

18. BONE MARROW FAILURE SYNDROMES

Mark Atlas, M.D.

1. What are the laboratory characteristics of stress erythropoiesis, and in which bone marrow failure syndromes are they common?

With stress erythropoiesis, erythrocytes are fetal-like and macrocytic, with increased hemoglobin F and i-antigen. These characteristics are common in Fanconi's anemia, aplastic anemia, dyskeratosis congenita and Blackfan-Diamond anemia (BDA), but not in transient erythroblastopenia of childhood (TEC).

2. Describe the inheritance patterns of the inherited bone marrow failure syndromes.

Inheritance Patterns of Inherited Bone Marrow Failure Syndromes

SYNDROME	GENETICS
Fanconi's anemia	AR
Dyskeratosis congenita	X-LR: 3/4), AR:1/8, AD:1/8
Shwachman-Diamond syndrome	AR
Amegakaryocytic thrombocytopenia	AR, X-LR
BDA	AR, AD, sporadic
Thrombocytopenia/absent radius	AR
Severe chronic neutropenia	AR

AD = autosomal dominant, AR = autosomal recessive, X-LR = x-linked recessive.

3. What are the different causes of acquired aplastic anemia?

- Radiation
- Drugs/toxins: benzene, chloramphenicol, anti-inflammatories, anti-epileptics, gold
- Viruses: Hepatitis, Epstein-Barr virus, parvovirus, HIV
- Thymoma
- Pregnancy
- Paroxysmal nocturnal hemoglobinuria
- Preleukemia
- Idiopathic

4. Name the theory for the pathophysiology of idiopathic aplastic anemia that has the most support.

Immune-mediated marrow failure has both direct and indirect support. Autologous reconstitution after bone marrow transplantation first stimulated this theory. Additionally, syngeneic transplantation from identical twin siblings usually requires immunosuppression, though this is typically not necessary when donor and recipient are genetically identical. Several trials have demonstrated the efficacy of immunosuppression in inducing clinical remission in aplastic anemia. One trial used high-dose cyclophosphamide without marrow transplant to successfully treat severe aplastic anemia.

5. What is the treatment of choice for idiopathic severe aplastic anemia?

Bone marrow transplantation is the treatment of choice, if there is an human leukocyte antigen–matched related donor. Such transplants have an event-free survival of greater than

80%. Every effort is made to proceed to transplant as rapidly as possible, ideally within 2 weeks. Transfusions should be avoided if at all possible, as they are associated with increased risk of graft rejection. For patients without a donor, immunotherapy—with or without cytokines—is the most common treatment.

6. What test is necessary to make the diagnosis of Fanconi's anemia?

Fanconi's anemia is characterized by abnormal chromosomal breakage. Chromosomes have a tendency toward breaks, rearrangements and endoreduplications. However, many of these abnormalities are not visible on standard karyotype analyses. Clastogenic studies, in which an agent such as diepoxybutane (DEB) or mitomycin-C is used to induce chromosomal breaks, are useful to assess whether breakage frequency is characteristic of Fanconi's anemia.

7. What are the most common physical anomalies in Fanconi anemia?

Physical Anomalies in Fanconi's Anemia

ANOMALY	PATIENTS AFFECTED (%)
Skin: café au lait spots, hyperpigmentation	60
Short stature	57
Arms: absent, bifid thumbs, absent radius	48
Genitourinary: hypogonadism, absent testes	37
Head: microcephaly, bird-like face	27
Eyes: microphthalmia, strabismus	26
Kidney: ectopic, dysplastic, absent	23
None	0

8. What is the natural history of Fanconi's anemia?

Patients are often diagnosed before onset of anemia because of physical anomalies or family history. This phase may last beyond the second decade but most commonly occurs later in the first decade of life. Therapy with androgens can reverse the cytopenias but does not cure the disease. Androgens do increase the median survival after onset of aplasia from 4–7 years. Patients die of complications of aplasia or from malignancy, as 10% of patients will progress to leukemia and an additional 5% will develop solid tumors. Bone marrow transplantation offers the only possible cure of aplasia and perhaps prevention of leukemia.

9. Why is the occurrence of malignancy in a patient with Fanconi's anemia such a poor prognostic factor? How does this affect the patient's potential therapy with stem cell transplantation?

Patients with Fanconi's anemia are predisposed to spontaneous breakage of DNA. They are also hypersensitive to bifunctional alkylating agents such as nitrogen mustard, platinum compounds and diepoxybutane. Even chemotherapeutic agents to which they are not "hypersensitive" affect these patients more severely, and toxicity is usually unmanageable. Successful therapy for cancer is rare, as it is almost impossible to deliver a normal chemotherapeutic regimen to patients because of significant toxicity. Stem cell transplantation, while potentially life-saving, must be performed with care. Reduced doses of chemotherapy and radiation are used to decrease risk of toxicity and second malignancy but increase risk of nonengraftment. Outcomes of stem cell transplantation are lower than with comparable patients, mostly because of transplant-related mortality.

10. What clinical characteristics differentiate TEC from BDA?

TEC is a presumably virally induced pure red cell aplasia that is self-limited, BDA is a presumably inherited disease. Some of the major differences are highlighted below:

Differences Between BDA and TEC

	BDA	TEC
Age	Typically < 1 year	Typically > 1 year
Antecedent history	None	Viral illness
Physical anomalies	~1/3	None
MCV at diagnosis	Increased	Normal
Hemoglobin F	Increased	Normal
i-antigen	Increased	Normal

11. What treatment options are available for Blackfan-Diamond anemia?

Corticosteroids are the initial treatment of choice. A reticulocytosis is typically seen within 2 weeks of starting therapy. Approximately 30–40% of patients are steroid refractory, and 10–15% of all patients will require long-term low-dose steroids; some will eventually remit completely. For steroid-refractory patients, transfusion and chelation is the mainstay of therapy. About 15% of refractory patients will respond to interleukin-3 therapy. Bone marrow transplantation also has been successfully used for the treatment of refractory BDA. Most patients become long-term survivors, with a median survival of 38 years.

12. Is therapy necessary for TEC?

No specific therapy is necessary. Close monitoring of the complete blood count and the reticulocyte count is important, and if the patient becomes hemodynamically unstable, packed red blood cell transfusion may be necessary.

13. What is the diagnostic triad of dyskeratosis congenita?

- Reticulated hyperpigmentation of the face, neck and shoulders
- Dystrophic nails
- Mucous membrane leukoplakia
- Approximately 50% of the cases will progress to aplastic anemia.

14. What is the underlying defect of paroxysmal nocturnal hemoglobinuria?

Clinically, the disorder is characterized by paroxysms of complement-mediated intravascular hemolysis. Patients may also have abdominal, musculoskeletal or back pain and are often iron deficient from blood loss. The underlying disorder, however, is a clonal stem cell defect that causes a decrease in membrane proteins requiring a glycosylphosphatidylinositol anchor. One is a delay-accelerating factor that normally inhibits complement-mediated cell lysis. This defect characterizes platelet, monocytes and granulocytes as well. Patients are prone to venous thrombosis and many develop aplastic anemia.

15. Discuss the clinical characteristics and course of the thrombocytopenia absent radii syndrome (TAR).

The diagnosis of TAR is based on the clinical findings of bilateral absence of the radii, with presence of thumbs and thrombocytopenia that is often initially severe. Other skeletal abnormalities are quite common. Bloody diarrhea and petechiae are the most common complications in infancy. Megakaryocytes are typically absent on bone marrow aspiration. Platelet counts usually rise slowly and are often above the levels predisposing to spontaneous hemorrhage after the first year. The pathophysiology is uncertain. Treatment is supportive, with platelet transfusions for significant bleeding. Orthopedic interventions are deferred until after platelet counts recover.

16. How do patients with severe chronic neutropenia (Kostmann's syndrome) present, and what is their clinical course?

Patients present with significant bacterial infections within the first 6 months of life and severe neutropenia with an absolute neutrophil count (ANC) of < 200. Neutrophil counts may be normal in the first week of life but then rapidly decrease. Untreated patients will have repeated bacterial infections and typically die from pneumonia or sepsis. With current therapy, patients are living longer, but an increased incidence of myeloid leukemias has been noted.

17. Describe the therapies available for severe chronic neutropenia.

Cytokine therapy with granulocyte-colony stimulating factor (G-CSF) is effective in improving the ANC of most patients with Kostmann's syndrome. Very high doses of G-CSF, up to 10 times the typical dose, may be necessary to achieve adequate neutrophil counts. Some patients may become refractory. There remains concern that as patients live longer, the incidence of leukemias will rise. Bone marrow transplantation offers a potential cure for patients with a suitable donor.

BIBLIOGRAPHY

1. Alter BP: Arms and the man or hands and the child: Congenital anomalies and hematologic syndromes. J Pediatr Hematol Oncol 19:287–291,1997.
2. Alter BP, Young NS: The bone marrow failure syndromes. In Nathan DG, Orkin SH (eds): Nathan and Oski's Hematology of Infancy and Childhood. Philadelphia,W.B. Saunders, 1998, pp 237-335.
3. Brodsky RA, Sensenbrenner LL, Jones RJ: Complete remission in severe aplastic anemia after high-dose cyclophosphamide without bone marrow transplantation. Blood 87:491–494,1996.
4. Guinan EC: Clinical aspects of aplastic anemia. Hematol Oncol Clin North Am 11:1025–1044,1997.
5. Horowitz MM: Current status of allogeneic bone marrow transplantation in acquired aplastic anemia. Semin Hematol 37:30–42, 2000.
6. Janov AJ, Leong T, Nathan DG, Guinan EC: Diamond-Blackfan anemia. Natural history and sequelae of treatment. Medicine (Baltimore) 75:77–88,1996.
7. Krijanovski OI, Sieff CA: Diamond-Blackfan anemia. Hematol Oncol Clin North Am 11:1061–1077,1997.
8. Kupfer GM, Naf D, D'Andrea AD: Molecular biology of Fanconi anemia. Hematol Oncol Clin North Am 11:1045–1060,1997.
9. Margolis DA, Casper JT: Alternative-donor hematopoietic stem-cell transplantation for severe aplastic anemia. Semin Hematol 37:43–55, 2000.
10. Mupanomunda OK, Alter BP: Transient erythroblastopenia of childhood (TEC) presenting as leukoerythroblastic anemia. J Pediatr Hematol Oncol 19:165–167,1997.
11. Young NS, Maciejewski J: The pathophysiology of acquired aplastic anemia. N Engl J Med 336:1365–1372,1997.
12. Young NS: Hematopoietic cell destruction by immune mechanisms in acquired aplastic anemia. Semin Hematol 37:3–14, 2000.

II. Oncology

19. PRINCIPLES AND PRACTICE OF PEDIATRIC ONCOLOGY

Michael A. Weiner, M.D.

1. What are the differences between cancer in children and adolescents versus that in adults?

Cancer in children and adolescents differs from cancer in adults in its histopathology, clinical manifestations, biology and responsiveness to treatment and outcome. Adult cancer of men and women originates commonly from an organ such as lung, breast, bowel, prostate or ovary. Pediatric cancers frequently originate from mesenchymal structures, such as bone and muscle. Tumors of the central nervous system (CNS) and cancers of hematologic origin are common in both children and adults.

2. Compare the incidence of childhood cancer to the incidence of cancer in adults.

The incidence of cancer from birth through 14 years of age is 14 cases per 100,000 per year. For patients between 15 and 19 years, the incidence approaches 20 cases per 100,000 per year. Thus, there are approximately 11,000–12,000 new cases of cancer per year diagnosed in children and teenagers. National Cancer Institute SEER (Surveillance, Epidemiology and End Results) data indicate that for every case of childhood cancer there are approximately 150 cases diagnosed in adults.

3. What are the genetic and congenital disorders that predispose patients to developing pediatric malignancies?

Approximately 15% of the cases of childhood cancer are associated with a genetic and/or congenital condition. Genetic disorders that have gene alterations that disrupt normal mechanisms of genomic repair, such as xeroderma pigmentosa, Bloom syndrome and ataxia telangiectasia, are associated with skin cancer, leukemia and lymphoma, respectively. Beckwith-Wiedemann syndrome, multiple endocrine neoplasia and neurofibromatosis are congenital conditions with dysfunctional cellular growth and proliferation and are associated with Wilms' tumor, hepatic tumors, adrenal cancers and CNS tumors, respectively.

4. What is the probability of children and teenagers developing cancer?

It has been estimated that before the age of 20 years, 1 of every 333 children and teenagers will develop cancer. The median age at which cancer is diagnosed is 6 years of age. Predicated on a cure rate (regardless of type) of 70% and a life expectancy of 77 years, it may be calculated that the number of person-years of life at risk from childhood cancer approaches 500,000.

5. Discuss the histologic prevalence of the various pediatric malignancies.

The chart on the following page indicates the incidence of childhood cancer (percent) by diagnosis, according to recent SEER data.

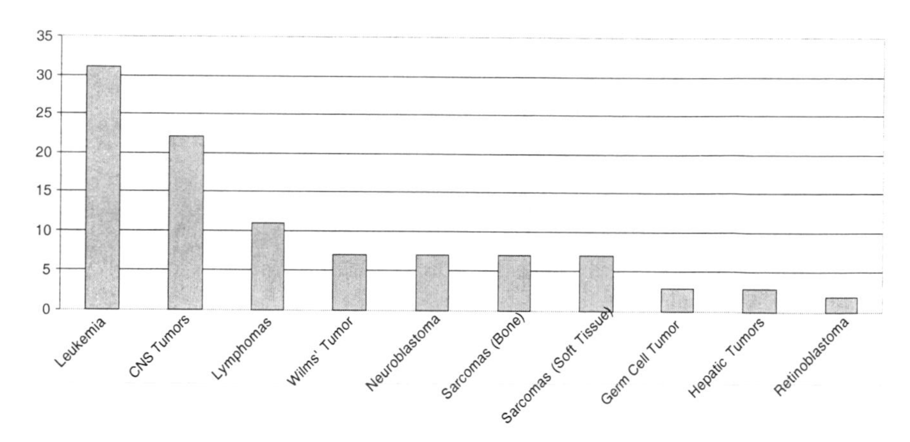

6. Give the projected survival for children diagnosed with cancer in the United States.

In 2000, the rate was 80%. This represents a reversal of outcome from 80% mortality to 80% survival in four decades. The mortality rates for leukemia, CNS tumors and all other pediatric malignancies combined decreased 52%, 20% and 59%, respectively. Significant decreases in death rates have been reported for lymphomas, Wilms' tumors and retinoblastoma. Thus, as the new millennium begins, it is estimated that 1 in every 1000 people is a childhood cancer survivor; by 2010, 1 in every 250 people will have been treated successfully for pediatric cancer.

7. Name the most important factor contributing to the improved survival of children diagnosed with cancer.

The ability to conduct clinical trials in a cooperative group setting is responsible for the improved survival of children and adolescents with cancer. Clinical trials are conducted at leading pediatric oncology centers under the auspices of the Children's Oncology Group, an international multi-institutional consortium that fosters translational research and utilizes a randomized study model to find the best treatment available. Today, 95% of all children diagnosed with cancer in the United Sates are enrolled in clinical trials. In contrast, only 2% of adults with cancer are entered in National Cancer Institute sponsored clinical trials.

8. What are the benefits derived by patients and families from participating in cooperative group clinical trials?

The benefits derived by patients and families from participating in clinical trials include:

- Access to the collective wisdom of leading experts in the treatment of pediatric cancer
- Access to state-of-the art therapies and technologies
- Access to unequaled expertise in translational research
- Access to specialized pediatric cancer centers that comprise the membership of the Children's Oncology Group

BIBLIOGRAPHY

1. Bleyer WA: What can be learned about childhood cancer from "Cancer Statistics Review 1973–1988." Cancer 71:3229–3236, 1993.
2. Bleyer WA: The U.S. pediatric cancer clinical trials programmes: International implications and the way forward. Euro J Cancer 33:1439–1447, 1997.
3. Li FP: Cancer families: Human models of susceptibility to neoplasia. Cancer Res 48:5381–5386, 1988.
4. Miller RW, Young JL Jr, Novakovic B. Childhood cancer. Cancer 75(suppl 1):395–405, 1995.
5. Quesnel S, Malkin D: Genetic predisposition to cancer and familial cancer syndromes. Pediatr Oncology, Pediatric Clin North Am 44:791–808, 1997.

20. GENETICS OF CHILDHOOD CANCER

Manuela Orjuela, M.D., Sc.M.

1. What percent of childhood cancer is attributable to inherited mutations?

In one review of 16,564 cases of childhood cancer diagnosed from 1971 to 1983 in Great Britain, only 4.2% of cases were thought to be secondary to inherited genetic syndromes. However, the total influence of heredity may be higher, as inherited genetic susceptibility to the effects of environmental mutagens may lead to the development of pediatric tumors that do not appear to be part of the classically described syndromes. With the exception of this small percentage of cases attributable to hereditary cancer syndromes (e.g., familial retinoblastoma) or genetic syndromes such as Down syndrome, the etiology of most childhood cancers is unknown.

2. Discuss the importance of rare cancers attributable to inherited mutations to the practice of pediatric oncology.

Despite their rarity, these syndromes and their underlying genetics permit a greater understanding of the processes underlying the development of malignancy. In addition, by identifying children at risk because of inheritance of a genetic defect, we can potentially screen these children for the tumors for which they are at risk and thus potentially decrease the morbidity and mortality from their malignancy.

3. A child referred to your service with presumed Wilms' tumor is found to have tumor present in both of her kidneys. Describe the underlying genetic changes present when patients have bilateral Wilms' tumor.

Wilms' tumor is thought to originate from pluripotent embryonic renal precursors. Five to ten percent of children diagnosed with Wilms' tumors present with bilateral disease and develop tumors at an earlier age (circa 2 yr) than children with unilateral disease (average age at diagnosis, 5 yr). Children with bilateral disease have persistent nephrogenic rests in their tumors. These nephrogenic rests (undifferentiated blast cells) may be present during kidney development, but they normally disappear shortly after birth; their persistence in Wilms' tumor suggests a constitutional abnormality in renal differentiation.

Most children with bilateral Wilms' tumor have de novo germline mutations in *WT1*. *WT1* is also inactivated in 15% of sporadic Wilms' tumors. *WT1* is a tumor suppressor gene located on chromosome 11p13 that encodes a zinc finger transcription factor and is inactivated in the germline of children with genetic predisposition to Wilms' tumor.

WT1 is a critical regulator of organ-specific differentiation; its inactivation or disruption triggers malignant transformation in embryonic cell types. *WT1* is expressed in glomerular precursors of the developing kidney, and mice who lack both copies of *WT1* do not develop kidneys. *WT1* encodes two major alternative splicing products: One isoform (2KTS) appears to mediate transcriptional activation of genes implicated in cellular differentiation, possibly also repressing proliferation-associated genes; the other isoform (1KTS, may be involved in some aspect of mRNA processing.

4. Name the genetic syndromes associated with Wilms' tumor. How should children with these syndromes be followed?

The WAGR and Beckwith-Wiedemann syndromes are both associated with a predisposition to the development of Wilms' tumor, and both are associated with developmental abnormalities, as well as with germline abnormalities involving gene loci on chromosome 11. (See question 10 as well.)

Patients with WAGR (Wilms' tumor, aniridia, genitourinary defects and mental retardation) have gross cytogenetic deletions at 11p13. This locus includes the *WT1* gene, as well as *PAX6*, a gene responsible for directing eye development. Loss of one copy of *WT1* in nephrogenic cells leads to genitourinary malformations, while Wilms' tumor (in 40% of these children) results from acquired point mutations occuring in the remaining WT1 allele in renal precursor cells. Loss of one allele for *PAX6* leads to aniridia. Children with WAGR should be followed closely for abdominal masses and should have renal ultrasonograms and urinalyses every 3 months until their 6th birthday.

Children with the Beckwith-Wiedemann syndrome (BWS), can present with asymmetric organomegaly, hypoglycemia and umbilical hernias; in addition, they are predisposed to developing adrenal cortical carcinoma, hepatoblastoma and Wilms' tumor. BWS is associated with abnormalities at the 11p15 gene locus. Fifteen percent of cases are familial. Some cases of BWS have a duplication of paternal 11p15 with no maternal contribution (uniparental isodisomy). These cases appear to have increased expression of *IGF2*, the insulin-dependent growth factor 2 gene, which is also located in this chromosomal region. Other cases of BWS with demonstrated maternal imprinting (paternal gene is not expressed) have inactivating mutations in p57, a cyclin-dependent kinase inhibitor (and therefore a cell cycle regulator), which is also located on 11p15. These children should also be followed with abdominal ultrasonograms and urinalyses every 3 months until they turn 6. In addition, they should have serum alpha fetoprotein (AFP) levels every 3 months until the age of 3 years.

5. What genetic lesion characterizes desmoplastic small round cell tumors?

Desmoplastic Small Round Cell Tumor (DSCRT) is an embryonic neoplasm that occurs primarily in adolescent boys and typically has an aggressive clinical course. These tumors typically arise within the abdomen, usually from the peritoneal lining. Their cells express markers suggestive of epithelial, muscle and neural lineages, suggesting that they derive from pluripotent progenitor cells. DSRCTs are characterized by the t(11;22) (p13;q12) chromosomal translocation which fuses the N-terminal domain of the Ewing sarcoma gene *EWS* to the three C-terminal zinc fingers of *WT1*. *WT1* is normally expressed at high levels in the mesothelial cells that line visceral organs and the pleural, peritoneal and pericardial surfaces. *WT1* is thought to play a role in regulating the mesenchymal-to-epithelial cell conversion, which is normally seen in these mesothelial cells. DSCRT is thought to arise in these mesothelial cells, which presumably lack normal *WT1* function because of the t(11;22) (p13;q12) translocation.

6. A school-age child in your care is diagnosed with juvenile chronic myeloid leukemia. On examination you notice that she has multiple café-au-lait spots which are greater than 5 mm. Her parents report that these spots have been present since infancy. She also has freckles in her axillae. What underlying genetic defect is this child likely to have? What other tumors is she at risk to develop?

This child is likely to have neurofibromatosis type 1 (NF1) or von Recklinghausen's disease. NF1 is an autosomal dominant inherited disorder that affects 1 in 4000 individuals and is due to mutations in the *NF1* gene located on 17q11.2. Most (50%) germline mutations in *NF1* in recently diagnosed patients are new (i.e., their parents don't have them in their germline) and are found to occur preferentially in the paternally inherited allele. *NF1* encodes several alternatively spliced transcripts and its product is neurofibromin, a cytoplasmic protein belonging to the *Ras* GTPase activating group of proteins, which acts as a tumor suppressor. Neurofibromin is expressed in most tissues, but it is found at highest levels in the central and peripheral nervous system and in the adrenal gland, which is consistent with the distribution of organs most frequently affected by this disease.

Diagnostic criteria for NF1 include having at least two of the following: six café-au-lait spots of at least 5 mm in diameter if prepubertal, (or >15 mm if postpubertal), axillary or inguinal freckling, two or more neurofibromas (originating from Schwann progenitor cells) or one plexiform neurofibroma, an optic nerve glioma, a distinctive osseous lesion (such as sphenoid wing dysplasia) or a first degree relative with NF1.

Children with NF1 are at increased risk for developing benign and malignant solid tumors, which also include iris hamartomas (Lisch nodules), glioblastoma multiforme, rhabdomyosarcomas, pheochromocytomas and carcinoid tumors, as well as hematologic malignancies, including de novo juvenile chronic myelogenous leukemia, monosomy 7 syndrome and acute myelogenous leukemia. In addition, 5% of plexiform neurofibromas progress to malignant peripheral nerve sheath tumors. The majority of gliomas found in patients with NF1 are pilocytic astrocytomas arising within the optic nerve. Children with NF1 can also be affected by scoliosis, short stature, macrocephaly, epilepsy, neuropathies, intellectual handicaps, hydrocephalus (secondary to aqueductal stenosis) and renal artery hyperplasia.

7. A teenage boy is found to have a thyroid nodule on routine examination. Endocrinologic studies reveal that his serum calcitonin levels are elevated. His younger brother has Hirschsprung's disease. They are foster children, and the foster parents have been told that the biological mother had a "kidney" tumor. Which genetic syndrome might this family have? What genetic test would you do on this child and his sibling? What would you recommend as follow-up for the younger brother if the test were positive?

This family history suggests that the older brother may have a medullary thyroid carcinoma, a malignant tumor derived from parafollicular C cells in the thyroid. If so, then these brothers may be affected by one of the multiple endocrine neoplasia type 2 (MEN2) syndromes, MEN2A or MEN2B, which are autosomal dominant genetic syndromes associated with specific germline mutations in the *RET* proto-oncogene. *RET*, located at chromosome 10q11.2, encodes a receptor functioning as a tyrosine kinase. Germline mutations in this gene are observed in 95% of patients with MEN2B and in 98% of those with MEN2A. The nature and location of these mutations correlates closely with the syndrome type. In more than 95% of MEN2B cases, a mutation in codon 918 (in exon 16) of the *RET* gene replaces a methionine with a threonine residue, which is part of the tyrosine kinase domain. Mutations in >90% of patient with MEN2A involve conserved cysteine residues of the extracellular domain, and 85% of these mutations occur in codon 634 (in exon 11).

Most familial cases (60%) are MEN2A. In addition to medullary thyroid carcinoma, the most frequently associated diseases in MEN2A are pheochromocytomas (in 50% of patients) and hyperparathyroidism, which can occur before or after the diagnosis of thyroid disease. In some families with MEN2A, children are at increased risk for Hirschsprung's disease in their first years of life.

MEN2B is an aggressive and rare disorder (5% of inherited medullary thyroid cancer), occurring early in life. The syndrome involves locally invasive thyroid tumors that can cause compressive symptoms and frequently have early mediastinal and lung metastases. MEN2B is associated with developmental abnormalities including marfanoid habitus; overgrowth of neural tissue of the lips, tongue and conjunctivae, and ganglioneuromatosis of the intestinal tract. Pheochromocytomas are also present, usually bilaterally, and are usually diagnosed after the thyroid disease. This form is not associated with primary hyperparathyroidism.

Familial screening for MEN2 is now offered to detect thyroid disease before clinical manifestations so that curative pre-symptomatic thyroidectomies can be performed. Screening is based on *RET* mutation detection in genomic DNA extracted from peripheral blood leukocytes. This genetic testing should be performed at birth in children suspected of having the MEN2B syndrome and before the age of 1 yr in those with possible MEN2A. If specific *RET* gene mutations are noted, total thyroidectomy is recommended as soon as the diagnosis is established. For MEN2A patients, thyroidectomy should be performed before 5 yr of age, whereas patients with MEN2B may need surgery during the first 6 months to 1 yr of life. Given this family history, the younger brother is most likely to have a genetic defect consistent with MEN2A; if so, then prophylactic thyroidectomy should be performed before he turns 5 yr.

8. A 12-yr-old girl presents with knee pain and is found to have an osteogenic sarcoma arising in the distal femur. She is brought by her father, because her mother is undergoing treatment for breast cancer. Her brother died at age 6 of a brain tumor. On further questioning, you discover that two maternal aunts also had breast cancer in their 30s. The patient's 10-yr-old sister is clinically well. What genetic syndrome do you suspect? What tumor suppressor protein is associated with this syndrome? How would you follow her and her sister?

This family appears to have Li-Fraumeni Syndrome (LFS), an autosomal dominant disorder characterized by germline mutations in the *P53* tumor suppressor gene which is located on chromosome 17p13. Patients with LFS are at increased risk for early onset of bone and soft tissue sarcomas, breast and adrenal cortex carcinomas, brain tumors (especially primitive neuroectodermal tumors and astrocytomas) and acute leukemia. The *P53* gene was first described as a result of studying families with this syndrome. It encodes a protein, p53, which is expressed at low levels in many cell types. This tumor suppressor protein plays a key role in controlling cell cycle progression, as well as DNA repair after oxidative damage or mutagenic DNA damage. Hypoxic and mutagenic DNA damage leads to a nuclear accumulation and activation of p53. In addition, p53 transcriptionally activates genes that induce cell cycle arrest and apoptosis. Mutant p53, such as that found in patients with LFS, is unable to suppress tumor development and can actually inhibit wild-type P53. Somatic *P53* mutations are also found in tumor cells in sporadically occurring tumors. The most common types of *P53* mutations in both LFS and in sporadically occurring tumors are point mutations causing cytosine-to-adenine transitions at CpG sites (G:C changes to A:T) and arise from deamination of 5-methylcytosine. Although these types of mutations can occur spontaneously, they are usually corrected by DNA repair mechanisms.

DNA from this child can be examined to look for mutations in *P53*. These would be expected to be present both in her tumor DNA as well as in her genomic DNA (and thus in her leukocytes). Once a *P53* mutation is found, then her sister's leukocytes could be examined to probe for the mutation. If her sister is found to have mutant *P53*, she can be counseled and followed closely to detect potential cancers at earlier stages. This patient will also need to be followed closely for early development of breast cancer. It is unknown whether avoidance of risk factors associated with development of sporadic breast cancer will decrease her probability of developing this disease.

9. A teenager presents in the emergency department with a history of severe headaches and a sudden loss of consciousness. He is found on magnetic resonance imaging (MRI) to have multiple cystic lesions in his cerebellum. His hemoglobin is 16 mg/dL. His father reports that the boy's grandfather died of a kidney tumor and that he himself was also recently diagnosed with a kidney tumor. The boy's 8-year-old sister is completely well. What genetic syndrome do you suspect in this family, and what do you expect these cystic lesions contain? How should this boy and his younger sister be followed?

This family probably has von Hippel-Lindau (VHL) disease, which is transmitted through autosomal dominant inheritance of a germline mutation of the *VHL* tumor suppressor gene located on chromosome 3p5-26. The VHL protein (pVHL) is involved in cell cycle regulation (it is involved in controlling the transition from G2 into G0, the quiescent phase) and angiogenesis (deficiency of pVHL is associated with overexpression of vascular endothelial growth factor). The *VHL* gene is expressed in epithelial cells in skin, gastrointestinal, respiratory and urogenital tracts, as well as in endocrine and exocrine organs. In the central nervous system, pVHL is found primarily in the Purkinje cells of the cerebellum.

The characteristic clinical findings in VHL disease include multiple capillary hemangioblastomas in the central nervous system (primarily in the cerebellum, brain stem and spinal cord and usually accompanied by cysts or syrinxes), retinal hemangioblastomas, renal cell carcinoma, pheochromocytomas, clear cell renal carcinoma and pancreatic and inner ear tumors. This youth therefore has a typical presentation that likely consists of multiple hemangioblastomas and adjacent cysts. The cysts can cause impaired cerebrospinal fluid flow and increased intracranial pressure, which can lead to the presenting symptoms. The hemangioblastomas themselves are often present in the walls of the large cysts. Because these tumors can produce erythropoietin, patients can present with secondary polycythemia.

Mortality in patients with VHL is primarily caused by effects secondary to the cranial hemangioblastomas. Therefore this boy and his sister (if affected) should undergo periodic MRI to detect the cranial lesions before they become symptomatic. Treatment is usually surgical or with gamma-knife radiation. Patients should also have regular ophthalmologic examinations to detect and remove retinal hemangioblastomas before they cause significant retinal damage. This boy and his sister (as well as his father and other paternal family members) should have genetic testing done to look for *VHL* mutations.

10. A child presents with newly diagnosed Wilms' tumor. You notice that the child is smaller than expected for her age and that she has malar hypoplasia and a telangiectatic rash on her cheeks. Her parents report that the rash worsens with sun exposure and that she has been small since birth. Describe the genetic defect this child might have.

This child may have Bloom's syndrome, a rare autosomal recessive disorder involving a mutation in the *BLM* gene, which is located at 15q26.1. The *BLM* gene encodes a DNA helicase, and functional mutations in this gene lead to defective DNA repair characterized by increased sister chromatid exchanges. Bloom syndrome is characterized by prenatal and postnatal growth retardation, photosensitivity (causing a facial telangiectatic rash) and malar hypoplasia. Twenty-five percent of persons with Bloom's syndrome develop some form of malignancy including leukemia, lymphoma or Wilms' tumor as children and breast, stomach or colon adenocarcinomas as adults (with an early age of onset).

11. An infant presents with hepatoblastoma. His maternal grandmother was diagnosed with colon cancer before she was 40, while his mother and maternal aunts have undergone prophylactic colectomies. Name the genetic syndrome this family is likely to have. What is the underlying genetic defect? What follow-up should this child and his siblings receive?

This family probably suffers from familial adenomatous polyposis (FAP), an autosomal dominant inherited syndrome characterized by the presence of adenomatous polyps in the colon and rectum and development of colorectal cancer. Children in these families are also at an increased risk for hepatoblastoma. FAP is caused by germline mutations in the adenomatous polyposis coli (*APC*) gene. The *APC* gene, located on chromosome 5q21-22, encodes a large multidomain protein that plays an integral role in the Wnt-signalling pathway, intercellular adhesion, stabilization of the cytoskeleton and possibly regulation of the cell cycle and apoptosis. *APC* mutations almost always result in a truncated protein product with abnormal function. Inheritance of *APC* germline mutations has a penetrance of almost 100%, but phenotypic expression of the disease is quite variable. Persons affected by FAP develop hundreds to thousands of adenomatous polyps in their colon and rectum. These polyps usually appear either by adolescence or by age 30. Colorectal cancer invariably develops by age 40. Colorectal tumours from FAP patients carry additional somatic APC mutations or loss of heterozygosity at this locus in addition to the original germline mutation.

One variant of FAP, Gardner's syndrome, is characterized by the presence of innumerable colonic polyps, in addition to epidermoid skin cysts and benign osteoid tumours of the mandible and long bones.

Follow-up for this child and his siblings should follow the recommended screening for children with APC, which includes colonoscopy starting at age 10 yr, prophylactic colectomy and serum alpha fetoprotein levels and abdominal ultrasound every 3 months until age 3 yr to screen for hepatoblastoma.

One additional familial syndrome involves retinoblastoma. Please see Chapter 32 for further details on this genetic disease.

BIBLIOGRAPHY

1. Clericuzio CL: Recognition and management of childhood cancer syndromes: A systems approach. Am J Med Genet (Semin Med Genet) 89:81–90, 1999.
2. Nicola S, Fearnhead NS, Britton MP, Bodmer WF: The ABC of APC. Hum Mol Genet 10(7):721–733, 2001.
3. Kleihues P, Cavenee WK (eds): Familial Tumor Syndromes in Pathology and Genetics of Tumours of the Nervous System. Lyon, IARC Press, 2000.
4. Lee SB, Haber DA: Wilms' tumor and the *WT1* gene. Exp Cell Res. 264:;74–99, 2001.
5. Modigliani E, Franc B, Niccolisire P: Diagnosis and treatment of medullary thyroid cancer. Baillieres Best Pract Res Clin Endocrinol Metab 14(4):631–649, 2000.

21. PRINCIPLES OF CHEMOTHERAPY

Julia Glade Bender, M.D.

1. What is the single most important determinant when choosing a treatment using anticancer drugs (chemotherapy)?

Prior to embarking on a treatment plan that involves the use of anticancer drugs, every effort should be made to ascertain an accurate histologic diagnosis. This involves pathologic examination of tumor tissue following surgical excision or a well-planned biopsy. Rarely, in the setting of a true oncologic emergency such as a mediastinal mass causing superior vena cava syndrome and superior mediastinal syndrome, empiric therapy prior to histologic diagnosis is permissible. Other critical factors in the determination of an appropriate chemotherapeutic regimen include the following:

- Histologic subtype: favorable or unfavorable in neuroblastoma, T or B cell leukemia/lymphoma
- Presence of adverse biological features: *MYC-N* amplification in neuroblastoma, and Ph+ chromosome in acute lymphoblastic leukemia
- Disease stage: extent of disease
- Patient age

2. What is meant by the terms *adjuvant* and *neoadjuvant chemotherapy* and what is the rationale behind them?

Adjuvant chemotherapy is given to patients without evidence of residual disease after local control of a malignant tumor has been achieved with surgery and/or radiation. Historically, patients treated with local measures alone had a high risk (60–95%) for tumor recurrence with distant metastases. The goal of adjuvant chemotherapy is to eliminate microscopic spread of the tumor or micrometastasis, which is assumed to have already occurred by the time of diagnosis. This strategy has been successful in the treatment of most pediatric solid tumors including Wilms' tumor, Ewing's sarcoma, osteosarcoma, rhabdomyosarcoma, medulloblastoma, and anaplastic astrocytoma.

Neoadjuvant chemotherapy, or primary chemotherapy, is given to patients prior to surgical resection or radiation to the primary site. Neoadjuvant chemotherapy has been used to decrease tumor bulk, thereby making the primary more amenable to surgery. Other rationale include the early eradication of micrometastasis, preempting costly delays in therapy from surgical or radiation-related morbidity, and the ability to assess tumor responsiveness to initial therapy, both clinically and histologically. The neoadjuvant strategy has been particularly important in treatment of osteosarcoma. Orthopedic surgeons are able to offer a larger number of patients limb-sparing procedures, in part due to tumor shrinkage and the extra time available to plan and obtain individualized prosthetic devices. Additionally, the histologic tumor response to initial therapy has proven to be a potent prognostic factor of relapse-free survival in this disease.

3. What does history tell us about the overall efficacy of single-drug regimens?

In the late 1940s and early 1950s, ALL was universally and rapidly fatal. The first single-agent trials were able to induce remarkable results with impressive complete remission rates of up to 60%. However, remissions were short lived, lasting only 6–9 months, despite continued therapy with the agent. Today, single agent trials are used to test the safety and efficacy of new agents under development in patients with advanced disease at diagnosis or with refractory disease.

4. What is the rationale behind the use of combination chemotherapy?

The rationale behind combination chemotherapy is twofold:

- Combination chemotherapy may be used to overcome inherent tumor resistance to a particular single agent. Since it is neither feasible, nor currently scientifically valid to test each individual tumor against a panel of cytotoxic agents, the concept is to treat with a combination of the most active agents for a given histologic diagnosis in order to increase the likelihood that any individual tumor will respond.
- Combination chemotherapy may be used to prevent acquired resistance in initially sensitive tumor. The assumption is that large, heterogeneous tumors harbor small populations of cells that are either naturally resistant or have undergone de novo mutation to acquire resistance. Single-agent therapy places selective positive pressure on these populations, while concurrent administration of other active drugs with different mechanisms of action may allow for independent cell killing.

5. What constitutes the ideal combination of agents for the treatment of a given neoplastic disease?

The ideal combination of agents would include drugs that

- Are the most active in the disease
- Have different, nonantagonistic, and preferably additive or synergistic mechanisms of action
- Are non–cross-resistant (i.e., are subject to different mechanisms of resistance)
- Have nonoverlapping toxicities so that each can be delivered at the dose and schedule that optimizes efficacy

6. Define dose intensity.

The concentration of a drug given over a specified period. Most chemotherapeutic agents have a very steep dose-response curve, and even small escalations in dose can have a profound effect on tumor cell kill. This is especially true of drugs that are not cell cycle dependent, particularly the alkylating agents, for which it has been shown that a two-fold increase in the dose of cyclophosphamide can increase therapeutic efficacy up to 10-fold. Numerous clinical studies have demonstrated that patients who receive greater dose intensity have superior response rates and disease-free survival. However, these gains must always be balanced against morbity and mortality from drug toxicity.

7. What is the fractional cell kill hypothesis?

The fractional cell kill hypothesis states that a given drug or drug combination at a given dose intensity kills a constant fraction of the tumor cell population, regardless of overall tumor burden. Thus, each cycle of chemotherapy will diminish the remaining tumor cell population by a fixed percent. The objective of curative therapy is complete eradication, or zero tumor cells. Thus, if there are 10^{11} tumor cells and each cycle has a 99% cell kill, it will take six cycles to diminish the tumor cell population to less than one cell, assuming no regrowth between cycles. While this hypothesis was initially derived for treatment of leukemia and lymphoma and may not be directly applicable to slow-growing solid tumors or treatment with cell cycle–dependent agents, the general principle regarding the need for frequent, repetitive therapy is a well-established paradigm.

8. List the most common anticancer drugs, by class, used to treat pediatric cancers and describe their mechanisms of action.

DRUG CLASS	EXAMPLES	MECHANISM OF ACTION
Alkylating agents		Cross-link DNA thereby preventing replication of DNA and transcription of RNA
	Mechlorethamine, cyclophosphamide, ifosfamide, melphalan, nitrogen mustard	DNA cross-linking via classic covalent bond of alkyl group to DNA template
	Carmustine (BCNU), lomustine (CCNU) (nitrosureas)	DNA cross-linking and inhibition of DNA repair
	Cisplatin, carboplatin	DNA cross-linking by platination
	Busulfan, thiotepa, dacarbazine, procarbazine	DNA cross-linking
Antimetabolites		Structural analogues of key molecules involved in DNA/RNA synthesis
	Methotrexate	Structural analogue of folic acid; inhibits dihydrofolate reductase (DHFR), depleting tetrahydrofolate and precursors for the synthesis of purines and thymidine
	6-Mercaptopurine, 6-thioguanine	Purine analogues; compete with endogenous purine bases
	Cytarabine	Pyrimidine analogue (deoxycytosine); incorporates into DNA and inhibits DNA polymerase leading to chain termination
Antitumor antibiotics		Naturally occurring products with various mechanisms
	Doxorubicin, daunomycin, idarubicin (anthracyclines)	DNA intercalation and inhibition of topoisomerases, altering the three-dimensional shape of DNA/RNA during replication and transcription leading to double- and single-strand breaks; free radical formation; interaction with cell membranes
	Dactinomycin	DNA intercalation and inhibition of topoisomerase II
	Bleomycin	Induction of DNA strand breaks by free radicals
Plant alkaloids		Derived from plant extracts
	Vincristine, vinblastine (vinca alkaloids)	Inhibitors of mitosis; bind to tubulin, interfering with microtubule assembly and formation of the mitotic spindle
	Etoposide (epidopophyllotoxins)	Topoisomerase II inhibitor
Miscellaneous	Prednisone, dexamethasone (corticosteroids)	Lympholysis, probably via binding of steroid receptor complex; also used as anti-inflammatory, immunosuppressant, and antiemetic
	L-asparaginase	Enzyme that depletes asparagine in cells

9. Describe the cell cycle and its critical phases.

The growth and division of cells must proceed through an orderly series of events termed the cell cycle. Normally, cell proliferation is regulated by checkpoints that control entry into the following phase. One such checkpoint is the *p53* gene that controls progression from G1 to S-phase.

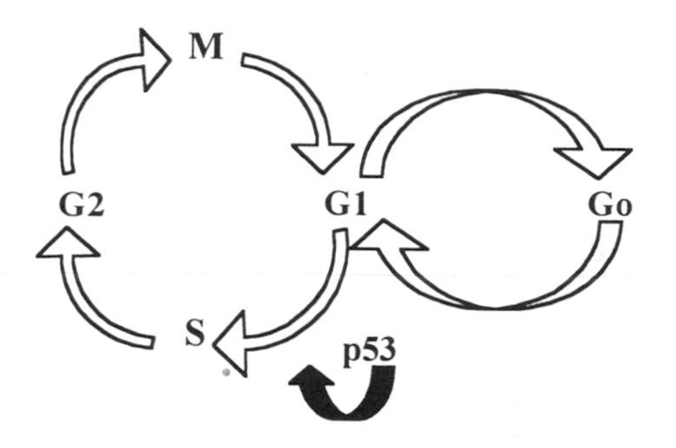

Go = resting phase: nonproliferation
G1 = Gap1or pre-DNA synthetic phase (12 hr-days):
DNA repair, no net DNA synthesis, diploid
RNA and protein synthesis
S = DNA synthesis (2-4 hr)
G2 = Gap2 or post-DNA synthesis (2–4 hr):
Two copies of each chromosome, tetraploid
RNA and protein synthesis
M = Mitosis (1–2 hr)

10. What are the implications for treatment with agents that are cell cycle dependent?

- Cell kill is limited with bolus dosing: Regardless of agent dose, only those cells active in the specific phase of the cell cycle at the time of drug administration will be killed.
- Prolonged continuous infusion or frequent intermittent dosing is required to increase cell kill: Administration using these principles at a fixed, effective dose represents a more rational intensification strategy than dose escalation, as cumulatively more cells will be exposed to drug during the sensitive phase of the cell cycle.
- "Recruitment" may increase cell kill: If more cells can be recruited into or arrested at the phase in which an agent is active, a greater number of cells will be killed.

11. Which chemotherapy agents are cell cycle dependent and what is the phase in which they are most active?

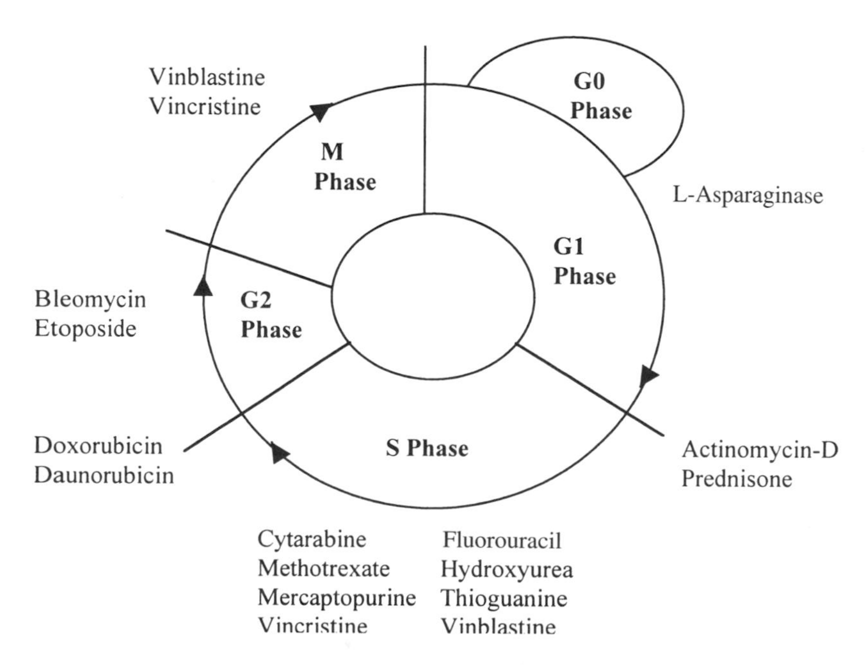

12. Why is drug toxicity such a major problem in cancer chemotherapy?

The agents used to treat cancer have a very narrow therapeutic index. In general, the mechanisms of action lead to nonspecific killing of rapidly dividing cells. Most conventional agents cannot differentiate between normal and tumor tissues. As a result, the dose needed to treat disease does not differ greatly from a dose that could cause potentially dangerous or even lethal damage to normal tissues. Normal cells most frequently affected include bone marrow, mucosal epithelium, hair, and detoxifying organs including the liver and kidney.

13. Describe the most common side effects of the major classes of chemotherapy agents.

- Myelosuppression: Critical depression of bone marrow production leading to reduced peripheral blood counts. Because of the short lifespan of granulocytes, neutropenia is the most significant effect, increasing the risk for severe infection. Thrombocytopenia and anemia may often precipitate the need for transfusion. The lowest counts (nadir) usually occur at 7–14 days after the initiation of chemotherapy, with complete recovery by 21–28 days.
- Mucositis: Inflammation, ulceration, and potential sloughing of the gastrointestinal mucosa. May occur anywhere from mouth to anus, impairing one's ability to eat, drink, swallow, or absorb nutrients. Also represents breakdown of an important barrier to infection. Most commonly occurs with the use of the antimetabolites, anthracyclines antibiotic agents, and the topoisomerase inhibitors.
- Nausea and vomiting: Rarely dose-limiting, but has a significant impact on quality of life. Can often be managed quite effectively with antiemetics, including the newer serotonin antagonists. The most emetogenic agents include the platinum analogs, nitrogen mustards, dactinomycin, irinotecan, cyclophosphamide, cytarabine, doxorubicin and methotrexate in higher doses.
- Alopecia: Total body hair loss. Predominantly caused by the alkylating agents, anthracyclines, and dactinomycin.
- Nephrotoxicity: Most often manifested as renal tubular damage. Dose-limiting with cisplatin and, to a lesser extent, carboplatin. Can also be a significant toxicity of ifosfamide and high-dose methotrexate. Managed with vigorous hydration and, potentially, amifostine.
- Syndrome of inappropriate antidiuretic hormone secretion: Leads to water retention and hyponatremia. Seen with high-dose cyclophosphamide and vincristine.
- Hepatotoxicity: Direct hepatocyte toxicity leading to elevation of transaminases, fibrosis, cholestasis, or hepatic venous outflow obstruction. Can be dose-limiting. Most commonly seen with the antimetabolites methotrexate, mercaptopurine, and thioguanine and the alkylating agents in myeloablative doses.
- Cardiotoxicity: Acute toxicity including arrhythmias, conduction abnormalities, and myopathy may be seen with the anthracyclines and cyclophosphamide or ifosfamide in high doses. Chronic, late cardiomyopathy is peculiar to the anthracyclines. Risk appears to increase with a cumulative dose of doxorubicin ≥ 450 mg/m^2, young age at exposure, and female sex. Dexrazoxane may be protective.
- Neurotoxicity: Commonly seen as the mostly reversible peripheral sensory/motor neuropathy and ileus that accompanies the use of vincristine. Central nervous system effects are more rare and include leukoencephalopathy with frequent intrathecal or high-dose methotrexate and cerebellar toxicity with high-dose cytarabine. Irreversible sensorineural hearing loss can be associated with cisplatin and to a lesser extent, carboplatin.
- Hypersensitivity: Anaphylactic response may limit use of asparaginase, paclitaxel, and, rarely, cisplatin or bleomycin.

14. What can be done to increase the maximum tolerated dose intensity without increasing the number of serious adverse events?

The best defense against toxicity includes aggressive supportive care with antiemetics, good hygiene and nutrition, blood component transfusions, and antibiotics. Recent innovations include specific chemoprotectants such as mesna, dexrazoxane, and amifostine; rescue agents such as leucovorin; and stem cell rescue with cytokine support that includes granulocyte colony–stimulating factor, erythropoietin, and interleukin-11.

15. Describe the mechanism of hemorrhagic cystitis with ifosfamide and cyclophosphamide and what can be done to prevent it.

Ifosfamide and cyclophosphamide undergo hepatic transformation to both active and inactive metabolites. One of these metabolites, acrolein, is believed to bind to and irritate the urogenic epithelium and can cause profuse bleeding of the bladder that may be dose-limiting. Mesna (sodium-2-mercaptoethane sulfonate) is rapidly oxidized in plasma to an inert disulfide compound that is resorbed by the kidney and only converted back to its active form in the renal tubules. Therefore, it combines and deactivates acrolein and acrolein-precursors by forming nontoxic thioethers only after these metabolites have been excreted in the urine. By giving ifosfamide and cyclophosphamide in conjunction with mesna, vigorous hydration, and frequent voiding, the incidence of hemorrhagic cystitis has been markedly reduced, even in the context of profound dose escalation.

16. How is leucovorin rescue used with methotrexate?

Methotrexate works by inhibiting DHFR, depleting cells of the reduced coenzyme tetrahydrofolate needed for the synthesis of purines, thymidine, and DNA. When high doses of methotrexate are used (usually >100 mg/m^2), leucovorin (folinic acid) supplies normal cells with reduced folate to prevent toxicity (gastrointestinal, bone marrow, renal, hepatic, and neurologic). Using this "rescue" strategy, doses in excess of 30 g/m^2, previously deemed lethal, may be delivered safely. To prevent rescuing tumor cells, the leucovorin is started 24 hr after the methotrexate is initiated. To prevent toxicity, the leucovorin is not discontinued until serum methotrexate levels fall below 0.1 μm.

17. What agents are most likely to cause morbidity from extravasation?

Extravasation, or leakage from a vessel into the surrounding normal tissue during the delivery of chemotherapy, can be particularly dangerous if the agent is an anthracycline or dactinomycin. Less severe injury can be caused by escape of nitrogen mustard, cisplatin, etoposide, or vincrisitine. Early symptoms include burning, discomfort, redness, or swelling. This may be followed by pain, edema, ulceration, and necrosis of involved tissues. Prompt recognition is extremely important. Interventions include stopping the infusion, withdrawing what may remain in the catheter and proximal vessel, applying ice to non-vinca alkaloids and heat to vinca alkaloid injuries, and the possible use of an antidote. Some antidotes are hyaluronidase (vinca alkaloid), sodium thiosulfate (nitrogen mustard), steroids, sodium bicarbonate, and dimethyl sulfoxide (anthracycline). As the use of an antidote can be controversial, local hospital and pharmacy policy should be consulted. To prevent extravasation, most children who will receive therapy containing frequent or continuous infusion vesicant are advised to have a secure central line placed with the position of the tip confirmed by X-ray or fluoroscopy.

18. Describe some of the most common biochemical mechanisms of drug resistance.

Drug resistance arises from spontaneous mutation or gene amplification in one generation of tumor cells that is passed on and expanded in subsequent generations, under the selective pressure of the drug. Most commonly, the mutation results in increased, decreased, or altered production of a gene product vital to a particular drug mechanism. For example, increased production of glutathiones by increased activity of the enzyme glutathione-S-transferase can detoxify the active metabolites of cyclophosphamide. Similarly, increased production of DHFR or an alteration of its affinity for methotrexate can decrease the efficacy of that drug.

Classic multidrug resistance was first noted in the late 1980s when it was found that a number of tumor cells developed cross-resistance to a seemingly unrelated but fixed constellation of naturally occurring cytotoxic agents. This phenomenon was subsequently attributed to a single gene, *MDR-1*, and gene product, the P glycoprotein (Pgp). Pgp appears to be a transmembrane efflux pump capable of ejecting numerous toxins but most notably the vinca akaloids, the anthracyclines, dactinomycin, the epipodophyllotoxins, and the taxanes.

Atypical multidrug resistance occurs when a cell acquires a mutation resulting in increased, decreased, or altered production of a gene product vital to a basic mechanism of cell upkeep. For example, both alkylating agents and topoisomerase inhibitors may be rendered ineffective by the enhanced function or production of DNA repair enzymes.

19. What can be done to overcome drug resistance?

Theoretically, once the biochemical mechanisms of drug resistance can be worked out, new agents can be developed or used in combination with standard agents to counteract or prevent resistance. For example, it is known that verapamil and cyclosporine can inhibit the Pgp efflux pump. However, they may also increase toxicity to normal cells. These and other agents in development are being used in clinical trials but as yet have not demonstrated significant benefit. Combination therapy with non–cross-resistant agents still appears to constitute the best approach.

20. Define so-called rationale drug development and give some examples of new agents.

Certain subsets of cancers have very characteristic biology. Rational drug development seeks to determine the genetic or immunologic signature of a given tumor cell and develop agents that can specifically target that aberrant cell. Examples of rational drug development include:

- Acute promyelocytic leukemia: Basic research identified t(15,17) as the cytogenetic marker of this histologically and clinically discreet form of acute myeloid leukemia. Subsequent work identified that the translocation occurred between the *PML* gene and one of the genes for the retinoic acid receptor RARα. Treatment with ATRA (tretinoin), an oral retinoid, has since been shown to confer considerable survival advantage for patients with this form of leukemia.
- B-cell non-Hodgkin's lymphoma: The neoplastic clones of some B-cell non-Hodgkin's lymphomas have been found to express the cell surface marker CD20. Rituximab, a humanized monoclonal antibody grown in mouse cells, can specifically target and lyse these malignant cells. Rituximab combined with conventional chemotherapy has proven effective in adults with specific types of refractory or recurrent non-Hodgkin's lymphoma without increasing toxicity. It has also shown promise in the treatment of post-transplant lymphoproliferative disease.

BIBLIOGRAPHY

1. Balis FM, Holcenberg JS, Poplack DG.: General Principles of Chemotherapy. In Pizzo PA, Poplack DG (eds), Principles and Practice of Pediatric Oncology, 3rd ed. Philadelphia, Lippincott-Raven, 1997, pp 215–272.
2. Chabner BA, Longo DL (eds): Cancer Chemotherapy: Principles and Practice, 2nd ed. Philadelphia, Lippincott-Raven, 1996.
3. Fischer DS, Knobf MT, Durivage HJ (eds): The Cancer Chemotherapy Handbook, 4th ed. St. Louis, Mosby, 1993.
4. Pratt WD, Ruddon RW: The Anticancer Drugs. Oxford, Oxford University Press, 1979.

22. PRINCIPLES OF PEDIATRIC SURGICAL ONCOLOGY

Jessica Kandel, M.D.

1. What are the surgical guidelines when treating neuroblastoma?

In an initial operation, the goals are

- To obtain adequate tissue for all diagnostic parameters, including molecular diagnostics
- To completely resect the tumor if feasible (complete resection may be delayed until after initial chemotherapy when removal of the primary tumor risks injury to vital structures)

2. When is second-look surgery for neuroblastoma performed?

After the completion of four or five cycles of chemotherapy in patients who have initially unresectable tumors. Complete resection is the goal.

3. Describe when lymph node sampling is performed in surgery for neuroblastoma.

At the time of initial surgery for staging purposes. It must be repeated at the time of delayed surgery as well.

4. When is a liver biopsy performed in surgery for neuroblastoma?

At the time of the initial exploratory surgery. It must be repeated at second-look surgery as well.

5. Describe the surgical guidelines for treating Wilms' tumor.

Complete resection of a unilateral Wilms' tumor without spillage and without biopsy prior to nephrectomy is the goal. The opposite kidney should be both palpated and visualized, if technically possible. Tumor-invading contiguous organs may be biopsied. If the tumor is not amenable to complete resection, chemotherapy is employed to shrink the tumor so that subsequent nephrectomy may be performed without compromise of other organs and vital structures. The extent of contamination by "spilled" tumor (e.g., limited spill, as after biopsy, versus widespread, as after tumor rupture) is important in Wilms' tumor surgery, because this will determine the extent of radiation therapy directed at the abdomen (e.g., flank versus whole abdominal irradiation).

6. Define the principles used for staging a Wilms' tumor.

Wilms' tumor is staged clinicopathologically by the surgeon at the time of operation and confirmed by the pathologist. National Wilms' Tumor Study staging guidelines are as follows:

- Stage I: Tumor confined to kidney
- Stage II: Tumor extends beyond kidney but is completely resectable
- Stage III: Residual gross tumor in the abdomen
- Stage IV: Distant metastases
- Stage V: Bilateral renal tumors at diagnosis

7. When is lymph node sampling performed in Wilms' tumor surgery?

Only clinically suspicious lymph nodes require excision.

8. Describe the surgical management of hepatoblastoma. How is hepatoblastoma staged?

The goal of surgery in hepatoblastoma is complete resection, if technically possible. If resection is not feasible and safe, an initial biopsy for diagnostic purposes is recommended. Patients with inoperable hepatoblastomas should receive chemotherapy in an attempt to shrink the tumor and render a previously inoperable tumor completely resectable.

Hepatoblastoma is staged by clinicopathologic criteria by the surgeon at the time of operation and confirmed by the pathologist. The following staging system is utilized:

- Stage I: Completely resected
- Stage II: Microscopic residual at the margins of resection but without tumor spillage and withnegative lymph nodes
- Stage III: Gross residual tumor and/or positive lymph nodes
- Stage IV: Distant metastases

9. List the guidelines for surgical management of testicular germ cell tumors.

- Stage I: Tumors are limited to the testis and completely resected by radical high *inguinal* orchiectomy with ligation of the spermatic cord. Retroperitoneal lymph nodes are free of tumor. Tumor markers, human chorionic gonadotropin (HCG) and alpha fetoprotein (AFP) fall to normal levels after surgery.
- Stage II: Microscopic extension to scrotum or spermatic cord, positive retroperitoneal lymph nodes less than 2 cm in greatest dimension and elevated tumor markers HCG and/or AFP. In addition, a primary *trans-scrotal* orchiectomy results in a stage II classification.
- Stage III: Positive retroperitoneal lymph nodes larger than 2 cm.
- Stage IV: Distant metastases.

10. How should tumor tissue be handled in the operating room?

Samples should be placed in sterile saline (NOT formalin) and immediately collected by the pathologist for transport to the laboratory. Fixatives, contamination and tissue decay compromise the retrieval of tissue for biological evaluation (e.g., mRNA for expression analysis and tissue for fluorescent in situ hybridization).

11. Give the guidelines for the use of minimally invasive surgical techniques in children with solid tumors of the chest or abdomen.

No data exist that allow direct comparison of such techniques with conventional "open" surgery. Thus, it appears prudent to use minimally invasive techniques in selected cases where such approaches may adhere to the previously established surgical guidelines. For example, a minimally invasive approach might be employed to biopsy an abdominal tumor where microscopic spillage is not of concern and where adequate tissue may be obtained (e.g., widespread nonlymphoblastic, non-Hodgkin's lymphoma of the abdomen).

12. What vascular access devices are available for pediatric patients with cancer, and how should the correct device be chosen?

The correct device for each child is that one that will most reliably permit infusion of therapeutic agents and sampling of blood, with a minimum of discomfort, restriction of normal activity and risk of infection. Considerations in choosing the correct device must include the age and size of the child, the diagnosis and the type and duration of therapy being contemplated. Devices may be separated into the following categories:

- Completely implanted, accessible units with subcutaneous reservoirs
- Externally accessed catheter devices with implanted "cuffs" allowing for tissue ingrowth
- Temporary percutaneous central venous catheters, including pheresis catheters

Clinical application of the various devices is demonstrated by the following examples:

- A completely implanted device with a reservoir might be most appropriate for an adolescent patient on the school swim team who has Hodgkin's disease involving unilateral cervical lymph nodes.
- A 2-year-old with acute lymphoblastic leukemia might best be managed with a double-lumen externally accessed catheter device.
- An infant with catheter sepsis during chemotherapy for neuroblastoma has the catheter removed but has poor peripheral access. A temporary percutaneous central venous catheter is placed.

13. What is typhlitis? How is it managed?

Typhlitis (or neutropenic enterocolitis) is a bacterial infection of the cecum and right colon, typically encountered in neutropenic patients. Patients are treated with broad-spectrum antibiotics directed at intestinal flora, including anaerobes. Treatment also involves bowel rest and careful serial examinations. Surgery in such patients is associated with significant morbidity; thus, it is reserved for patients who display evidence of uncontrolled disease, such as free intraperitoneal air, gastrointestinal hemorrhage and systemic sepsis with cardiovascular collapse.

14. Discuss special considerations involved in wound healing in patients with cancer.

Cytotoxic and antiproliferative treatment including radiation therapy impairs tumor cell growth and prohibits the physiologic proliferation of the cells that support normal healing, including fibroblasts, endothelial cells and enterocytes. Thus, children who will or have undergone such therapies must be monitored for alterations in healing, including

- Increased incidence of wound infection
- Increased incidence of device infection
- Failure of healing in a setting where it would normally be expected, such as the closure of the abdominal wall after laparotomy or intestinal anastomosis

15. What is the role of staging laparotomy in Hodgkin's disease?

Treatment for Hodgkin's disease requires a careful balance between the expected high cure rates and the avoidance of late effects of therapy. Current approaches rely on combined modalities; this permits lower cumulative doses of chemotherapy and radiation and limited fields of irradiation. These approaches do not require the precise staging achieved by laparotomy to achieve the goals of therapy. Instead, patients are staged clinically by noninvasive means such as computed tomography, magnetic resonance imaging and gallium scans. For patients who are not candidates for or who refuse chemotherapy, staging laparotomy may be useful in defining the anatomic extent of disease to allow delivery of precise radiotherapy.

BIBLIOGRAPHY

1. Adzick NS, Nance ML: Pediatric surgery: Second of two parts. N Engl J Med 342(23):1726–32, 2000.
2. Haase G, Wiener E, et al: Surgical Guidelines of the Children's Cancer Group. Distributed by the Children's Cancer Group, CCG Group Operations Center, Arcadia, CA.
3. Haase GM, Perez C, Atkinson JB: Current aspects of biology, risk assessment, and treatment of neuroblastoma. Semin Surg Oncol 16(2):91–104, 1999.
4. Schellong G: Pediatric Hodgkin's disease: Treatment in the late 1990s. Ann Oncol 9 (suppl 5):S115–119, 1998.

23. PRINCIPLES OF RADIATION ONCOLOGY FOR PEDIATRIC MALIGNANCIES

Karen Fountain, M.D., F.A.C.R.

1. What is ionizing radiation?

Electromagnetic radiation includes x-rays, gamma rays, ultraviolet and visible light, infrared radiation or heat, radio waves and electric waves. These radiations are made up of bundles of energy or photons, which travel like waves, but may behave like particles in certain interactions. The wavelength of a photon, its frequency and its energy are intimately related. When the energy per photon is greater than the binding energies of electrons in a target, the interaction of the photon and the target atom ejects an electron from its orbit, causing ionization. Photons with energies above 10 electron volts (eV) are ionizing radiation; those with energies below 10 eV are nonionizing radiation. Photons capable of ionization interact with material in three ways, dependent on their energy. The photoelectric effect depends on the atomic number of the target and may be seen in radiation utilized to produce diagnostic x-rays. Compton scattering is seen at higher energies, is not dependent on atomic number and explains why "port films" from cobalt units and linear accelerators show little anatomic detail. Pair production predominates in interactions over 20 megaelectron volts (MeV), and would be applicable only in high-energy accelerators.

2. Describe how radiation dose is measured in clinical practice.

One centigray in SI units (cGy) is equal to one rad (radiation absorbed dose), which is defined as the deposition of 100 ergs per gram in the tissue or medium of interest.

3. What is the mechanism of action of ionizing radiation?

Once radiation has caused ionization in the molecules of cells, especially in DNA and intracellular water, interactions take place that cause sublethal damage. If enough "hits" occur, cellular repair may no longer be possible and inactivation or cell death may occur. The sensitivity of a cell to radiation depends on its position in the cell cycle; cells that are actively dividing are most susceptible. As a result, tissues composed of rapidly growing, rapidly cycling cells such as bone marrow, the lining of the gut, hair follicles and rapidly growing tumors, are the most sensitive to radiation. Mature resting cells such as myocytes and neurons would be more resistant, as would tissues composed of such cells; for example, muscle and brain, which could therefore tolerate higher doses of radiation safely.

4. Name the factors that influence the response to fractionated treatments.

Experiments with cell cultures and animal models demonstrated four factors that are important. They are the "Four Rs":

1. Repair of radiation damage
2. Repopulation by proliferation of surviving cells
3. Redistribution of proliferating cells through the cell cycle
4. Reoxygenation of hypoxic cells

5. What types of ionizing radiation are used in clinical practice, and how are they produced?

Gamma rays are produced by the nuclear disintegration of an artificial isotope, cobalt-60. X-rays are produced when a high-energy electron beam strikes a gold target in a linear accelerator. Both are energy beams. If the gold target is removed, the electron beam itself may be utilized for radiation therapy in a wide range of energies. An electron beam is a particle beam.

6. Name the members of the radiation oncology team and describe their functions.

The *radiation oncologist* is a physician specialist whose area of expertise includes clinical oncology, radiation biology and radiation physics. It is the responsibility of the radiation oncologist to approve the final plan involving the tumor volume, appropriate margins, critical normal tissues and organs and acceptable tissue tolerances. The responsibility of the *radiation oncology physicist* is to ensure the accuracy, calibration and quality assurance of the therapy units, the simulator and computerized dosimetry. A *dosimetrist* obtains all pertinent measurements of the patient and the intended treatment volume, including computed tomography scans for treatment planning and performs sophisticated computerized dosimetry calculations. The *radiation oncology nurse* has special expertise in nursing assessment and symptom management of patients receiving radiation therapy. The *simulator technologist* operates a diagnostic x-ray machine mounted in a replica of a therapy unit. Diagnostic-quality x-rays are taken that replicate the intended treatment volume.

7. Define brachytherapy.

The temporary or permanent placement of radioactive material in the form of tubes, seeds, needles or catheters into tissue (interstitial) or body cavities (endocavitary). It is utilized to deliver a focused dose of radiation as primary treatment, as a boost following external beam radiation therapy or as postoperative adjuvant treatment to improve local control and lessen the risk of local recurrence while sparing surrounding normal tissues. Brachytherapy procedures may be characterized as low dose rate (LDR) or high dose rate (HDR). LDR procedures may occur over several days; HDR procedures may take only a few minutes. To minimize radiation dose to hospital support staff, nursing staff, visitors and families, remote after-loading units may be employed for brachytherapy procedures. The radioactive materials are withdrawn into a special safe while interventions are performed and reinserted via special catheters when indicated. According to the inverse square law, if the distance from the radioactive source is doubled, the radiation dose is divided by four. Therefore, there is rapid falloff of radiation dose the farther away one moves from a brachytherapy implant.

8. How is treatment planning performed?

After a patient is seen in consultation and treatment options have been discussed, informed consent is obtained. The patient is brought to the simulation suite and positioned as if for treatment. Immobilization devices to ensure reproducibility of daily treatment setup are constructed. Such devices include plaster body casts, heat sensitive rapid-setting styrofoam molds, vacuum immobilization bags, thermoplastic face masks and head frames. Preliminary diagnostic films are taken at the same angle and distance as the intended treatment beams. A special computed tomography scan or other imaging studies may be performed with or without appropriate contrast agents with the patient in the treatment position. The tumor volumes, required margins, critical organs, areas at risk and normal tissues are outlined and defined. Computerized treatment planning is utilized to optimize the treatment volume. When indicated, three-dimensional conformal techniques may be used. Custom Cerrobend blocks are fabricated to shape the fields; alternatively, multileaf collimators may directly shape the treatment beams. Cone-down fields to boost an area of high risk or to avoid a structure that has received tolerance dose levels are also incorporated into the final plan. The attending radiotherapist and physicist and the dosimetrist must review and approve each customized treatment plan.

9. Discuss the biological effects of radiation therapy.

Radiation is more effective in the presence of oxygen; conversely, hypoxic, necrotic tumors are more resistant and require higher doses of radiation to obtain local control. Fractionation (using divided doses) allows delivery of higher total doses of radiation by permitting repair of sublethal damage sustained by normal tissues after each treatment. As tumor cells have lost the ability to repair such damage, the therapeutic ratio is thereby improved. Standard fractionation is one treatment per day, five days per week, until the appropriate dose has been reached. Hyperfractionation is treating more than once per day to try to increase the total dose. Accelerated fractionation is treating to the same dose in a shorter period of time. All these methods try to modify the therapeutic ratio between normal tissue tolerance, local control of the tumor and tissue necrosis. Areas of investigation include radiation protection agents and radiation-sensitizing agents. The former lessen radiation effects on normal tissues as opposed to tumor cells, whereas the latter heighten radiation damage to tumor tissue, sparing normal cells and thereby increasing the therapeutic ratio.

10. What happens to bones when they are included in the radiation field?

Inhibition or impairment of skeletal growth is an important toxicity of ionizing radiation, especially in younger children who have not yet completed their growth. Axial skeletal growth arrest may occur at doses above 2000 cGy, resulting in disproportionate sitting and standing heights. Scoliosis may be caused by partial inclusion of vertebral bodies in the radiation field. Abnormalities of craniofacial growth may cause cosmetic or functional deformities.

11. Define gamma knife.

A gamma knife treatment unit is an external-beam radiation therapy machine that uses multiple high-energy cobalt 60 sources to treat very small focused tumor volumes to high doses. Such treatments may be given at a single session or as multiple fractions. Appropriate indications for gamma knife treatment include small primary brain neoplasms, small metastases to the brain, arteriovenous malformations and acoustic neuromas.

BIBLIOGRAPHY

1. DeVita VT Jr, Hellman S, Rosenberg SA (eds): Cancer: Principles and Practice of Oncology, 3rd ed. Philadelphia, Lippincott Williams and Wilkins, 2000.
2. Hall E: Radiobiology for the Radiobiologist, 4th ed. Philadelphia, Lippincott-Raven, 1994.
3. Halperin EC (ed):. Pediatric Radiation Oncology, 3rd ed. Philadelphia, Lippincott Williams and Wilkins, 1999.
4. Khan FM: The Physics of Radiation Therapy, 2nd ed. Baltimore, Lippincott Williams and Wilkins, 1994.
5. Khan FM: Treatment Planning in Radiation Oncology. Baltimore, Maryland, Williams & Wilkins, 1998.
6. Khan, FM: Treatment Planning for Radiation Oncology, Baltimore, Williams and Wilkins, 1997.
7. Leibel S, Phillips T: Textbook of Radiation Oncology. New York, W. B. Saunders, 1998.
8. Pazdur R, Cola LR, Hoskins WJ, Wagman LD (eds): Cancer Management: A Multidisciplinary Approach—Medical, Surgical & Radiation Oncology, 3rd ed. Melville, NY, PRR, 1999.
9. Perez CA, Brady LW: Principles and Practice of Radiation Oncology. Philadelphia, Lippincott-Raven, 1998.
10. Rubin P, Constine LS, Fajardo LF, et al: Late effects of normal tissues (LENT) scoring system. Intl J Radiat Oncol Biol Phys 31(5):1041–1091, 1995.

24. ACUTE LYMPHOBLASTIC LEUKEMIA

Kara M. Kelly, M.D.

1. Describe the frequency of acute lymphoblastic leukemia (ALL) of childhood.

Acute leukemias are the most common type of childhood cancer in the United States, representing 31% of cancer cases in children < 15 years, of which 75% are classified as ALL. The age-adjusted annual incidence rate is 3.1/100,000 children. All together, nearly 2500 children are diagnosed with ALL each year in the United States.

2. What is the cause of ALL?

The etiology for the majority of cases of ALL remains unknown. There is an increased risk for development of ALL in individuals with Down syndrome, Shwachman syndrome, Bloom syndrome and ataxia-telangiectasia, but these individuals represent the minority of cases of ALL. Factors that have consistently been associated with an increased risk for ALL include male gender, age 2–5 yr, Caucasian race, higher socioeconomic status, in utero radiation exposure and postnatal exposure to radiation from atomic bomb exposure or therapeutic radiation treatments. Less proven risk factors include increased birth weight, maternal history of fetal loss and advanced maternal age. There has been no proven association with low-frequency electromagnetic field or indoor radon exposure. Infectious agents are hypothesized to be involved, but to date there has been no strong evidence implicating a common infection. The interaction of multiple environmental and host factors is likely involved in the etiology of ALL.

3. List the common presenting signs and symptoms of a child with ALL.

The signs and symptoms of ALL reflect the degree of bone marrow infiltration by leukemic cells and the extent of disease outside the bone marrow. The inability to continue normal hematopoiesis with resultant anemia, thrombocytopenia and neutropenia leads to the most common signs and symptoms. Fatigue, pallor, petechiae, purpura, bleeding and fever are typically observed. Lymphadenopathy and hepatosplenomegaly are signs of extramedullary involvement. Leukemic infiltration of the periosteum and bone results in bone pain and associated limp or refusal to walk in up to 25% of children. Infiltration of the joint may cause arthralgia and make distinction of ALL from juvenile rheumatoid arthritis or osteomyelitis difficult.

4. What diagnostic studies are necessary in a child suspected of having ALL?

A complete blood count with differential may provide the first clues that a child has ALL. An elevated leukocyte count is seen in 50% of cases, and it is > 50,000/μl in 20%. Anemia is observed 80% of the time, and platelet counts < 100,000/μl are seen in 75%. Morphologic assessment of the peripheral smear may reveal lymphoblasts, although it occasionally may be misleading. Therefore, to definitively establish a diagnosis of ALL, a bone marrow aspirate is necessary. The finding of at least 25% blast cells in the bone marrow confirms the diagnosis of leukemia. The diagnosis of ALL is then established by cytochemical analysis of the bone marrow slides with differential stains such as periodic acid schiff, and sudan black B and immunophenotyping using a panel of monoclonal antibodies directed against early B or T cell antigens that are expressed on the blast surface. Cytogenetic analysis of the leukemic blasts provides important prognostic information. A lumbar puncture is necessary to screen for central nervous system (CNS) leukemia. Cerebrospinal fluid is examined after cytocentrifugation, to concentrate the leukemic cells and increase the diagnostic sensitivity. Evidence of CNS leukemia is present in < 5% of children at the time of diagnosis. A chest radiograph to ascertain the presence of mediastinal involvement, which is most prevalent in patients with T cell ALL, should be obtained.

5. Define the morphologic subtypes of ALL.

The French-American-British (FAB) classification defines three main types of ALL based on morphology:

	L1	*L2*	*L3*
Size of nucleus	Small	Large	Large
Nuclear pattern	Regular with homogeneous chromatin	Irregular with clumped chromatin	Regular with homogeneous chromatin
Nucleoli	Inconspicuous	Prominent	Prominent
Cytoplasm	Scant	Moderately abundant	Moderately abundant; basophilic with prominent vacuoles
Frequency of occurrence	85%	14%	1%

6. Describe the National Cancer Institute Risk Groups for ALL.

ALL is generally classified into two main risk groups:

Risk	*Definition*	*Percentage of B-precursor Patients*
Standard*	Age 1–9.99 yr and WBC count < 50,000/μL	68
High	Age ≥10 years or WBC count ≥ 50,000/μl	32

*Patients with poor risk genetic features, such as presence of t(9;22), or t(4;11), would be classified as high risk.

WBC = white blood cell.

7. List the prognostic factors for ALL.

Host Related	*Disease Related*	*Treatment Related*
	Predictive of Outcome	
Age	White blood cell count	Protocol
Gender	T-cell or B-cell lineage	Early response
Race	Karyotype: t(9;22), t(4;11), balanced t(1;19)	
	Hyper/Hypodiploidy	
	TEL/AML1	
	Possible Predictive of Outcome	
Down syndrome	CNS disease	Day 7 marrow
Immunodeficiency	Mediastinal mass	Day 14 marrow
Nutrition	Splenomegaly	Day 28 marrow
Compliance	Hepatomegaly	Peripheral blasts
Access to healthccare	Immature T-cell lineage	Minimal residual disease
Pharmacogenetics	CD10 negativity	CDRIII PCR
Glutathione S-transferase polymorphisms	Karyotype: +4, +10, del 9p, +17, +18, 13q12-14, 15(q13-15), other t(11q23), t(1;19), MLLr	T-cell receptor PCR

Prognostic Factors for ALL (Continued)

Pharmacogenomics	Immunologic fingerprint Fluorescent in situ hybridization Leukemic colony-forming units Prednisone response Red blood cell thioguanine nucleotides Systemic methotrexate or thiopurine exposure Methotrexate polyglutamates MTT assay
No Longer Considered Predictive of Outcome	
Enlargement of kidneys Testicular disease Hgb > 10 g/dL or platelets < 100,000/mL Visible adenopathy FAB morphology PAS positivity Labeling index Myeloid antigen positivity LDH Glucocorticoid receptor number	

Modified from Lange BJ: The ultra low-risk child with acute lymphoblastic leukemia. Hematology x: 287, 2000.

LDH = lactate dehydrogenase; MTT = methyltetrazolium; PAS = periodic acid Schiff; PCR = polymerase chain reaction.

8. List the characteristics of T-cell ALL.

- Massive splenomegaly
- Massive lymphadenopathy
- Large anterior mediastinal mass
- Increased risk for initial CNS involvement or relapse
- Initial leukocyte count ≥ 50,000 /mL
- Hemoglobin ≥ 10 g/dL
- L2 morphology
- Focal paranuclear positivity of acid phosphatase staining
- Expression of CD2, CD3, CD5, CD7
- Rearrangements of the T-cell receptor gene in leukemic cells

9. Why do infants have a particularly poor prognosis?

Infants tend to have a type of leukemia that is biologically different than the usual ALL seen in older children. The leukemic blasts are more likely to have an unfavorable translocation, such as t(4;11) that involves chromosome 11q23, the location of the MLL fusion gene. Immunophenotyping is usually consistent with an early B-cell precursor origin, with CD10 (common ALL antigen) negativity. Infants often present with elevated leukocyte counts and CNS disease and frequently have massive hepatosplenomegaly, an indication of significant extramedullary disease. The prognosis is particularly poor in infants < 6 months.

10. What is the prognosis for children with ALL?

Children with standard risk ALL have an 85% long-term event-free survival, whereas even patients with high-risk ALL have an event-free survival that approaches 75%. Nevertheless, there do exist some subgroups of patients (e.g., infants and patients whose blasts cells possess the Philadelphia chromosome) that continue to have a very poor prognosis.

11. What are the phases of therapy for the treatment of ALL?

Since ALL is a heterogeneous disease, the stratification of children into risk groups has a significant impact on outcome. Despite this risk-based approach, the treatment is still divided into four main phases: induction, CNS preventative therapy, consolidation and maintenance. The goal of induction chemotherapy is to attain remission. Remission is defined as the absence of leukemia by physical examination and morphologic assessment of the bone marrow. The bone marrow must be of normal cellularity and have fewer than 5% blasts. Most protocols utilize vincristine and a glucocorticoid (prednisone or dexamethasone), in combination with L-asparaginase with or without an anthracycline. Remission is attained in 95% of children with ALL. However, since remission is not always synonymous with overall freedom from relapse, additional therapy is needed. CNS preventative therapy is used to eradicate subclinical CNS leukemia and consists primarily of intrathecal chemotherapy (typically methotrexate alone or in combination with cytarabine and hydrocortisone) with or without cranial irradiation. An early consolidation phase is designed to kill residual leukemic cells, and its use has resulted in an improved outcome across all risk groups. The choice of agents varies among protocols but typically utilizes more intensive and myelosuppressive drugs. Maintenance therapy is used to continue to suppress leukemic cell growth, reduce the leukemic cell burden and prevent the emergence of a drug-resistant clone. 6-Mercaptopurine and methotrexate provide the basis for most maintenance regimens, with further agents added according to the risk group and particular protocol. The total duration of therapy is variable among protocols, with a range of 24–38 months. Boys often receive therapy for a longer duration because of the increased risk for relapse.

12. Describe the role of CNS preventative therapy.

CNS preventative therapy is based on the concept that the CNS is a sanctuary site for previously undetected leukemic cells to be protected by the blood-brain barrier from therapeutic concentrations of systemically administered chemotherapy. As these cells are partially treated at best, resistant leukemic cells are selected out and can ultimately lead to CNS or bone marrow relapse. The choice of therapy for presymptomatic CNS therapy is a balance between the risk of CNS relapse and the late effects of the therapy. For standard-risk patients, treatment with intrathecal methotrexate or methotrexate in combination with cytarabine and hydrocortisone, administered periodically throughout the course of therapy, results in CNS relapse rates < 5%. For patients at an intermediate risk for CNS relapse, intrathecal chemotherapy in conjunction with moderate- or high-dose intravenous methotrexate appears to afford good protection. For high-risk patients, such as those with a slow response to initial chemotherapy or unfavorable cytogenetic features including t(9;22), cranial radiation using a dose of 1800 cGy is often employed.

13. Why is trimethoprim-sulfamethoxazole prescribed for children with ALL?

Children with ALL receiving maintenance chemotherapy are at high risk for development of a potentially life-threatening pneumonia with *Pneumocystis carinii*. The prophylactic use of trimethoprim-sulfamethoxazole administered as infrequently as 2–3 days each week is highly effective in reducing the incidence of this complication. In addition, it has been suggested that patients who receive trimethoprim-sulfamethoxazole also have reduced intercurrent infections.

14. A child with ALL is exposed to a child with chicken pox while in daycare. What steps should be taken?

If the child with ALL does not have prior immunity to varicella zoster, he or she is at risk for disseminated varicella, a potentially life-threatening infection in immunocompromized patients. Significant exposure is defined by the Centers for Disease Control as a continuous household contact, a playmate contact (>1 hour indoor play) or a hospital contact. Administration of varicella zoster immunoglobulin within 72–96 hr of exposure may reduce this risk and ameliorate the severity of the illness. The dose is 1 vial per 15 kg body weight. The exposed patient should be considered potentially infectious for 10–28 days following the exposure and should be isolated from other nonimmune children. If the child develops signs of infection, high-dose intravenous acyclovir therapy should be administered until all lesions are crusted.

15. Identify and describe the management of the fourth most common type of childhood cancer.

Relapsed ALL is the fourth most common diagnosed pediatric malignancy. Although the majority of patients can attain a second remission with further chemotherapy, the probability of sustaining this second remission depends on the length of the first remission and the site of relapse. Factors associated with a poor outcome after relapse include first remission < 24 months, bone marrow relapse, older age, T-cell ALL and male sex. Patients with a late occurring extramedullary relapse, typically CNS or testicular, have an improved prognosis and may be treated according to an intensified chemotherapy regimen with local radiotherapy to sites of extramedullary disease. The management of relapsed ALL is summarized below:

Poor Risk	Early bone marrow relapse (< 24 mos)	5–15% EFS	Sibling or unrelated stem cell transplant
	Early CNS or testicular relapse (< 18–24 mos)	20–25% EFS	Sibling or unrelated stem cell transplant Local irradiation
Standard Risk	Late bone marrow relapse (> 24 mos)	40–60% EFS	Sibling transplant if available Intensified chemotherapy
	Late CNS or testicular relapse	60–80% EFS	Intensified chemotherapy Local irradiation

16. Describe the type of relapse boys are at risk for.

Overt testicular involvement by leukemic cells may be seen in up to 10% of boys who have completed a full course of chemotherapy for their disease. The risk is higher in boys with a high initial leukocyte count, T-cell disease, prominent lymphadenopathy or hepatosplenomegaly or an initial platelet count > 30,000/μl. The testes have been considered a "sanctuary site," in that leukemic cells are protected from therapeutic doses of systemic chemotherapy by the "blood-testes" barrier. However, recent studies have disputed this concept.

17. What are the late sequelae associated with treatment for ALL?

The use of anthracycline chemotherapy (daunorubicin, doxorubicin) has been associated with cardiomyopathy, especially when given in high cumulative doses to young girls. Acute myeloid leukemia is a rare complication that has developed in children receiving intensive treatment with epipodophyllotoxins (etoposide, teniposide). Cranial radiotherapy is rarely associated with brain tumors, neuropsychological deficits and endocrine abnormalities (obesity, short stature, precocious puberty). The intensive use of glucocorticoids has resulted in avascular necrosis of bone, particularly in adolescent males.

BIBLIOGRAPHY

1. Biondi A, Cimino G, Pieters R, Pui C-H: Biological and therapeutic aspects of infant leukemia. Blood 96:24–33, 2000.
2. Chessells JM: Relapsed lymphoblastic leukaemia in children: a continuing challenge. Br J Hematol 102:423, 1998.
3. Margolin JF, Poplack DG: Acute lymphoblastic leukemia. In Pizzo PA, Poplack DG (eds): Principles and Practice of Pediatric Oncology. Philadelphia, Lippincott-Raven, 1997, pp 409–462.
4. Pui C-H: Acute lymphoblastic leukemia. Pediatr Clin North Am 44:831–846, 1997.
5. Pui C-H, Evans WE: Acute lymphoblastic leukemia. N Eng J Med 339:605–615, 1998.

25. ACUTE MYELOID LEUKEMIA

Kara M. Kelly, M.D.

1. How often is childhood acute myeloid leukemia (AML) diagnosed in the United States each year?

There are approximately 400–500 new cases of AML diagnosed in children and adolescents in the United States each year; the incidence is 5.2 cases per million children. AML represents about 20% of all newly diagnosed cases of childhood leukemia and acute lymphoblastic leukemia represents 75–80% of new cases. Interestingly, there is an increased incidence of AML seen in children < 1 year of age.

2. Which disorders are associated with an increased risk for development of AML?

- Down syndrome
- Fanconi's anemia
- Bloom syndrome
- Blackfan-Diamond anemia
- Neurofibromatosis type I
- Shwachman-Diamond syndrome
- Kostmann syndrome

3. Which carcinogens have been associated with an increased risk for development of AML?

- Benzene
- Ionizing radiation
- Maternal drug use
- Maternal ethanol use
- Maternal smoking
- Maternal topoisomerase II inhibitor intake
- Alkylating agents
- Topoisomerase II inhibitors

4. In what situation is a twin at risk for development of AML?

A monozygotic twin of an infant with AML has a one in five risk for development of AML. This is hypothesized to be due to an in utero twin-twin transfusion of a premalignant clone that undergoes malignant transformation in each individual sibling.

5. List the signs and symptoms of AML and their frequency of occurrence.

- Fever: 35%
- Bleeding: 35%
- Pallor: 25%
- Anorexia: 20%
- Fatigue: 20%
- Bone and/or joint pain: 20%
- Lymphadenopathy: 15%
- Gastrointestinal symptoms: 15%
- Neurologic symptoms: 10%
- Swollen gingivae: 10%

6. Define the French American British (FAB) histologic classification of AML.

FAB Subtype	*Percent of Total*	*Prominent Features*	*Unique Clinical or Laboratory Features*
M0	2	Large and agranular blasts with minimal myeloid differentiation; negative myeloperoxidase and Sudan black B by cytochemistry; expression of at least one myeloid antigen (e.g., CD13, CD33)	Blasts often express CD34 and terminal deoxynucleotidyl transferase (TdT)
M1	10–18	Poorly differentiated myeloblasts with occasional Auer rods	
M2	27–29	Myeloblastic with differentiation (< 20% monoblasts) and prominent Auer rods	Myeloblastomas (especially orbital)
M3	5–10	Hypergranular abnormal promyelocytes with bundles of Auer rods and often reniform or bilobed nuclei; M3 variant characterized by deeply notched nucleus, a few fine granules and infrequent Auer rods	Disseminated intravascular coagulation
M4	16–25	Myeloblastic and monoblastic differentiation (20–80% of nonerythroid cells are monoblastic); M4Eo variant associated with > 5% dysplastic eosinophilic precursors in marrow	Infants, extramedullary leukemia
M5	13–22	Monoblastic differentiation; M5a subtype has predominant monoblasts (≥ 80% of leukemic cells) and M5b subtype shows differentiation (< 80% leukemic cells as monoblasts)	Infants, extramedullary leukemia, second leukemia after epipodophyllotoxins
M6	1–3	Erythroleukemic with bizarre dyserythropoiesis and megaloblastic features	
M7	4–8	Megakaryoblastic with bone marrow fibrosis	Down syndrome

From Ebb DH, Weinstein HJ: Diagnosis and treatment of childhood acute myelogenous leukemia. Pediatr Clin North Am 44:849, 1997; with permission.

7. How is the diagnosis of AML confirmed?

Since AML is a morphologically heterogeneous disorder, multiple methods are used to confirm the diagnosis and sub-classify according to the FAB criteria. Standard morphologic assessment with interpretation of stained specimens using the Romanowsky method, demonstrating that at least 30% of bone marrow cells are blasts, is necessary to make a diagnosis of AML. Although the morphologic diagnosis is straightforward in most cases, other malignancies may mimic AML. Undifferentiated leukemia, metastatic alveolar rhabdomyosarcoma and L2 ALL may resemble M7 AML. Neuroblastoma and alveolar rhabdomyosarcoma may also be confused with M5 AML. The demonstration of the staining of blasts with the cytochemical stains, myeloperoxidase, Sudan black or nonspecific esterase, will help to distinguish from these other disorders and confirm the diagnosis in up to 80% of cases. Further confirmation is done with immunophenotyping using a panel of monoclonal antibodies recognizing B-cell, T-cell and myeloid antigens, and this has become standard practice at most institutions. The antigens, CD13, CD14 and CD33 are expressed on AML blasts in more than 90% of pediatric patients. Karyotyping and molecular genetics (detection of gene fusions such as PML-RARα that may not be seen with standard cytogenetics) are useful adjunct studies that may provide prognostic information.

8. List the favorable and unfavorable prognostic variables in childhood AML.

- Favorable
  - Chromosomal changes: t(8;21), inv(16), t(9;11), t(15;17)
  - Remission after one cycle of chemotherapy
  - FAB M4 with eosinophilia
- Unfavorable
  - Chromosomal changes: monosomy 7
  - Initial leukocyte count > 100,000/μL
  - Secondary AML
  - Myelodysplasia associated AML

9. What are the major components of therapy for pediatric AML?

The treatment of AML begins with a remission induction regimen and central nervous system prophylaxis and continues with consolidation and intensification therapy. Some protocols also include a maintenance phase. The goals of induction are to reduce the leukemic burden in the bone marrow to < 5% and clear any extramedullary disease (which defines remission) and to restore normal hematopoiesis. The use of a cytarabine- and daunomycin-based induction has led to improved remission rates. The use of intensive consolidation therapy has decreased relapse rates. If available, bone marrow transplantation with a familial matched donor is generally recommended for consolidation. There is variability in the conditioning regimen, source of stem cells and graft-versus-host disease prophylaxis. Busulfan and cyclophosphamide or total body irradiation with a cyclophosphamide-based chemotherapy regimen are most commonly used to eradicate any residual leukemia, make space for the donor stem cells and provide immunosuppression to prevent rejection of the donor stem cells. If a familial matched donor is not available, consolidation and intensification chemotherapy is administered, using high-dose cytarabine based regimens. Unrelated donor transplants are not recommended in first remission because the risks of graft-versus-host disease outweigh any potential benefit from a graft-versus-leukemia effect. Autologous bone marrow transplantation for intensification is incorporated in protocols by the United Kingdom Medical Research Council, but this approach was not shown to be of benefit in studies by the Children's Cancer Group (CCG) and the Pediatric Oncology Group (POG) in the United States and the French Cooperative AML Group (LAME). Maintenance chemotherapy is part of the German BFM AML trials, but maintenance therapy has been shown to possibly decrease event-free survival and overall survival in studies by the CCG and LAME. Most importantly, aggressive supportive care, especially with blood product support, empiric antibiotics, anti-fungal therapy and nutritional support, has allowed intensification of therapy to be possible, as AML therapy is associated with a high rate of mucositis, infection and prolonged bone marrow suppression. With these components, approximately 40–50% of children with AML can be cured.

10. Which vitamin has become part of the standard treatment for acute promyelocytic leukemia?

A form of vitamin A, all-trans retinoic acid (ATRA) is used as an adjunct to cytarabine- and daunomycin-based chemotherapy for the treatment of acute promyelocytic leukemia (APL). A reciprocal translocation between chromosomes 15 and 17 is found in APL cells, and this translocation results in a fusion of the PML gene and one of the receptors for retinoic acid, the RARα gene. ATRA leads to differentiation of leukemic cells in vitro and in vivo. ATRA has been associated with a reduction in serious bleeding from coagulopathy and a significant improvement in event-free survival for this particular subtype of AML.

11. Define the "retinoic acid syndrome."

A syndrome of unexplained fever with fluid retention, leading to pleural effusions, pericarditis and pulmonary edema may occur in an APL patient receiving ATRA. As it is believed to be a response to the differentiating effect of ATRA, the risk for development of the syndrome is greater in patients with a high leukocyte count. Symptoms improve with the use of steroids.

12. What is a granulocytic sarcoma?

A granulocytic sarcoma is a discrete solid collection of AML cells. It may arise in bones or soft tissues, and is more frequently found in the epidural area or around the orbits. The term *chloroma* is also sometimes used, because the presence of the enzyme myeloperoxidase gives the collection a green appearance on the cut surface.

13. Which subtype of AML is observed most frequently in children with Down syndrome?

Infants with Down syndrome most frequently develop acute megakaryoblastic leukemia (M7).

14. What complications may develop in a child with a leukocyte count that exceeds 200,000/μL?

Hyperviscosity with intravascular clumping of blasts and subsequent hypoxia, hemorrhage and infarction of affected tissue may occur. Sludging in the brain is manifested by somnolence, stroke and coma. Tachypnea and a reduction in partial pressure of arterial oxygen may develop in patients with lung involvement. The leukocyte count may be transiently lowered with leukopheresis or exchange transfusion, but cytotoxic therapy needs to be initiated promptly. In a child with ALL and a high leukocyte count, the development of tumor lysis syndrome is a major concern. The risk for development in a child with AML is substantially lower because of the slower cytotoxic response to chemotherapy and the less-frequent occurrence of renal infiltration. Empiric measures, including hydration, initiation of an agent to promote uric acid excretion (allopurinol or urate oxidase) and close monitoring of laboratory values are usually undertaken. The need for hemodialysis is extremely rare.

15. What chromosomal changes are observed in secondary AML?

Chromosomal changes involving band 11q23 are common in secondary leukemias resulting from exposure to the topoisomerase II inhibitors etoposide and teniposide. This region is involved in a translocation with several different partner genes such as *t(9;11)*, *t(10;11)*. The translocation results in the disruption of a single gene, the mixed-lineage leukemia (MLL) gene. Secondary leukemias have also been described after exposure to alkylating agents such as nitrogen mustard, chlorambucil, cyclophosphamide and melphalan and are associated with karyotypic changes involving chromosomes 5, 7 and 8.

16. Describe the major differences between AML and ALL.

	AML	*ALL*
Common presenting signs/symptoms	Constitutional symptoms more pronounced: fever, pallor, anorexia, weight loss, fatigue Oral bleeding, epistaxis, purpura or petechiae Lymphadenopathy	Fever common Extramedullary disease frequent as manifested by hepatosplenomegaly or lymphadenopathy Petechiae or purpura Bone pain
Morphology of blasts in more common sub-types	Large Nucleus often irregular Open nuclear chromatin	Small Large nucleus Homogeneous nuclear chromatin

Major Differences between AML and ALL (Continued)

	AML	*ALL*
	Cytoplasm more prominent	Scant cytoplasm
	Granules and Auer rods in cytoplasm	
Cytochemical stains	Myeloperoxidase	Periodic acid-Schiff
	Sudan black	Acid phosphatase (T-cell)
	Nonspecific esterase	
Immunophenotyping	CD13, CD14, CD 33	B cell origin: CD10, CD19, CD22, TdT
		T cell origin: CD3, CD7, CD5, CD2, TdT
Treatment	Intensive chemotherapy	Less-intensive chemotherapy
	Stem cell transplant in first remission (if matched familial donor available)	Stem cell transplant reserved for relapse (unless very high risk cytogenetics)
	Short duration (< 9 mo)	Long duration (2–3 yr)
Prognosis (event-free survival)	Human leukocyte antigen–matched donor: 65%	Standard risk: 85%
		High risk: 75%
	No donor: 40–50%	Infants: < 50%
	Infants: no difference	

BIBLIOGRAPHY

1. Aplenc R, Lange B: Pediatric acute myeloid leukemia. In Bast RC Jr, Kufe DW, Pollock RE, et al (eds): Cancer Medicine, 5th ed. Hamilton, B.C. Decker, 2000, pp.2151–2156.
2. Bhatia S, Neglia JP: Epidemiology of childhood acute myelogenous leukemia. J Pediatr Hematol Oncol 17:94, 1995.
3. Biondi A, Rambaldi A: Molecular diagnosis and monitoring of acute myeloid leukemia. Leukemia Res 20:801, 1996.
4. Chopra R, Goldstone AH: Modern trends in bone marrow transplantation for acute myeloid and acute lymphoblastic leukemia. Curr Opin Oncol 4:247, 1992.
5. Ebb DH, Weinstein HJ: Diagnosis and treatment of childhood acute myelogenous leukemia. Pediatr Clin North Am 44:847–862, 1997.
6. Golub T, Weinstein H, Grier H: Acute myeloid leukemia. In Pizzo PA, Poplack DG (eds): Principles and Practice of Pediatric Oncology, 3rd ed. Philadelphia, Lippincott-Raven, 1997, pp 463-482.
7. Grignani F, Fagioli M, Alcalay M, et al: Acute promyelocytic leukemia: From genetics to treatment. Blood 83:10, 1994.
8. Lange B: Progress in acute myelogenous leukemia: The one hundred years' war. J Pediatr Hematol Oncol 17:91, 1995.

26. MYELOPROLIFERATIVE DISORDERS IN CHILDREN

Mark Atlas, M.D.

1. Name the chromosomal abnormality associated with adult-type chronic myelogenous leukemia (CML). How commonly is it found in patients with CML?

Adult-type CML demonstrates a translocation of chromosomes 9 and 22 [t (9;22)]. This creates the bcr/abl fusion protein (P210). While the t(9;22) can be demonstrated in only 90% of patients with CML, the bcr/abl fusion protein can be detected in virtually all patients using molecular probes.

2. How does the activity of the P210 bcr/abl fusion protein differ from normal abl (P145)?

Both proteins have tyrosine kinase activity, but the P210 has increased activity and the ability to autophosphorylate. Additionally, the P210 is translocated to the cytoplasm from the nucleus. This increases the substrates on which it may work. One potential protein substrate is CRKL, which may play a role in differentiation and normally is nonphosphorylated. Phosphorylation blocks its function, potentially blocking differentiation and allowing increased proliferation of immature myeloid precursors.

3. Describe the different phases of CML.

Most patients present in the chronic phase that is characterized by fever, splenomegaly, elevated white blood cell (WBC) count and thrombocytosis. Patients occasionally have leukostasis but often are only minimally symptomatic. There are fewer than 5% blasts in the marrow. Treated or untreated, this phase may last several years.

The accelerated phase is characterized by hematologic abnormalities and refractoriness to therapy. There may be increased basophilia, anemia, splenomegaly and leucocytosis. New chromosomal abnormalities may appear.

The blast phase is essentially indistinguishable from acute leukemia. Approximately two thirds of the cases are myeloid, and one third lymphoid. There may be additional cytogenetic abnormalities. Lymphoid transformation may respond better to therapy, but both phenotypic variants are almost uniformly fatal.

4. What is the preferred medical therapy for CML?

Busulfan, hydroxyurea and interferon-α are all effective. Busulfan is equi-effective with hydroxyurea, but is disfavored because of side effects such as hyperpigmentation and rare interstitial pneumonitis.

Interferon-α can normalize hematologic parameters in about 3/4 of patients, similar to hydroxyurea. However, in contrast to hydroxyurea, it can also normalize bone marrow cytogenetics, although bcr/abl remains detectable by polymerase chain reaction (PCR). In one study, interferon was associated with a > 2-yr delay in progression to accelerated phase with a significantly prolonged survival. Many practitioners therefore prefer interferon as initial therapy, though a clear consensus is lacking.

5. Is there a curative therapy for CML?

Hematopoietic stem cell transplantation (SCT) remains the only potentially curative therapy for patients with CML. In adults, the indications for SCT remain controversial, as transplant is more toxic and patients potentially have 5–7 yrs of good-quality life with medical therapy. In pediatrics, however, because of the potential to extend life significantly, 5–7 yr survival is not considered sufficient; thus, SCT is the therapy of choice for patients with a related donor. The use of unrelated donors is also reasonable, though toxicity is higher. Currently, efforts to use chimera-mediated immunotherapy, in which less-aggressive conditioning regimens are employed, will likely improve results and should increase the feasibility of SCT for adults as well.

6. Why is hematopoietic stem cell transplant potentially curative while chemotherapy is not?

CML is basically a relatively chemotherapy resistant disease. While symptoms may be controlled for a period of time, the initial clonal defect is so early in hematopoietic ontogeny that it is unlikely to be cured with cytotoxic therapy. The curative potential of SCT likely results from its properties as immunotherapy. The donor graft possesses a potent graft-versus-leukemia effect, a T-cell–mediated process in which the graft attacks and destroys host hematopoietic cells. This can result in sustained hematologic and molecular remissions, in which the bcr/abl transcript is no longer detectable by PCR techniques.

7. Are there therapeutic options for advanced/refractory or relapsed patients with CML?

For patients in blast crisis, SCT can be curative, but the results are significantly inferior to transplant in chronic phase. Patients who demonstrate relapse after SCT can frequently be salvaged using adoptive immunotherapy with donor lymphocyte infusions. These infusions augment graft-versus-leukemia and can reinduce remission. This is frequently done if patients who become bcr/abl negative have a "molecular" relapse, when retrieval is easier. Nonetheless, a significant risk of associated graft-versus-host disease must be considered.

8. Differentiate adult-type CML from juvenile CML.

	CML	*JCML*
Age	> 4 yr	< 4 yr
WBC > 100 x 10^9/L	Typical	Unusual
Anemia	Variable	Mild-moderate
Platelet count	Increased	Decreased
Lymphadenopathy	Unusual	Typical
Splenomegaly	Present	Present: less pronounced
Fever	Common	Common
Infection	Rare	Common
Bleeding	Rare	Common
Bcr/abl fusion protein	Present	Absent
Fetal hemoglobin	Normal	Increased (median, 38%)
Leucocyte alkaline phosphatase	Decreased	Variable

9. What is the probable underlying biologic defect in Juvenile Chronic Myelogenous Leukemia (JCML)?

Patients appear to have a hypersensitivity to granulocyte-macrophage colony-stimulating factor (GM-CSF). Colony-forming units-GM (CFU-GM) are significantly increased in vitro when cultured with marrow from patients with JCML. JCML monocytes do not, however, secrete increased amounts of GM-CSF. This appears to be related to the myeloproliferation in JCML.

10. What is the clinical course of JCML?

Patients with JCML present with significant lymphadenopathy and organomegaly, though splenomegaly is typically less than in adult CML. Signs of stress erythropoiesis are characteristic. Despite therapy, there is progression of disease, typically without a blast crisis. Infection, bleeding or other complications from disease progression are usually the cause of death within 1–2 yr of diagnosis.

11. What therapy is available for JCML?

Juvenile CML is an extremely aggressive and refractory disease. While there may be transient responses to hydroxyurea or interferon-α, these drugs generally will induce only short-term control of symptomatology. One small study demonstrated improvement of most symptoms when patients were treated with cis-retinoic acid. Hematopoietic stem cell transplant remains the only potential cure for JCML, but cure rates do not appear to be as high as with the adult type of CML.

12. How does secondary polycythemia differ from primary polycythemia vera?

Secondary polycythemia is an increase in red blood cell (RBC) mass that results from an increase in the level of erythropoietin. This may be a reactive increase induced by tissue hypoxia or secretive from a tumor. Primary polycythemia vera is an idiopathic clonal expansion of erythroid progenitors whose proliferation is erythropoietin independent.

13. What are the clinical diagnostic criteria for Polycythemia vera?

*Diagnostic Criteria**

CATEGORY A	CATEGORY B
1. Increased RBC volume	Thrombocytosis (> 400 x 10^9/L)
2. Arterial O2 saturation ≥ 92%	Leukocytosis (> 12 x 10^9/L)
3. Splenomegaly	Increased leukocyte alkaline phosphatase
	Increased vitamin B_{12} (> 900 pg/mL)

*Diagnosis requires three from category A or numbers 1 and 2 from category A and any two from category B.

14. What is the most important process in diagnosing essential thrombocythemia?

To confirm a diagnosis of primary thrombocytosis, it is important to rule out other causes of secondary thrombocytosis. Essential thrombocythemia is a clonal myeloproliferative disorder that is quite rare in childhood; its diagnosis requires a very detailed work-up to evaluate other causes of thrombocytosis. This includes evaluation to exclude other myeloproliferative disorders, such as CML and polycythemia vera.

BIBLIOGRAPHY

1. Altman AJ: Chronic leukemias of childhood. In Pizzo PA, Poplack DG (eds): Principles and Practice of Pediatric Oncology. Philadelphia, Lippincott-Raven, 1997, pp 483–504.
2. Gale RP, Hehlmann R, Shang MJ et al: Survival with bone marrow transplantation versus hydroxyurea or interferon for chronic myelogenous leukemia. Blood 91:1810–1819, 1998.
3. Grier HE, Civin CI: Myeloid leukemias, myelodysplasia, and myeloproliferative diseases in children. In Nathan DG, Orkin SH (eds): Nathan and Oski's Hematology of Infancy and Childhood. Philadelphia, W.B. Saunders, 1998, pp 1286–1321.
4. Kelemen E, Masszi T, Remenyi P, et al: Reduction in the frequency of transplant-related complications in patients with chronic myeloid leukemia undergoing BMT preconditioned with a new, non-myeloblative drug combination. Bone Marrow Transplantaton 21:747–749, 1998.
5. Nichols GL, Raines MA, Vera JC, et al: Identification of CRKL as the constitutively phosphorylated 39-kd tyrosine phosphoprotein in chronic myelogenous leukemia cells. Blood 84:2912, 1994.

27. NON-HODGKIN'S LYMPHOMA IN CHILDREN AND ADOLESCENTS

Kiery A. Braithwaite, M.D., and Mitchell S. Cairo, M.D.

1. What is the incidence of childhood non-Hodgkin's lymphoma (NHL) in the United States?

Lymphomas comprise an estimated 12% of all childhood cancers, ranking third behind acute leukemias and brain neoplasms as the leading pediatric malignancies. Sixty percent of all childhood lymphomas are classified as NHL, representing a yearly incidence of 8% of all childhood cancers. This translates into an estimated 500 cases of childhood NHL annually.

2. Describe the demographic and geographic differences in the incidence of NHL.

Pediatric NHL occurs worldwide; however, there are significant geographic variations in its distribution and frequency. NHL represents 50% of all pediatric malignancies in equatorial Africa, secondary to the high occurrence of Burkitt's NHL. There is also an increased incidence of Burkitt's NHL in northeastern Brazil. On the other hand, NHL is relatively rare in Japan. Within the United States, childhood NHL occurs two to three times more often in male than in female patients; and caucasians have twice the incidence than that in African Americans. NHL's relative incidence increases throughout childhood, and it is unusual in children younger than five years.

There is also an increased prevalence of NHL, especially B cell lymphomas, in children with both inherited and/or acquired immunodeficiencies. In fact, NHL is the leading cause of malignancy in the immunocompromised pediatric patient. This includes patients with congenital immunodeficiencies, such as severe combined immune deficiency (SCID) and Wiskott-Aldrich syndrome (WAS), as well as secondary immunodeficiencies such as HIV/AIDS or immunosuppression following solid organ or allogeneic stem cell transplantation.

3. What are the major pathological subtypes of childhood NHL? Discuss some important morphological features of each.

- Small non–cleaved cell lymphoma: The small non–cleaved cell lymphomas constitute 40% of all pediatric NHLs in the United States. This group is divided into Burkitt's and non-Burkitt's based on the degree of pleomorphism. Small non–cleaved cell lymphomas have a mature B cell phenotype and express surface-bound monoclonal immunoglobulin as well as B cell–associated surface antigens. Morphologically, these lymphomas are composed of sheets of intermediate-size lymphoid cells with multiple nucleoli and a distinct rim of basophilic cytoplasm. A "starry sky" pattern is commonly described secondary to the scattering of reactive macrophages throughout the tumor. Small noncleaved cells are morphologically similar to those in acute lymphoblastic leukemia (ALL), and when greater than 25% bone marrow involvement exists, they are classified as ALL, L3 subtype, also called B cell ALL.
- Lymphoblastic lymphoma: Lymphoblastic lymphoma comprises 30% of the NHLs in children in the United States. Ninety-five percent of these tumors are derived from immature T cells and display the immunophenotype of differentiating cortical thymocytes. The tumor cells frequently express the enzyme terminal deoxytidyl transferase, which is involved in the generation of T and B cell receptor diversity. Morphological examination reveals small lymphoblasts with round or convoluted nuclei,

absent or inconspicuous nucleoli, and a rim of slightly basophilic cytoplasm. A starry sky pattern, as with small non–cleaved cell lymphomas, also may exist. Cytologically, these tumors are indistinguishable from ALL, and when greater than 25% bone marrow involvement exists, they are classified as ALL.

- Large cell lymphoma: This heterogeneous group of tumors, which phenotypically includes B cell, T cell and indeterminate neoplasms, comprises 20% of pediatric NHLs in the United States. The three phenotypes occur with equal frequency among pediatric patients. The B cell large cell lymphomas express mature B cell–associated surface antigens and have a variety of morphological appearances, including large noncleaved and cleaved cells as well as immunoblastic cells. The majority of the T cell and null cell types are classified as anaplastic large cell lymphomas (ALCLs). These anaplastic lymphomas express CD30 (Ki-1) and vary in morphology. A characteristic t(2;5)(p23;q35) translocation commonly noted in ALCL adjoins a nucleolar phosphoprotein gene (NPM1) with the ALK (anaplastic lymphoma kinase) tyrosine kinase gene.

4. Describe some of the classic clinical presentations for each pathological subtype of childhood NHL.

Small non–cleaved cell lymphomas vary in their mode of clinical presentation depending on their geographic origin: endemic versus sporadic. Children in Africa typically present with head and neck disease, including jaw, orbital, and paraspinal involvement. A painless jaw mass is the classic endemic presentation, especially in younger children. On the other hand, 80% of children in North America and Europe present with abdominal disease that is manifested by abdominal pain, nausea and vomiting and/or signs of bowel obstruction or intussusception. Symptoms may also be occasionally confused with appendicitis. Involvement of the bone marrow and central nervous system (CNS) is common in children with small non–cleaved cell lymphomas.

Pediatric lymphoblastic lymphomas typically manifest as mediastinal or intrathoracic tumors. The clinical presentation includes respiratory distress and signs and symptoms associated with the superior vena cava syndrome, such as swelling of the neck, face and arms. Tumors also may present as painless, nontender masses in the head and neck region, but abdominal involvement is rare. Spread to the CNS and bone marrow may occur but less frequently than in small non–cleaved cell lymphomas.

Large cell lymphomas in children can present in almost any anatomic location. B cell large cell lymphomas have a predilection for the abdomen and mediastinum and rarely involve the CNS or bone marrow. Anaplastic large cell lymphomas also manifest in the mediastinum, as well as involving the skin, lymph nodes, testes and bone.

5. What are some of the main differences between NHL in children and adults?

Adult NHL has traditionally been classified into low, intermediate or high grade based on clinical aggressiveness; however, this distinction is unwarranted in pediatrics, as 90% of NHLs in children are high grade. Conversely, low- and intermediate-grade tumors predominate in adults. This difference is thought to reflect maturational differences in the immune system. Similarly, the majority of pediatric NHLs are considered aggressive, compared with the indolent nature of adult lymphomas. Paradoxically, the more aggressive NHLs have a much higher sensitivity to chemotherapy, which translates into a better prognosis in children, compared with adults. This improved prognosis and sensitivity to chemotherapy is especially significant because the majority of children have locally advanced or metastatic disease at the time of diagnosis. Finally, an important clinical distinction is that adults present with lymph node disease, while children typically have extranodal disease.

6. List and discuss the three characteristic chromosomal translocations associated with Burkitt's lymphoma.

The three chromosomal translocations associated with Burkitt's lymphoma involve the *c-myc* proto-oncogene located on chromosome eight (8q24) and include t(8;14), (8;22) and (2;8). The myc-encoded protein is involved in cell cycle progression and as a result of these translocations is juxtaposed with one of the immunoglobulin constant region sequences. The t(8;14)(q24;q32) translocation is the most common, occurring in 80% of Burkitt's lymphomas, and places the *c-myc* gene adjacent to immunoglobulin heavy chain genes. Translocations t(8;22)(q24;q11) and t(2;8)(p11;q24) comprise the remaining 20% of Burkitt's lymphomas and involve the lambda and kappa light-chain genes, respectively.

7. Discuss the difference between endemic and sporadic Burkitt's lymphomas.

Endemic Burkitt's lymphoma is analogous to the African type of small non–cleaved cell lymphoma, while sporadic Burkitt's lymphona is the prevailing type in North America and Europe. Clinical and molecular differences are significant between the two varieties, although they are histologically indistinguishable. As mentioned previously, the endemic type presents classically in the head and neck, most commonly with a painless jaw mass, while sporadic Burkitt's has a predilection for the abdomen. Another significant distinction between endemic and sporadic varieties is the association with the Epstein-Barr virus. In endemic or African Burkitt's, there is a 95% presence of the virus, as compared with only a 15–20% correlation in the sporadic or North American type. Lastly, there is a disparity in the breakpoint region in the *c-myc* proto-oncogene between the types. In the endemic type, there is a common area of breakpoint rearrangements that occur on chromosome 8 upstream to the *c-myc* gene; in the sporadic type, the rearrangements occur within the *c-myc* gene itself.

8. Describe the most widely used staging systems for childhood NHL.

St. Jude's staging classification applies to all histological types of pediatric NHL. It accounts for the more classic presentations of childhood NHL and separates patients into two categories, limited-stage disease and more advanced disease. Limited-stage disease, stages I and II, is defined as one or two masses on one side of the diaphragm; more advanced disease, stages III and IV, includes disease on both sides of the diaphragm, extensive intrathoracic and/or intraabdominal disease and metastatic disease to the CNS and bone marrow.

St. Jude's Staging for Pediatric Non-Hodgkin's Lymphoma

STAGE	DESCRIPTION
I	A single tumor (extranodal) or single anatomic area (nodal), excluding the mediastinum or abdomen.
II	1) A single extranodal tumor with regional node involvement 2) Two or more nodal areas on the same side of the diaphragm 3) Two single extranodal tumors on the same side of the diaphragm, with or without regional node involvement 4) A primary gastrointestinal tract tumor grossly and completely excised, with or without associated mesenteric nodes only
III	1) Two single extranodal tumors on opposite sides of diaphragm 2) Two or more nodal areas on opposite sides of diaphragm 3) All of the primary intrathoracic tumors (mediastinal, pleural, thymic) 4) All extensive primary intra-abdominal disease 5) All paraspinal or epidural tumors, regardless of the other tumor site(s)
IV	Any of the above with initial CNS and/or bone marrow involvement (< 25% malignant cells)

*The FAB Classification System for Pediatric Non-Hodgkin's Lymphoma**

GROUP	DESCRIPTION
A	Completely resected stage I (St. Jude) or completely resected abdominal stage II (St. Jude)
B	All patients not eligible for group A or group C
C	Any CNS involvement, defined as any L3 blast, cranial nerve palsy or compression, intracerebral mass and/or parameningeal compression and bone marrow involvement, defined as ≥ 25% blasts

*The FAB (French, American and British) classification system was developed after the St. Jude's classification. This system sought to resolve some ambiguities in the St. Jude's system and to improve on the accuracy of staging.

9. What laboratory and radiographic studies are important in newly diagnosed patients with NHL?

Initial laboratory studies indicated in any child diagnosed with NHL include a complete blood count, serum electrolytes, lactic dehydrogenase, uric acid and HIV serology. Examination of the cerebrospinal fluid and bone marrow are essential to accurately determine the stage of disease. Bilateral bone marrow aspirations and biopsies are recommended to minimize the risk of missing disseminated disease and the possibility of erroneously underestimating the stage of disease. Radiographic assessment should include ultrasound, computed tomography (CT), magnetic resonance imaging and nuclear medicine studies such as gallium and positron-emission tomography scans. CT scans of the chest, abdomen and pelvis are routine; however, abdominal and pelvic ultrasound may sometimes be superior to CT, especially in younger children who have minimal retroperitoneal fat. Gallium scanning provides a thorough whole-body screen, especially in small non–cleaved cell lymphomas that readily absorb the isotype. Positron-emission tomography scans may be valuable for follow-up studies in NHL secondary to their ability to distinguish residual active tumor from fibrosis and necrosis.

10. Discuss the role of surgery in the diagnosis and treatment of childhood NHL.

Surgical biopsies are performed to establish a diagnosis of childhood NHL when other means, such as examination of the cerebrospinal, pleural and peritoneal fluid or the bone marrow, are not available. Complete or major resection of a childhood NHL tumor usually is not required; however, a few possible exceptions exist. First, complete resection is required in patients with stage I or group A disease. Second, if intensive chemotherapy is unavailable, such as in countries with limited resources, a total resection of an abdominal Burkitt's tumor may be curative. Third, surgical resection is occasionally performed if an emergency laparotomy is indicated for complications arising from the tumor mass, such as in patients with an intussusception or intestinal perforation. In the latter case, it is only appropriate if total resection is feasible without any major organ compromise. However, in the majority of cases, there is little role for surgery in the treatment of pediatric NHL.

11. What is the role of radiation therapy in the treatment of childhood NHL?

Radiation is rarely required in the treatment of pediatric NHL. Studies indicate that radiation, alone or combined with chemotherapy, provides no therapeutic advantage over present regimens of intensive, multiagent chemotherapy. Radiation is occasionally utilized in acute conditions, such as paraplegia secondary to spinal cord compression, and in patients who present acutely with the superior vena cava syndrome.

12. Why is rapid diagnosis and initiation of therapy important in childhood NHL?

Childhood lymphomas are extremely fast-growing neoplasms; for example, the potential doubling time in African or endemic Burkitt's lymphoma can range from 12 hours to a few days. Depending on the anatomic location of the tumor, this rapid growing time can result in severe symptoms due to sheer bulk, such as airway compromise secondary to tracheal compression. Similarly, abdominal tumors may precipitate an acute intestinal obstruction or perforation, and epidural masses can cause spinal cord compression and paraplegia. Lastly, any delay in diagnosis may worsen prognosis, secondary to the aggressive nature of childhood NHLs.

13. Discuss the prognosis of children diagnosed with NHL.

With the advent of multiagent chemotherapy in the past two decades, the prognosis for children with NHL has improved dramatically. Overall, there is a greater than 70% cure rate for all children diagnosed with NHL. Children with limited-stage disease have an excellent prognosis, with cure rates approaching 85–95%. Prognosis is generally poorer in patients who relapse, especially those who initially received intensive multiagent chemotherapy. A main determinant of prognosis on diagnosis is the tumor burden, which is reflected by clinical stage. Other predictive factors, such as lactic dehydrogenase (LDH), serum interleukin-2 receptor, uric acid, lactic acid and β_2-microglobulin, that are associated with tumor burden may additionally be indicative of prognosis.

14. Discuss the role of stem cell transplantation (SCT) in pediatric NHL.

There are limited data available on the utilization of autologous and allogeneic SCT in the management of children with newly diagnosed NHL. Small studies have shown promise, especially in children with relapsed disease. Autologous SCT coupled with intense chemotherapy has been effective in children with relapsed Burkitt's lymphoma or large-cell NHL. Allogeneic SCT may be considered for children with relapsed lymphoblastic lymphoma or Burkitt's lymphoma with bone marrow involvement.

15. What is the role of immunotherapy in childhood NHL?

Rituximab (IDEC-C2B8) is an anti-CD20 chimeric monoclonal antibody used to target the CD20 antigen expressed by B cell tumor cells. CD20 is an antigen expressed on the surface of both normal as well as malignant B cells. Rituximab has both specificity and affinity for the CD20 antigen and when bound induces complement-dependent cytotoxicity, antibody-dependent cytotoxicity and apoptosis. This depletes B cells from the peripheral blood, lymph nodes and bone marrow without affecting stem cells, which do not express CD20. Furthermore, it additionally sensitizes lymphoma cells to the cytotoxic effects of chemotherapy. Rituximab has proven to be well tolerated and efficacious in adult NHL clinical trials. Its efficacy has been extended to children in a recent study involving B cell lymphoma, as well as in children with post-transplant lymphoproliferative syndrome. Currently, Rituximab is being tested in a phase II study for children with newly diagnosed high-grade B cell leukemia and lymphoma.

16. Discuss the presentation, prognosis and treatment of ALCL.

This lymphoma represents a distinct entity, with more unique clinical features than the other subtypes of pediatric NHL. An estimated half of the pediatric large cell lymphomas are anaplastic, representing 10–15% of all childhood NHL cases. The anaplastic tumors are referred to as Ki-1+ due to their expression of CD30, which is recognized by Ki-1 monoclonal antibodies. Phenotypically, most are either T cell or null and consist morphologically of large, pleomorphic cells. As mentioned previously, they are additionally associated with the t(2;5)(p23;q35) translocation that is characteristic of, but not completely unique, to the anaplastic variety. This translocation results in an NPM-ALK oncoprotein. These tumors are quite diverse in clinical presentation and much less predictable than the other pediatric NHLs. They have a predilection for extranodal tissues, such as skin, bone, gastrointestinal tract, soft tissue and the thorax, as well as lymph nodes.

The prognosis for anaplastic large cell tumors is slightly poorer than in large B cell tumors. Patients with localized disease have a better prognosis compared with those having advanced disease, although two thirds of all pediatric cases are advanced at diagnosis. The increased occurrence of late relapse in these children reduces the long-term survival rate, compared with children with the other subtypes of pediatric NHLs. Traditionally, treatments include a variety of multiagent chemotherapies adopted from other lymphoma regimens, although at present, an optimal course of therapy has not been completely determined. Poorer prognostic factors that have been identified include skin involvement, mediastinal involvement, and any visceral involvement at diagnosis, as well as relapse.

BIBLIOGRAPHY

1. Brugières L, Deley MC, Pacquement H, et al: CD30(+) anaplastic large-cell lymphoma in children: Analysis of 82 patients enrolled in two consecutive studies of the French Society of Pediatric Oncology. Blood 92:3591–3598, 1998.
2. Cairo MS, Perkins S: Non-Hodgkin's lymphoma in children. In Bast RC Jr, Kufe DW, Polock RE, et al (eds): Cancer Medicine, 5th ed. London, B.C. Decker Inc, 2000, pp 2162–2167.
3. Coiffier B, Haioun C, Ketterer N, et al: Rituximab (anti-CD20 monoclonal antibody) for the treatment of patients with relapsing or refractory aggressive lymphoma: A multicenter phase II study. Blood 92: 1927–1932, 1998.
4. Faye A, Quartier P, Lutz P, et al: Anti-CD20 monoclonal antibody in the treatment of post-transplant lymphoproliferative disorders (PTLD) occurring after bone marrow transplantation (BMT) in children [abstract]. Blood 94:2842, 1999.
5. Jerusalem G, Beguin Y, Fassotte MF, et al: Whole-body positron emission tomography using 18F-fluorodeoxyglucose for posttreatment evaluation in Hodgkin's disease and non-Hodgkin's lymphoma has higher diagnostic and prognostic value than classical computed tomography scan imaging. Blood 94:429–433, 1999.
6. Link MP, Donaldson SS: The lymphomas and lymphadenopathy. In Nathan DG, Orkin SH (eds): Hematology of Infancy and Childhood. Vol. 5th ed. Philadelphia: W.B. Saunders, 1998, pp 1324–1339.
7. Press OW: Monoclonal antibody therapy for indolent non-Hodgkin's lymphoma. In The ASH Education Program Book, 1999. Published by the American Society of Hematology, Washington, DC, pp. 305–311.
8. Sandlund JT, Downing JR, Crist WM: Medical progress: Non-Hodgkin's lymphoma in childhood. N Eng J Med 334:1238–1248, 1996.
9. Shad A, Magrath I: Malignant non-Hodgkin's lymphomas in children. In Pizzo PA, Poplack DG (eds): Principles and Practice of Pediatric Oncology, 3rd ed. Philadelphia, Lippincott-Raven Publishers, 1997, pp 545–587.
10. Veerman AJP, Nuijens JH, Van der Schoot CE, et al: Rituximab in the treatment of childhood B-ALL and Burkitt's lymphoma. Report on three cases [abstract]. Blood 94:4414, 1999.

28. HODGKIN'S DISEASE IN CHILDREN AND ADOLESCENTS

Michael A. Weiner, M.D.

1. Briefly describe the incidence and epidemiology of Hodgkin's disease in children and adolescents.

There are approximately 1.5 cases of Hodgkin's disease diagnosed in children and adolescents per 100,000 population. A bimodal age distribution exists, with one peak during the second to third decade of life and a second peak during the fifth and sixth decades. Hodgkin's disease is more common in male than in female patients (2:1). It represents 5% of all childhood malignancies; thus, there are approximately 600 cases diagnosed each year in children and adolescents younger than 21 years.

2. What is the epidemiologic relationship between the Epstein-Barr virus (EBV) and Hodgkin's disease?

Epstein-Barr virus has been linked to Hodgkin's disease by epidemiologic and serologic studies. Molecular techniques such as in situ hybridization and the polymerase chain reaction have demonstrated EBV genome products within Sternberg-Reed cells (SRCs) and Hodgkin's cells. The presence of EBV fragments is most prevalent in patients with the mixed cellularity subtype and unusual in patients with lymphocyte-predominant subtypes.

3. What is the SRC, and what is its cell of origin?

The SRC is a multi-nucleated giant cell that is surrounded by benign-appearing inflammatory cells such as lymphocytes, eosinophils, histiocytes and granulocytes. The SRC originates from "B lineage" lymphocytes that arise in the germinal center of an affected lymph node. Immunophenotypically, the SRC is likely to be CD15 (Leu M1) and CD30 (Ki-1/Ber H2) positive.

4. Describe the histopathologic classification of Hodgkin's disease.

The Rye modification of the Lukes-Butler histopathologic classification of Hodgkin's disease has been utilized for more than 30 years. It includes four subtypes: nodular sclerosis, mixed cellularity, lymphocyte predominance and lymphocyte depleted. Recently, a panel of experts suggested another classification system, the Revised European-American Classification (REAL) system, which suggests two categories, classic Hodgkin's disease and lymphocyte predominance. The following table compares the two classification systems:

Comparison of REAL and RYE Classification Systems of Hodgkin's Disease

REAL	RYE
Lymphocyte predominance, nodular, ± diffuse	Lymphocyte predominance
Classic	
Lymphocyte rich	Nodular sclerosis
Nodular sclerosis	Mixed cellularity
Mixed cellularity	Lymphocyte depleted

Modified from DeVita VT Jr, et al: Hodgkin's disease. In Devita VT Jr., Hellman S, Rosenberg SA (eds): Cancer Principles and Practice of Oncology. Philadelphia, Lippincott-Raven, 1997, pp 2242–2283.

5. Describe the common presenting signs and symptoms of patients with Hodgkin's disease.

SIGNS AND SYMPTOMS	PERCENTAGE OF PATIENTS
Lymphadenopathy	90
Mediastinal mass	60
"B" symptoms	30
Fever > 101[5]	
> 10% weight loss	
Night sweats	
Hepatosplenomegaly	25

6. What is the frequency of initial sites of involvement in children with Hodgkin's disease?

SITE	PERCENTAGE
Cervical, supraclavicular	75
Mediastinum	60
Spleen	25
Axilla	24
Pulmonary hilum	24
Para-aortic, celiac, splenic hilum	22
Lung	15
Iliac	7
Bone marrow	5
Bone	2
Liver	2

7. Describe the common laboratory features at the time of diagnosis in children and adolescents with Hodgkin's disease.

Hematologically, many patients with Hodgkin's disease present with a mild normochromic, normocytic anemia. Approximately 15–20% of patients manifest mild to moderate eosinophilia. Biochemically, most patients demonstrate heightened acute-phase reactants, such as an elevated erythrocyte sedimentation rate, serum copper, serum ferritin, fibrinogen, serum alkaline phosphatase and β^2-macroglobulin.

8. Hodgkin's cells and SRCs manufacture proteins referred to as cytokines that may be responsible for the signs and symptoms of patients with Hodgkin's disease. Enumerate the cytokines produced and their clinical and biologic manifestations.

CYTOKINES PRODUCED BY RSC	CLINICAL AND BIOLOGIC FEATURES
Interleukin 1 (IL-1)	Lymphoproliferation, fever, night sweats
IL-2	T-cell immunodeficiency
IL-5	Eosinophilic infiltration
IL-6	Thrombocytosis
IL-9	Lymphoproliferation
Tumor necrosis factor (α and β)	Weight loss
Granulocyte colony–stimulating factor	Myeloproliferation
Transforming growth factor β	Lymph node fibrosis

9. Describe the diagnostic evaluation of a newly diagnosed patient with Hodgkin's disease.

1. Physical examination
2. Blood work: complete blood count, serum chemistries, liver function studies, LDH, erythrocyte sedimentation rate, serum copper, serum ferritin, serum immunoglobulins

3. EBV serology
4. Chest radiograph
5. Computed tomography of the neck, chest, abdomen, pelvis
6. Radionuclide ^{67}gallium citrate scan including single photon emission computed tomography
7. The following tests are optional and/or indicated in certain circumstances: bone marrow aspirate and biopsy, ^{99}technetium bone scan, magnetic resonance imaging positron emission tomography scans, staging laparotomy
8. Baseline assessment of the following systems:
   - Cardiac (echocardiogram, electrocardiogram)
   - Pulmonary function tests
   - Thyroid function tests
   - Lutenizing hormonc, follicle-stimulating hormone

10. What is a staging laparotomy, and what are the indications for surgical staging?

A staging laparotomy is a procedure designed to assess the presence of Hodgkin's disease below the diaphragm. Radiographic staging techniques may fail to detect occult disease of the abdomen and pelvis in as many as 30% of patients; thus, the staging laparotomy is performed to identify disease in these patients. The procedure involves multiple lymph node biopsies (para-aortic, mesenteric, celiac, porta hepatis, pancreatic, splenic hilum, inguinal); liver biopsy, needle and wedge, from both lobes; bilateral bone marrow biopsies; and midline transposition of the ovaries in female patients.

Patients who require a staging laparotomy include those with early-stage clinical disease who are not candidates for chemotherapy and who receive involved field radiation therapy alone as their primary treatment modality.

11. Describe the "Ann Arbor" staging classification and subclassification for patients with Hodgkin's disease.

- Stage I: Involvement of a single lymph node region
- Stage II: Involvement of two or more lymph node regions on the same side of the diaphragm
- Stage III: Involvement of lymph node regions on both sides of the diaphragm
- Stage IV: Diffuse or disseminated involvement of extra-lymphatic sites (e.g., lung, liver, bone, bone marrow)
- A: Denotes no specific symptoms
- B: Denotes specific symptoms
  1. Unexplained weight loss of > 10% of premorbid weight
  2. Unexplained recurrent fever > 101[5]
  3. Unexplained night sweats

12. Describe the prognostic factors that predict outcome in children and adolescents with Hodgkin's disease.

FACTOR	FAVORABLE	UNFAVORABLE
Stage	I, II	III, IV
"B" symptoms	(-)	(+)
Mediastinal to thoracic ratio	< 1/3	> 1/3
Bulk disease (> 6 cm)	(-)	(+)
ESR (mm/hour)	< 50	> 50
Response to initial therapy	Rapid complete response	Delayed complete response

13. Describe the treatment modalities employed for children and adolescents with Hodgkin's disease.

Appropriate treatment for patients with Hodgkin's disease depends on the stage of disease, presence or absence of "B" symptoms, assessment of bulk disease and gender. Therapy may be chemotherapy, radiotherapy, or combined modality therapy. Numerous multiagent chemotherapy regimens have been reported to be effective; the number of cycles of chemotherapy depends on the prognostic group of the patient at the time of diagnosis. Radiotherapy should be delivered utilizing megavoltage irradiation with a 4–8 MeV linear accelerator. Fields of radiotherapy are defined as involved field, extended field, or total lymph node irradiation. Dosages of radiotherapy may be either low dose (2100–2500 cGy) or standard dose (3500–4400) cGy).

14. Describe a therapeutic approach for Hodgkin's disease patients with favorable and unfavorable prognostic characteristics.

Clinical trials are in progress for patients with both early-stage and advanced-stage Hodgkin's disease that employ a reduced number of dose-intensified chemotherapy cycles administered over a compressed interval of time. The number of cycles of chemotherapy may be individually tailored predicated on the response to initial chemotherapy. Male patients with favorable, early-stage disease should receive DBVE (doxorubicin, bleomycin, vincristine, etoposide) for two to four cycles followed by low-dose involved-field radiotherapy; female patients may receive four to six cycles of chemotherapy without radiotherapy. Male patients with unfavorable, advanced-stage disease should receive four cycles of BEACOPP (bleomycin, etoposide, doxorubicin, cyclophosphamide, vincristine, procarbazine, prednisone) plus two cycles of ABV (doxorubicin, bleomycin, vinblastine), followed by low dose involved-field radiotherapy. Female patients with unfavorable, advanced-stage disease should receive four cycles of BEACOPP plus four cycles of alternating COPP (cyclophosphamide, vincristine, procarbazine, prednisone) and ABV without radiotherapy.

15. Utilizing contemporary therapeutic modalities, what are the expected event-free survival (EFS) and overall survival (OS) rates for children and adolescents with Hodgkin's disease?

For patients with favorable prognostic factors and early-stage disease, the predicted EFS is between 85% and 90% at 5 years, and the OS approaches 95%. Patients with unfavorable variables and advanced disease have an EFS and OS of 80–85% and 90%, respectively.

16. Describe the management of children and adolescents with relapsed/recurrent Hodgkin's disease.

Most relapses in patients with Hodgkin's disease occur within the first 3 years from the original diagnosis; however, late relapses up to 10 years from initial diagnosis have been reported. Prognosis after relapse is dependent on several factors: first, the time from completion of treatment to recurrence; second, the site of relapse (nodal vs. extra-nodal); third, the prescence of systemic "B" symptoms at relapse. Patients who relapse beyond 1 year from completion of therapy and who have an asymptomatic nodal recurrence have the best outcome with re-treatment. Numerous conventional salvage regimens exist, and if radiotherapy may be safely added, it may improve long-term survival up to 60–70%. Patients who relapse within 1 year from the completion of initial therapy and who have "B" symptoms or extra-nodal disease have a poor prognosis. They require dose-intensive reinduction with ICE (ifosfamide, cisplatin, etoposide), followed by ablative chemotherapy, an autologous peripheral blood stem cell transplant and radiotherapy, if feasible. Long-term survival in this subset of patients is between 40% and 50%.

17. Describe the potential complications of therapy in survivors of Hodgkin's disease.

ORGAN	ETIOLOGY/CAUSE	COMPLICATION
Pulmonary	Bleomycin, radiotherapy	Pneumonitis, abnormal pulmonary function tests
Cardiac	Doxorubicin (anthracyclines), radiotherapy	Cardiomyopathy, arrhythmias
Gonadal function	Cyclophosphamide (alkylating agents), radiotherapy	Infertility in male patients, amenorrhea in female patients
Thyroid	Radiotherapy	Hypothyroidism

18. What is the risk of developing a second malignant neoplasm (SMN) in children and adolescents who survive Hodgkin's disease?

The development of SMNs in survivors of Hodgkin's disease is a major concern to patients, families and health care professionals. The overall risk of developing a SMN is approximately 2% at 5 years from the completion of treatment, 5% at 10 years, and 9% at 15 years. The incidence of a secondary leukemia or non-Hodgkin's lymphoma is 1–3%. With respect to solid tumors the risk is 0.4%, 2% and 6% at 5 years, 10 years and 15 years respectively. There appears to be a singularly heightened incidence of breast cancer in young women who have received standard dose radiotherapy (3500–4400 cGy) to their mediastinum/chest; the incidence increases with time and may approach 20% at 20–25 years from the time of treatment.

The risk of SMNs is greatest in patients who have received combined modality therapy including alkylator chemotherapy agents such as cyclophosphamide, procarbazine and nitrogen mustard as their initial therapy. In addition, patients who relapse and subsequently receive high dose–intensive regimens have an increased risk of second cancers. Today, as we enter the new millennium, contemporary therapeutic regimens attempt not only to maintain the high cure rate for patients treated for Hodgkin's disease, but also to devise treatment plans that will reduce the incidence of therapy-related complications in general and SMN in particular.

BIBLIOGRAPHY

1. Bhatia S, Robison LL, Oberline O, et al: Breast cancer and other second neoplasms after childhood Hodgkin's disease. N Engl J Med 334:754–751, 1996.
2. Chauvenet A, Schwartz CL, Weiner MA: Hodgkin's disease in children and adolescents. In Holland JF, Frei E, Bast RC, et al (eds): Cancer Medicine, 5th ed. Ontario, Canada, B.C. Decker Inc, 2000.
3. Constine LZ, Quazi R, Rubin: Malignant lymphomas. In Rubin P, McDonald S, Quazi R (eds): Clinical Oncology:A Multidisciplinary Approach for Physicians and Students. Philadelphia, W.B. Saunders, 1993, pp 217–250.
4. DeVita VT Jr, Mauch PM, Harris NL: Hodgkin's disease. In DeVita VT Jr, Hellman S, Rosenberg SA (eds): Cancer Principles and Practice of Oncology. Philadelphia, Lippincott-Raven, 1997, pp 2242–2243.
5. Glanzmann C, Kaufman P, Jenni R, et al: Cardiac risk after mediastinal irradiation for Hodgkin's disease. Radiother Oncol 46:51–62, 1998.
6. Harris NL: Hodgkin's disease: Classification and differential diagnosis. Mod Pathol 12:159–175, 1999.
7. Ilhan I, Sarialioglu F, Bilgic H, et al: Long-term pulmonary function in children with Hodgkin's disease. Acta Paediat 85: 324–326, 1996.
8. Lukes RJ, Butler JJ: The pathology and nomenclature of Hodgkin's disease. Cancer Res 26: 1063–1083, 1966.
9. Mackie EJ, Radford M, Shalet SM: Gonadal function following chemotherapy for childhood Hodgkin's disease. Med Pediatr Oncol 27:74–78, 1996.
10. Mauch PM, Weinstein H, Botnick L, et al: An evaluation of long-term survival and treatment complications in children with Hodgkin's disease. Cancer 51:925–932, 1988.
11. Schellong G: Pediatric Hodgkin's disease: Treatment in the late 1990's. Ann Oncol 5(suppl): 115–119,1998.

29. LYMPHOPROLIFERATIVE DISORDERS

Manuela Orjuela, M.D., Sc.M.

1. What infectious agent plays a central role in the development of most lymphoproliferative diseases and why?

Epstein-Barr virus (EBV), a ubiquitous human herpesvirus transmitted primarily via saliva, is causally involved in most lymphoproliferative disease. Initial infection with EBV occurs during childhood but persists as a latent infection throughout life. EBV colonizes antibody-producing (B) cells and thus evades recognition and destruction by cytotoxic T cells. EBV infection is largely controlled by memory cytotoxic T cells (EBV-CTL) and remains an asymptomatic infection in B cells. EBV carries a set of latent genes that induce cellular proliferation when expressed in resting B cells. This cell proliferation when unregulated or accompanied by additional genetic events can lead to malignant transformation.

EBV infection in patients with compromised T cell immunity following transplantation leads to the development of post-transplant lymphoproliferative disease (PTLD) (see question 2). Other DNA viruses such as human immunodeficiency virus (HIV) (HTLVIII), human herpes virus 8 (HHV8, also known as Kaposi's sarcoma–associated virus), cytomegalovirus (CMV), and hepatitis C virus have also been associated with the development of lymphoproliferative diseases.

2. How does PTLD present clinically?

PTLD comprises a diverse spectrum of symptoms, including isolated adenopathy, hepatitis, lymphoid interstitial pneumonitis, meningo-encephalitis, an infectious mononucleosis-like syndrome or a septic shock–like presentation. Although PTLD can arise after any organ transplant, the cells of origin in patients who have undergone a bone marrow transplant are usually donor cells, while in patients who have undergone solid organ transplants (SOT), PTLD arises in cells that are of host origin. However, clinical manifestations do not appear to differ by cell of origin.

PTLD appears to arise as a defective response to a viral infection, most commonly EBV. This defective response is due in part to immune dysregulation, stemming from an absence of EBV-specific cytotoxic T cells (EBV-CTL). This inability to clear EBV-infected B cells leads to B cell proliferation with the potential for malignant transformation.

3. What histologic and genetic changes are described in PTLD?

The histologic presentation of PTLD ranges from benign hyperplasia with polymorphic cellular infiltration (with EBV-positive Reed-Sternberg–like cells) to lesions with monomorphic, lymphoblastic cell populations. These lesions can be polyclonal, oligoclonal or monoclonal, even within different lesions in the same patient. Though PTLD may appear histologically identical to non-Hodgkin's lymphoma (NHL) or even Hodgkin's disease (HD), it is genetically distinct. The EBV gene expression in PTLD is like that seen in EBV-positive large cell lymphoma, not Burkitt's lymphoma or HD. Cytogenetic abnormalities commonly found in Burkitt's or HD, such as those involving *c-myc, N-, H-* and *K-ras, p53, bcl-2*, and *bcl-6* are rare in PTLD.

4. Describe the period after transplant associated with the highest incidence of occurrence of PTLD.

Incidence of PTLD occurs primarily during the first 6 months after transplantation, coinciding with the period of greatest immunosuppression. More than 90% of early (<6 months after transplant) cases of PTLD are EBV positive, when EBV CTL immunity is lowest. PTLD at this stage is more often polymorphic and often responds to decreased immunosuppression without additional therapy. A second peak in incidence of PTLD occurs 2 yr after transplant. These cases of PTLD are frequently EBV negative, can be of T cell origin, require more aggressive therapy, and have a much poorer prognosis. These late PTLD may be a different disease and appear more akin to lymphoproliferative disorders observed in other immunodeficient states (e.g., acquired immunodeficiency syndrome and primary immunodeficiencies) which are not always of B cell origin or associated with EBV.

5. How frequent is PTLD and what factors increase the likelihood of developing the disorder after SOT?

In 1998, there were estimated to be more than 400 new cases of PTLD following SOT in the United States, and about 100 cases in children and adolescents. Risk factors for developing PTLD in SOT recipients include: type of organ transplanted (1–5% in renal, heart and liver transplants; 10–30% in lung, small bowel and multiple organ grafts), frequency of rejection episodes requiring intensified immunosuppression (especially the use of T cell antibody therapy), EBV seronegativity at time of transplant and younger age of recipients (especially < 5 yr of age, at which time children are more likely to be EBV seronegative in industrialized countries).

6. Describe how PTLD is treated.

Treatment of PTLD requires controlling the EBV-induced B cell proliferation and facilitating the development of an appropriate EBV-CTL response. The initial step for treating PTLD is reduction of immunosuppression to enhance alloreactive T cell immunity and thus the development of EBV-specific CTLs. However this increases the risk of organ rejection and graft loss. Decreased immunosuppression can be sufficient for controlling PTLD, especially when localized or polyclonal. Anti-viral agents (acyclovir or ganciclovir), and/or intravenous immunoglobulin have also been used as initial therapy and may be useful in prophylaxis or delaying primary EBV infection or reactivation. Surgery can be used to cure disease only when it is localized. Chemotherapy (modified NHL regimens) has been used in patients who fail reduction of immune suppression by not resolving the PTLD and/or developing rejection. More recently, anti–B cell monoclonal antibodies have also been used to treat PTLD to decrease B cell proliferation. Adoptive T cell therapy (i.e., donor leukocyte infusion), has also been used in an attempt to boost CTL activity. In BMT, donor leukocytes from the marrow donor can be used; however, in solid organ transplant, the donors are often no longer available. In addition, the lymphocyte proliferation occurs in host, not donor cells, so the immunologic recognition, specificity and efficacy of donor leukocytes are uncertain. One alternative for SOT has been to give patients EBV-CTLs, which are generated ex-vivo; however, because these take several weeks to generate, this can only be used as a second line of therapy.

7. What is X-linked lymphoproliferative syndrome (XLP)?

X-linked lymphoproliferative syndrome (XLP) is a familial disorder affecting males characterized by a rapidly fatal course following infection with EBV. XLP is clinically characterized by three major phenotypes: fulminant infectious mononucleosis (seen in 50% of pediatric patients with XLP), B cell lymphomas (20%) and dys-gammaglobulinemia (30%). Additionally, aplastic anemia, vasculitis and pulmonary lymphomatoid granulomatosis are often associated with the syndrome. The B cell lymphomas associated with XLP are usually extra-nodal non-Hodgkin's lymphomas (primarily Burkitt's) and frequently involve the intestines, especially the ileo-cecal region. Mortality for patients with XLP is 80% by the age of 10 yr, and 100% by 40 yr. Death occurs as a result of uncontrolled lymphocyte proliferation with organ infiltration and T cell cytotoxic activity leading to multiorgan failure.

8. Discuss the genetic defect and associated immunologic manifestations responsible for the clinical picture of XLP.

DSHP, also known as SH2D1A, or SLAM (signaling lymphocytic activation molecule)–associated protein, is mutated in XLP, a sex-linked inherited immunodeficiency. DSHP is expressed primarily in T and natural killer (NK) cells. Defects in both T and NK cells have been reported. Some cases present with a decreased population of NK cells or with NK cells that have lost the ability to lyse their target cells. Patients with XLP also have an increased cytotoxic T cell response to EBV-infected B cells. XLP patients with fulminant infectious mononucleosis appear to have abnormal T and B cell proliferation in response to EBV-induced lymphoblasts. The resultant polyclonal T and B cell proliferation infiltrates many organs, leading to fulminant hepatitis and bone marrow failure. The cellular mechanisms that lead to the B cell expansion are not understood. Dysgammaglobinemia and B cell lymphomas have been detected in XLP patients after an EBV infection, but they have also been observed in XLP patients who are EBV seronegative and/or have negative polymerase chain reaction results for EBV genes. XLP appears to be an immunodeficiency that is manifested progressively after viral infections but which can be accelerated clinically by EBV in the case of the fulminant infectious mononucleosis.

9. Describe how Castleman's disease presents.

Castleman's disease (angiofollicular lymphoid or giant lymph node hyperplasia) is a rare polyclonal lymphoproliferative disorder that can be found in both nodal and extranodal sites. It is characterized by faulty immunoregulation mediated by interleukin-6 overexpression that results in excessive proliferation of B lymphocytes and plasma cells in lymphoid organs. There are two distinct histopathological variants with different clinical characteristics: the hyaline vascular type and the plasma cell variant. The hyaline vascular type usually presents as a solitary mass in the mediastinum or retroperitoneum and is frequently curable by surgical resection. The rarer plasma cell variant often presents with generalized lymphadenopathy, B symptoms and immunological abnormalities and is also known as multicentric Castleman's disease (MCD). Patients with MCD have an increased risk for developing Kaposi's sarcoma and B cell lymphomas .

10. Which herpesvirus has been causally associated with Castleman's disease?

HHV-8 also called Kaposi's sarcoma–associated herpesvirus, infects lymphoid cells in MCD. Its transmission is thought to occur primarily via saliva. Infection by HHV8, unlike most other herpesviruses, is not ubiquitous. HHV8 was first reported in MCD biopsies from HIV-seropositive French patients with MCD. These included patients with plasma cell, hyaline vascular and mixed variants, as well as among HIV-seronegative cases. HIV-seronegative patients who are infected with HHV8 tend to experience a worse clinical prognosis and frequently develop autoimmune hemolytic anemia and polyclonal gammopathies.

In MCD, HHV8 is present in cells belonging to the B cell lineage, including a subset that have a centroblastic/immunoblastic morphology (so-called plasmablasts) that is not present in HHV8-negative MCD. HHV8-positive MCD is considered a plasmablastic variant of MCD. In MCD, both lytic and latent HHV-8 antigens are produced by lymphoid cells. Both vascular endothelial and lymphoid cells proliferate in response to the viral infection. Infected endothelial cells in MCD may be the reservoir for HHV-8.

11. What retroviruses can precipitate lymphoproliferative disorders and how do these lymphoproliferative disorders manifest themselves?

The retroviruses HTLV1 and HIV are both tropic for CD4 helper T cells. Children and adolescents infected with these viruses can manifest lymphoproliferative disease. Patients infected with HIV characteristically develop generalized adenopathy. Non-Hodgkin's lymphoma can develop after prolonged (>6 month) periods of CD4 cell depletion. This risk is particularly elevated for Burkitt's lymphoma (unusual in other immunocompromised patients), primary brain lymphoma (diagnosed as early as infancy) and immunoblastic lymphoma.

The primary mode of transmission of HTLV1 to children is through infected breast milk. Children infected early in life are at risk for developing acute T cell lymphoblastic leukemia, an aggressive lymphoproliferative disorder. Although the disease can occur in HTLV1-infected individuals during childhood, the mean age for onset of clinical symptoms is 20–30 yr after infection.

BIBLIOGRAPHY

1. Boshoff C, Chang Y: Kaposi's sarcoma–associated herpesvirus: A new DNA tumor virus. Ann Rev Med 52:453–470, 2001.
2. Crawford DH: Biology and disease associations of Epstein-Barr virus. Philos Trans R Soc Lond B Biol Sci 356(1408):461–473, 2001.
3. Gross TG: Treatment of Epstein-Barr virus–associated post-transplant lymphoproliferative disorders. J Pediatr Hematol Oncol 23(1):7–9, 2001.
4. Morra M, Howie D, Grande MS, et al: X-linked lymphoproliferative disease: A progressive immunodeficiency. Ann Rev Immunol 19:657–682, 2001.
5. Nichols KE: X-linked lymphoproliferative disease: Genetics and biochemistry. Rev Immunogenet 2(2): 256–266, 2000.

30. LANGERHANS CELL HISTIOCYTOSIS

Kara M. Kelly, M.D.

1. What was the former name for Langerhans cell histiocytosis (LCH) and what was its significance?

The term *histiocytosis X* was proposed in 1953, with "X" standing for unknown, to represent the lack of understanding of the disorder. With the recognition that the disorder is a proliferation of abnormal Langerhans cells, the term *Langerhans cell histiocytosis* was chosen to replace histiocytosis X as well as the syndromes eosinophilic granuloma, Hand-Schüller-Christian disease and Letterer-Siwe disease. The clinical spectrum of LCH is wide so that the prognosis relates to the extent of disease. Single system disease, affecting the bones, skin or lymph nodes, has a favorable prognosis, whereas multisystem disease, particularly involving the liver or bone marrow, has an unfavorable prognosis.

2. What is the cause of LCH?

The etiology is unknown. It is considered to be a reactive disorder, although clonal expansion of Langerhans cells is observed. An exaggerated activation of cytokines or loss of control of cytokine activation may be involved in the pathogenesis. An abnormal immune response to a viral infection has been postulated, but research has not supported this hypothesis to date.

3. What is the typical clinical presentation of single system disease?

Single system disease tends to occur in the older child. It is usually confined to bone and may involve multiple sites. The skull is most often affected. Pain or lumps are the most common symptoms, and pathologic fracture may occur in weight-bearing bones. Skin involvement is noted in approximately one third of children with LCH. The classic lesion is an erythematous papule that may ulcerate or depigment and resolve. Lymph node involvement occurs in < 10% of children.

4. Describe the typical presentation of multisystem disease.

The aggressive presentation of multisystem disease is usually seen in children younger than 2 yr. The presentation is often similar to an acute leukemia, with evidence of bone marrow suppression, massive hepatosplenomegaly and constitutional symptoms. Organ dysfunction is hypothesized to develop as a result of excessive cytokine production by the abnormal Langerhans cells and subsequent fibrosis. Involvement of lungs may be manifested by respiratory distress with tachypnea, retractions, and persistent cough. Chronic respiratory failure may ensue as a result of widespread cyst and bullae formation. Rupture of a bullous lesion may lead to pneumothorax. Involvement of the skin, bones and lymph nodes usually coexists with a presentation similar to single system disease. Gingival disease will be marked by early loss of deciduous teeth and hypertrophy of the gums. Auditory canal involvement is manifested by persistent ear drainage, which is nonresponsive to antibiotic therapy. Both the small and large colon may be infiltrated with abnormal Langerhans cells, resulting in failure to thrive, hematochezia and stools streaked with mucus.

5. What is the most frequent endocrinopathy in LCH?

Diabetes insipidus, which may occur either before the diagnosis of LCH is established, concurrently with the diagnosis or subsequent to the development of the disease in other sites, especially in association with bone lesions of the skull.

6. What feature must be observed to make a definitive pathologic diagnosis of LCH?

The diagnosis of LCH is confirmed by either the demonstration of Birbeck granules in the cytoplasm of the Langerhans cells by electron microscopy or staining positive for CD1a antigen on the lesional cell.

7. Discuss the therapeutic options for single system disease.

Bone lesions of the skull, spine and long bones may remit spontaneously, so observation alone may be warranted if the lesions are nontender and not cosmetically deforming. Surgical curettage with or without local injection of corticosteroids is often effective in obtaining a complete response. In areas inaccessible to surgery or in places that might compromise vital structures such as the spinal cord, optic nerve or sella turcica, treatment with low-dose radiation is usually effective. Multiple bone or lymph node lesions may resolve with a short course of systemic therapy, using corticosteroids in conjunction with oral methotrexate or intravenous vinblastine, or other agents. Skin lesions may occasionally respond to topical or systemic corticosteroids. Topical nitrogen mustard has been effective for refractory cases.

8. What are the therapeutic options for multisystem disease?

Multiagent chemotherapy is most often used, typically with regimens containing etoposide, vinblastine and corticosteroids. The purine analogue 2-chlorodeoxyadenosine has demonstrated efficacy in some refractory patients. Immunosuppressive therapy with cyclosporin A or antithymocyte globulin has been tried in poor responders with mixed results. Immunomodulation with thalidomide has resulted in some objective responses in adults with LCH. Allogeneic bone marrow transplantation following myeloablative conditioning is being evaluated for very high risk patients.

9. Discuss the most important prognostic factors.

Without treatment, LCH may resolve spontaneously or disseminate, causing organ dysfunction, leading to chronic problems and possibly death. There have been a few studies that have identified prognostic factors to better guide therapy. In a review of 83 patients treated with chemotherapy by the Children's Cancer Study Group, organ dysfunction (i.e., involvement of the bone marrow, liver or lungs) was an important adverse factor. In a retrospective study of 155 children by the Southwest Oncology Group, organ dysfunction and age younger than 2 yr were important risk factors. More recent studies, the Austrian-German DAL-HX 83/90 and the LCH-1 trial, have determined that response to initial therapy can be used to identify patients most at risk for death.

10. What are potential late sequelae from LCH?

Inactive lesions may have late sequelae that significantly impact the quality of life of survivors of LCH. The risk for development of these complications must be considered in the planning of initial therapy. These late effects of the disease include:

- Orthopedic problems
- Short stature
- Poor dentition
- Deafness
- Diabetes insipidus
- Pulmonary fibrosis
- Hepatic cirrhosis

BIBLIOGRAPHY

1. Arico M, Egeler RM: Clinical aspects of Langerhans cell histiocytosis. Hematol Oncol Clin North Am 12:247–258, 1998.
2. Broadbent V, Egeler RM, Nesbit ME Jr: Langerhans cell histiocytosis—clinical and epidemiological aspects. Br J Cancer 70:S11–S16, 1994.
3. Egeler RM, D'Angio GJ: Langerhans cell histiocytosis. J Pediatr 127:1–11, 1995.
4. Gadner H, Heitger A, Grois N, et al: Treatment strategy for disseminated Langerhans cell histiocytosis. Med Pediatr Oncol 23:72–80, 1994.
5. Howarth DM, Gilchrist GS, Mullan BP, et al: Langerhans cell histiocytosis: Diagnosis, natural history, management and outcome. Cancer 85:2278–2290, 1999.
6. Kelly KM, Friedman DF: The histiocytosis syndromes. In Burg FD, Wald ER, Ingelfinger JR, Polin RA (eds): Gellis & Kagan's Current Pediatric Therapy, 16th ed. Philadelphia, W.B. Saunders, 1999, pp 1129–1131.

31. TUMORS OF THE CENTRAL NERVOUS SYSTEM

James H. Garvin, Jr. M.D., Ph.D.

1. How common are childhood brain tumors?

Approximately 2200 cases of central nervous system (CNS) tumors are diagnosed each year in the United States in children from birth to age 19 years, an incidence of 2.8 per 100,000. Brain tumors account for one fifth of all childhood cancers, second only to leukemia and about equal to acute lymphoblastic leukemia (the most common type of childhood leukemia).

2. What is the peak age group for childhood brain tumors? Give the usual location and histology and the current survival rate.

The peak age for childhood brain tumors is 3–7 years. Unlike adults and older children, who have primarily cerebral hemispheric tumors, young children most often have infratentorial tumors (brain stem, cerebellum) or occasionally tumors in midline supratentorial locations (optic chiasm, suprasellar region, pineal). About half of childhood brain tumors are supratentorial or cerebellar astrocytomas; next most common are medulloblastomas and brain stem tumors. Five-year survival is about 65% overall, highest for cerebellar astrocytomas but considerably lower for high-grade astrocytomas and especially brain stem tumors.

Location and Frequency of Pediatric Brain Tumors

Hemispheric
- Low-grade astrocytoma: 23%
- High-grade astrocytoma: 11%
- Other CNS tumors: 3%

Midline
- Chiasmal gliomas: 4%
- Craniopharyngiomas: 8%
- Pineal region tumors: 2%

Posterior Fossa
- Brain-stem gliomas: 15%
- Medulloblastomas: 15%
- Ependymomas: 4%
- Cerebellar astrocytomas: 15%

3. Why is the incidence of childhood brain tumors increasing?

The incidence of childhood brain tumors in the United States increased by 35% between 1973 and 1994, due mainly to increased numbers of supratentorial low-grade gliomas and brain stem gliomas diagnosed annually starting in the mid-1980s. Although there has been concern that this could be due to new environmental or dietary exposures, the most likely reason is increased diagnostic capability with the introduction of magnetic resonance imaging (MRI) in the mid-1980s. Evidence for any increased risk associated with specific exposures such as to electromagnetic fields or N-nitroso compounds in food, remains inconclusive.

4. You are asked to see a child because of headache and vomiting. What additional findings might raise suspicion for the presence of a brain tumor?

Persistent vomiting, morning headache, diplopia, neurologic abnormalities (ataxia, head tilt, vision loss, papilledema), endocrine disturbance (growth deceleration, diabetes insipidus) and stigmata of neurofibromatosis should all prompt further evaluation for the presence of a CNS tumor. In infants, symptoms may be nonspecific but can include irritability, loss of appetite and developmental delay or regression. Tumor location will determine symptoms. Supratentorial tumors primarily cause headache, motor weakness, sensory loss, seizures, and/or deterioration in school performance. Infratentorial tumors typically present with headache, vomiting, diplopia and gait imbalance.

5. Is a child's risk of a brain tumor increased if a parent or sibling has a brain tumor?

Having a parent or sibling with a brain tumor is associated with a three- to ninefold increased risk. Nearly all of these cases (about 5% of all childhood CNS tumors) represent associations with specific inherited genetic disorders, such as neurofibromatosis, and there is increasing information about the specific gene mutations involved. The table demonstrates the association between inherited genetic disorders and tumors of the CNS.

CNS Tumors Associated with Inherited Genetic Disorders

GENETIC DISORDER	TUMOR TYPE	CYTOGENETIC FEATURES
Neurofibromatosis type 1	Astrocytoma Optic pathway glioma	NF gene maps to 17q11.2; allelic loss occurs in 25% of pilocytic astrocytomas
Neurofibromatosis type 2	Bilateral vestibular Schwannomas	22q deletions and NF2 gene mutations in 50% of tumors
Tuberous sclerosis	Subependymal giant cell astrocytoma	TS gene map to 9q and 16p; allelic loss is seen in tumors
Von Hippel-Lindau disease	Hemangioblastoma Choroid plexus carcinoma	Loss of 3p sequence in one case of choroid plexus carcinoma
Li-Fraumeni syndrome	Glioma	P53 tumor suppressor gene mutations
Turcot syndrome	Medulloblastoma Glioblastoma	Germ line mutations in adenomatous polyposis coli gene or mismatch repair genes hMLH1 or hPMS2

6. Why is MRI preferred to computed tomography (CT) for imaging of CNS tumors in the pediatric age group?

Compared with CT, MRI is more sensitive, especially for nonenhancing infiltrative tumors and leptomeningeal involvement. Images can be generated in any plane and are not compromised by bone artifact in the posterior fossa. Magnetic resonance imaging of the spine has replaced myelography as the standard procedure for evaluation of spinal cord lesions and leptomeningeal involvement. Spine imaging and lumbar cerebrospinal fluid examination are specifically recommended for children with malignant brain tumors (medulloblastoma/PNET, high-grade astrocytoma, ependymoma, pineoblastoma and germ cell tumors).

7. Should children with seizures be evaluated by MRI for the presence of a brain tumor?

Seizures are an uncommon presenting symptom of childhood brain tumors and in the absence of other symptoms are not indicative of a CNS tumor. However, among children with intractable epilepsy, occult temporal lobe tumors have been described and may be discovered in nearly 20% of the cases.

8. Name some recent advances in neurosurgery for childhood brain tumors.

Surgery is the mainstay of treatment and can be curative for benign tumors. Total resection is attempted for most malignant tumors, with the exception of intrinsic brain stem tumors and lesions in deep structures such as the thalamus. Intraoperative monitoring of sensory and other evoked potentials can facilitate surgery. Stereotactic (MRI- or CT-guided) techniques are used increasingly for biopsy or subtotal resection in difficult areas such as the basal ganglia. When tumors cause obstructive hydrocephalus, the newer technique of endoscopic ventriculostomy may obviate the need for permanent ventriculoperitoneal shunting.

9. When is radiation therapy indicated in the treatment of childhood brain tumors?

Radiation therapy is an important treatment for nearly all malignant CNS tumors and certain benign lesions as well. Depending on histology, the volume irradiated may include only the area involved by the tumor or the entire brain and spine (with an increased dose or "boost" to the primary tumor). Presymptomatic craniospinal irradiation is routinely given for medulloblastoma because of the risk of neuraxis dissemination. Newer techniques intended to optimize radiation delivery to the tumor while sparing normal brain include stereotactic irradiation ("radiosurgery") and three-dimensional ("conformal") treatment planning.

10. When is chemotherapy used in treating childhood brain tumors?

Chemotherapy is used as an adjunct to radiation therapy, as primary postsurgical treatment in infants and toddlers and for recurrent or progressive tumors in all age groups. There is evidence that chemotherapy improves survival for children with medulloblastoma, high-grade astrocytoma and germ cell tumors. Chemotherapy may be effective in delaying the need for radiation therapy in infants and young children with these and other malignant tumors. Chemotherapy is generally given systemically. Regional delivery of drugs (intra-arterial, intrathecal or intratumoral), although potentially affording higher drug concentration within the tumor, has not yet been shown to be generally effective.

11. A 10-year-old boy presents with vision loss, headache and diabetes insipidus. What is the likely diagnosis and what are the treatment options?

Craniopharyngiomas may appear at any age, arising in the suprasellar region from rests of embryonic tissue located in Rathke's pouch, which forms the anterior pituitary gland. In this case, the differential diagnosis would include optic chiasm glioma and suprasellar germinoma. Craniopharyngiomas may be treated by surgery or radiation therapy. Total removal can be difficult because of invasion of adjacent structures. Radical surgery is likely to be accompanied by panhypopituitarism, whereas radiation therapy has fewer endocrine sequellae but may result in cognitive deficits, particularly in young children. Recurrence rates are similar—about 20–25%.

12. You are asked to see a 12-year-old boy because of clumsiness, unsteady gait, headache and vomiting. Magnetic resonance imaging shows a lateral cerebellar hemispheric tumor. What is the likely diagnosis?

This child probably has a benign juvenile pilocytic astrocytoma. Medulloblastoma is a possibility, but these usually arise in the midline cerebellar vermis. Cerebellar astrocytomas are usually resectable, with survival exceeding 90% following surgery alone.

13. A 6-year-old girl has slowly progressive cranial neuropathy, motor weakness and disturbance of speech and swallowing. Give the likely diagnosis and outcome.

Diffuse intrinsic brain stem gliomas carry the worst prognosis of any childhood brain tumor, being nearly uniformly fatal within 18–24 months. Surgery is not warranted, given the accuracy of radiologic diagnosis and the negligible impact of surgery on survival. Standard treatment is involved field radiation therapy. Chemotherapy and immunotherapy have been unsuccessful, although new approaches continue to be studied.

14. Optic pathway tumors may be diagnosed as early as infancy, especially when associated with neurofibromatosis. How should these very young patients be managed?

Visual pathway tumors tend to spread to contiguous structures. Radiation therapy may be considered if useful vision persists, but the adverse endocrine and neurocognitive effects of radiation therapy in such young children can be substantial. Chemotherapy has been effective as initial treatment in children younger than 5 years with progressive optic pathway tumors, delaying the need for radiation therapy by a median of about 4 years. Infants with neurofibromatosis should have periodic surveillance MRI because of the risk of developing an optic glioma.

15. You are asked to see a 14-year-old girl with headache, motor weakness and personality change of 4 weeks' duration. Magnetic resonance imaging reveals a frontoparietal tumor. What is the likely diagnosis and prognosis?

High-grade astrocytomas (anaplastic astrocytoma and glioblastoma) account for about 10% of childhood brain tumors. Symptom duration tends to be brief. Major resection, postoperative radiation and adjuvant chemotherapy all improve survival, currently about 30–35%. There may be a benefit of consolidative high-dose chemotherapy with hematopoietic stem cell rescue in patients with minimal residual disease following surgery and radiation therapy, based on experience in patients with recurrent high-grade astrocytomas.

16. A 5-year-old boy presents with progressive vomiting, morning headache, unsteadiness and diplopia of 4 weeks' duration. Magnetic resonance imaging shows a contrast-enhancing tumor filling the 4th ventricle, with evidence of obstructive hydrocephalus. Discuss the likely diagnosis and recommended treatment.

Medulloblastoma (cerebellar primitive neuroectodermal tumor) represents the most common malignant CNS tumors of childhood. Isochrome 17q is seen in one third of medulloblastomas, possibly indicating inactivation of a tumor suppressor gene. Standard treatment includes surgical resection and postoperative craniospinal irradiation. Overall survival exceeds 50%. Children with incompletely resected or disseminated medulloblastoma benefit from adjuvant chemotherapy. For children with complete resection, chemotherapy may be useful in permitting reduction of the neuraxis radiation dose and associated late sequellae. Chemotherapy is also used as primary postsurgical treatment in infants and for recurrent medulloblastoma (including high-dose chemotherapy with hematopoietic stem cell rescue).

17. You are asked to see a 5-year-old girl with headache, vomiting and cranial neuropathy. Magnetic resonance imaging reveals a tumor filling the 4th ventricle but also extending into the upper cervical spinal cord, with evidence of obstructive hydrocephalus. What is the likely diagnosis?

This is most likely an ependymoma, a glial neoplasm derived from ependymal cells. Posterior fossa ependymomas may extend inferiorly through the foramen magnum into the upper cervical cord in about one third of cases. Magnetic resonance imaging will demonstrate the caudal extent of the tumor more clearly than CT. Complete resection of ependymoma affords greater than 60% survival but is limited in the posterior fossa by tumor infiltration of the brain stem and involvement of cranial nerve nuclei. After incomplete resection, the majority of tumors will recur despite radiation therapy and chemotherapy; newer treatment approaches are being studied.

18. A child with HIV infection has symptoms and signs of a brain tumor. What is the most likely diagnosis?

Central nervous system lymphomas have been associated with both congenital and acquired immunodeficiency. Primary CNS lymphomas are most often located in the cerebral cortex. This child's symptoms could also represent leptomeningeal or brain parenchymal metastasis of lymphoma. Treatment is intensive chemotherapy with or without brain irradiation.

19. Nine months after radiation treatment of a supratentorial high-grade astrocytoma, a child develops seizures and progressive neuropsychological impairment, indicating possible tumor recurrence. Biopsy shows brain necrosis, without evidence of viable tumor. How should this problem be managed?

Although uncommon, brain necrosis is a serious complication of radiation therapy for primary CNS tumors. Surgical resection should be attempted, and unresectable lesions may be treated medically with corticosteroids. Positron emission tomography may be helpful in distinguishing tumor recurrence from brain necrosis.

20. What types of endocrine dysfunction may follow radiation therapy for tumors of the hypothalamus and pituitary region?

Treatment doses are typically in the range of 5400 cGy. But doses as low as 1800 cGy may cause growth hormone deficiency, and doses above 3600 cGy may cause hypothyroidism and gonadal dysfunction. There may be precocious or delayed puberty. Frank adrenal insufficiency is uncommon.

BIBLIOGRAPHY

1. Albright AL: Pediatric brain tumors. CA Cancer J Clin 43:272–288, 1993.
2. Garvin JH Jr, Feldstein NA: Congenital and childhood central nervous system tumors. In Rowland LP (ed): Merritt's Neurology, 10th ed. Hagerstown, MD, Lippincott Williams & Wilkins, 2000, pp 354–367.
3. Gurney JG, Smith MA, Bunin GR: CNS and miscellaneous intracranial and intraspinal neoplasms. In Ries LAG, Smith MA, Gurney JG, et al (eds): Cancer Incidence and Survival Among Children and Adolescents: United States SEER Program, 1975–1995. NIH Pub. No. 99-4649. Bethesda, MD, National Cancer Institute, 1999, pp 51–64.
4. Kun LE: Brain tumors: Challenges and directions. Pediatr Clin North Am 44:907–917, 1997.
5. Schold SC, Burger PC, Mendelsohn DB, et al: Primary Tumors of the Brain and Spinal Cord. Boston, Butterworth-Heinemann, 1997.

32. RETINOBLASTOMA

Manuela Orjuela, M.D., Sc.M.

1. Describe is the underlying genetic defect in retinoblastoma.

Retinoblastoma, a primitive neuroectodermal cell tumor, develops as a result of an absence of pRb, the retinoblastoma protein, which functions as a regulator of the cell cycle by modifying transcription factors, which allow progression into S phase. Lack of functional pRb occurs primarily as a result of mutations in *RB1*, the retinoblastoma gene. These mutations can occur in either germline or somatic cells. As predicted by Knudson's elegant two-hit hypothesis, both *RB1* alleles must be affected for a tumor to develop.

2. What are the presenting signs for retinoblastoma?

Most (>50%) children with retinoblastoma present with leukocoria (cat's eye reflex). Children with more advanced tumors can present with a dilated pupil in their affected eye. In these patients, the leukocoria is more easily visible. Leukocoria is usually first noted by the parents or another close relative. It is best visualized when the pupil is dilated and light strikes the eye obliquely, such as when it is dark and there is electric lighting, or in photographs in which flash has been utilized. Families will often notice that in recent photographs, one eye has a white pupil (the affected eye) and the other one has a red pupil. Less frequently, children can present with esotropia, exotropia or amblyopia. These symptoms are due to visual loss in the affected eye. Rarely, children can present with heterochromia, or rubeosis iridis. Children with retinoblastoma rarely complain of pain unless they have developed secondary glaucoma (increased intraocular pressure). Discomfort from increased intraocular pressure can cause anorexia. Children with increased intraocular pressure usually have poor vision in the affected eye at diagnosis and usually require prompt enucleation (see below). The pain and anorexia resolve immediately after enucleation.

3. Describe the staging classification for retinoblastoma.

There are two types of staging classification systems for retinoblastoma. One (Reese-Ellsworth) is used by ophthalmologists to stage intraocular disease. The second (St. Jude's Classification System) is used to stage extraocular disease.

The Reese-Ellsworth classification system groups retinal tumors by size and location in the retina, from group I (unifocal small tumor) through group V (massive tumor occupying more than half the retina, or vitreous seeding). This staging system predicts the probability for saving vision and avoiding enucleation (see below). Although a new intraocular staging system has recently been proposed, the Reese-Ellsworth system is still the most widely used.

The St. Jude's Classification system classifies stage I as disease involving only the retina. Stage II disease is restricted to the ocular globe and is subclassified by region of involvement: vitreous seeding (IIA), invasion of the choroidal vessels (IIC), involvement of the optic nerve head (IIB), or both choroidal and nerve head involvement (IID). Subclassification of stage II disease requires an enucleated specimen. Stage III includes extraocular disease with localized spread, including orbital involvement, scleral involvemen, and optic nerve involvement beyond the surgical margin. Stage IV includes disease metastatic to brain (usually extending through the optic nerve), meninges or bone marrow.

4. How do you evaluate a child who presents with possible retinoblastoma?

The diagnosis of retinoblastoma is made clinically, as tissue diagnosis is unnecessary if a child is evaluated by an ophthalmologist familiar with the disease. Initial evaluation includes an examination under anaesthesia, an ultrasonogram looking for characteristic calcifications and an magnetic resonance imaging to evaluate optic nerve involvement, extraorbital extension, and central nervous system involvement. If there is concern that the disease may have spread to the optic nerve or extraocular tissues (such as orbital soft tissue or pre-uricular lymph nodes), a lumbar puncture and bilateral bone marrow aspirates and biopsies are also indicated.

5. What proportion of retinoblastoma is unilateral? At what age does unilateral disease usually present?

Sixty-five percent of retinoblastoma is unilateral. The mean age at diagnosis is 24 months. Most children affected by retinoblastoma are diagnosed before the age of 6 years.

6. Discuss how bilateral retinoblastoma is genetically different from unilateral retinoblastoma.

Children with bilateral retinoblastoma usually have *RB1* mutations in their germline. Therefore all cells (including retinal cells) have one defective RB1 allele. Ninety percent of children with bilateral retinoblastoma have new germline mutations occurring preferentially on the paternally inherited allele. Only 15% of children with unilateral disease have germline mutations. Most children with unilateral disease have *RB1* mutations present only in their retinal cells.

7. How does this biologic difference manifest itself clinically?

Children with bilateral disease present at an earlier age. Although disease can be present from birth (cases have been detected prenatally), the mean age at diagnosis is 11 months. These children usually present with multifocal tumors that do not necessarily develop simultaneously in both eyes; therefore, each eye must be staged separately. Tumors can begin to develop as late as 28 months of age and can continue to develop until age 7 yr. A small proportion of children with bilateral retinoblastoma develop pineal tumors (trilateral retinoblastoma).

8. What proportion of retinoblastoma is familial?

Only 10% of newly diagnosed cases of retinoblastoma occur in children with a prior family history of retinoblastoma. However, each child of a patient with a germline *RB1* mutation has a 45% risk of developing bilateral disease.

9. How is intraocular disease treated?

The goal of treating intraocular disease is to eliminate tumor and save vision. If there is no salvageable vision at diagnosis, ophthalmologists usually recommend enucleation. If however, there is still salvageable vision, small tumors are treated with combinations of laser therapy, cryotherapy and surgically placed radioactive plaques, as well as systemic chemotherapy (usually carboplatin and etoposide). Some tumors are also treated with subconjunctival carboplatin.

10. Describe the options for therapy for extraocular disease.

Orbital disease (stage III) requires enucleation followed by chemotherapy, usually 6 cycles of carboplatin and etoposide, sometimes followed by radiation therapy. If localized soft tissue spread is noted at diagnosis, chemoreduction may be attempted prior to enucleation to avoid orbital exenteration. Metastatic disease (stage IV) requires intensive chemotherapy and, frequently, consolidation with autologous bone marrow transplantation. Survival rates for metastatic disease are below 50%; survival rates for ocular and orbital disease are above 85%, and those for retinal disease are above 95%.

11. Children with bilateral retinoblastoma are at risk for developing secondary malignancies as they get older. Which tumors do they develop? When are they at risk for developing these tumors?

Patients who have germline mutations of *RB1* and survive their retinoblastoma are at increased risk of dying from sarcoma (bone or soft tissue), melanoma or brain tumors. This increased risk results from the acquisition of a second (somatic cell) mutation in their one remaining normal RB1 allele, thereby leading to an absence of pRb-dependent regulation in that particular cell. This risk is particularly increased in areas exposed to radiation. The risk of osteogenic sarcoma is highest between the ages of 10 and 20 yr. The risk for developing brain tumors is highest between the ages of 25 and 35. Carriers of *RB1* mutations also have an increased risk for developing early-onset (before age 55) smoking-induced lung cancers.

12. Discuss how the age at which children receive radiation therapy affects their chance for development of secondary malignancies.

Risk for secondary malignancies is greatest when children with germline mutations receive radiation therapy before their first birthday. These children are at greatly increased risk for developing sarcomas in the soft tissues of their heads (between the ages of 5 and 25), as well as in the bones of their skulls (the highest risk occurring between ages 12 and 25). They also have a lower but still increased risk for developing brain tumors. Children with germline mutations who receive radiation after their first birthday are still at increased risk for developing all of these tumors, but their risk is significantly less than that of those who receive radiation as infants.

BIBLIOGRAPHY

1. Abramson DH, Frank CM, Susman M, et al: Presenting signs of retinoblastoma. J Pediatr 132(3, pt. 1): 505–508, 1998.
2. Eng C, Li FP, Abramson DH, et al: Mortality from second tumors among long-term survivors of retinoblastoma. J Natl Cancer Inst 85:1121–1128, 1993.
3. Wong FL, Boice JD Jr, Abramson DH, et al: Cancer incidence after retinoblastoma. Radiation dose and sarcoma risk. JAMA 278(15):1262–1267, 1997.
4. Zheng L, Lee WH: The retinoblastoma gene: A prototypic and multifunctional tumor suppressor. Exp Cell Res. 264(1):2–18, 2001.

33. HEPATIC TUMORS

Gustavo del Toro, M.D.

1. What are the pediatric tumors that commonly present with liver metastases?

Neuroblastoma and lymphoma. Liver metastases from a distant primary tumor may be more common than primary liver tumors.

2. Name the common benign liver tumors.

Hemangioendothelioma is the most common benign hepatic tumor. Other benign liver tumors arc hemangioma, hamartoma, focal nodular hyperplasia, and liver adenoma.Benign liver tumors will usually be detected by 6 months of age.

3. Why is it problematic to label liver hemangioendothelioma as a benign tumor?

- In 15–20% of patients, liver hemangidendothelioma works as AV fistula, leading to high-output cardiac failure.
- Multifocal liver hemangioendothelioma is unresectable: All treatment options are experimental.
- Multifocal liver hemangioendothelioma can degenerate into angiosarcoma.

4. Describe the common malignant primary liver tumors.

Hepatoblastoma and hepatocellular carcinoma are by far the most common ones. Others include rhabdomyosarcoma, undifferentiated sarcoma, angiosarcoma, and germ cell tumors.

Germ cell tumors present a diagnostic problem, as they could secrete alpha-fetoprotein (AFP), making it impossible to differentiate them from hepatoblastomas without a tissue diagnosis.

5. Which pediatric liver tumor is associated with familial adenomatous polyposis?

Familial adenomatous polyposis (FAP) families have an increased risk of hepatoblastoma. The FAP gene, located in chromosome 5, is thought to be a mutated tumor suppressor gene.

The risk of hepatoblastoma in the offspring of a person with FAP is less than 1%. However, those offspring that do dcvclop hepatoblastoma and are cured will have a 50% chance of developing FAP. Therefore, they must be screened regularly.

6. Name the pediatric liver tumor strongly associated with hepatitis B.

Hepatocellular carcinoma is strongly associated with hepatitis B virus. Children with chronic hepatitis B virus infection need frequent screening for hepatocellular carcinoma with serial AFPs and liver ultrasound.

7. Cite differences in the clinical presentation of hepatoblatoma and hepatocellular carcinoma.

Clinical Presentations of Hepatoblastoma and Hepatocellular Carcinoma

HEPATOBLASTOMA	HEPATOCELLULAR CARCINOMA
Median age at diagnosis = 1 yr	Median age at diagnosis = 12 yr
Usually an asymptomatic abdominal mass	Usually symptomatic: anorexia, weight loss, emesis, fever, abdominal pain/distention

Continued next page

Clinical Presentations of Hepatoblastoma and Hepatocellular Carcinoma (continued)

HEPATOBLASTOMA	HEPATOCELLULAR CARCINOMA
Thrombocytosis	Polycythemia
Acute abdomen due to tumor rupture: rare	Acute abdomen due to tumor rupture: more common
Jaundice in 5%	Jaundice in 25%
AFP elevation in 90%	AFP elevation in 50%

8. What is the most important determinant of prognosis in hepatoblastoma?

The histopathology. There are two major histological types in hepatoblastoma:

- Pure epithelial type
- Mixed epithelial and mesenchymal type

It is the degree of differentiation of the epithelial type that determines malignant potential. The presence of any embryonal cells provides a much worse prognosis when compared with tumors in which the epithelial tissue is strictly composed of fetal cells.

9. Describe how hepatic tumors are staged.

Stage I	Complete tumor resection
Stage II	Microscopic residual disease
Stage III	Gross residual disease
Stage IV	Distant metastases

10. What are the most effective chemotherapy agents in the treatment of hepatoblastoma?

Cisplatin and doxorubicin have shown excellent effects in the treatment of hepatablastoma.

11. Discuss the role of liver transplantation in the treatment of malignant liver tumors.

Liver transplantation can cure patients whose tumors are unresectable after neoadjuvant chemotherapy (preoperative chemotherapy). Active metastatic disease will preclude liver transplantation.

12. Does radiation therapy have any role in the treatment of malignant hepatic tumors?

Only in the management of incompletely resected, localized, chemoresistant lung metastases.

13. Discuss the controversy regarding the timing of definitive surgery for patients with malignant hepatic tumors.

Different pediatric oncology cooperative groups differ in their approach to timing of surgical resection, with some experts favoring initial surgery (if possible), as complete surgical resection of malignant liver tumors gives the best prognosis. Other experts prefer neoadjuvant chemotherapy, as there is no delay in treatment of micrometastases and it ensures the best chances of complete surgical resection, even in tumors judged to be inoperable at diagnosis.

BIBLIOGRAPHY

1. Greenberg M, Filler RM. Hepatic tumors. In Pizzo PA, Poplack DG (eds): Principles and Practice of Pediatric Oncology. Philadelphia, Lippincott-Raven, 1997, pp 717–732.
2. Pinkerton CR. Hepatoblastoma and hepatocellular carcinoma. In Pinkerton CR, Michalski AJ, Veys PA (eds): Cinical Challenges in Paediatric Oncology. Oxford, Isis Medical Media, 1999, pp 157–162.

34. KIDNEY TUMORS IN CHILDREN AND ADOLESCENTS

Darrell Yamashiro, M.D., Ph.D.

1. What is the most common renal cancer in children younger than 15 yr?

Renal cancers represent 6.3% of cancer diagnoses among children younger than 15 yr, with an incidence of 7.9 per million. Wilms' tumor or nephroblastoma is by far the most common primary renal tumor in children younger than 15 yr, representing approximately 95% of diagnoses. In the United States, approximately 500 children are diagnosed with Wilms' tumors each year. Rhabdoid tumors of the kidney and clear cell sarcoma represent 1% and 1.6% of renal cancers, respectively. Carcinoma of the kidney, the most common form of renal cancer in adults, represents only 2.5% of renal cancers in children younger than 15 yr.

2. At what age is a child most commonly diagnosed with Wilms' tumor?

Wilms' tumor occurs most commonly in children younger than 5 yr, with a very low incidence in children 10–14 and 15–19 yr.

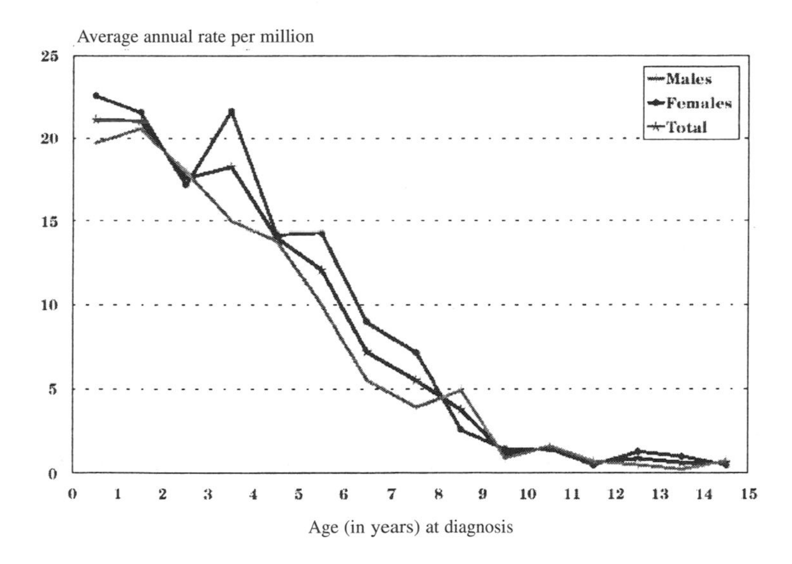

Wilms' tumor age-specific incidence rates by sex, all races, SEER, 1976–84 and 1986–94. From Ries et al., Cancer Incidence and Survival Among Children and Adolescents: United States SEER Program 1975–1995. Bethesda, MD, NIH, Pub. No. 99-4649. (Copyright information: All material in this report is in the public domain and may be reproduced or copied without permission; citation as to source, however, is appreciated.)

3. What are the three different clinical scenarios in which Wilms' tumor arises?

The majority of Wilms' tumors occur in children with no unusual physical features or positive family history. These cases of Wilms' tumor are termed **sporadic**. The second clinical scenario is Wilms' tumor arising in children with **congenital anomalies or syndromes**. About 7.6% of cases of Wilms' tumor have associated congenital anomalies. The third scenario is Wilms' tumors arising in more than one person in a family—**familial Wilms' tumor**—and occurs in 1–2% of cases.

4. List the congenital anomalies and syndromes most commonly associated with Wilms' tumor.

The congenital anomalies associated with Wilms' tumor include

- Aniridia
- Hemihypertrophy
- Cryptorchidism
- Hypospadias
- Other genitourinary anomalies

The syndromes associated with Wilms' tumor include

- WAGR syndrome: Wilms' tumor, aniridia, genitourinary malformations, mental retardation
- Beckwith-Wiedemann syndrome (BWS): visceromegaly, macroglossia, omphalocele, hemihypertrophy, mental retardation
- Denys-Drash syndrome: nephropathy, macrosomia, organomegaly
- Perlman syndrome: macrocephaly, macrosomia, organomegaly, characteristic facies
- Sotos' syndrome: large size at birth, excessive growth during childhood, dysmorphic craniofacial features, developmental delay
- Simpson-Golabi-Behmel syndrome: x-linked syndrome with pre- and postnatal overgrowth, coarse facies, visceromegaly, heart defects, diaphragmatic hernia and gastrointestinal malformations

5. What genes are associated with the development of Wilms' tumor?

WT1 gene at chromosome 11p13: Children with the WAGR syndrome have constitutional deletions encompassing chromosome 11p13, resulting in loss of a number of contiguous genes. These include the aniridia gene *Pax6* and the Wilms' tumor suppressor gene *WT1*. Loss of one copy of *Pax6* is responsible for aniridia, whereas mutations in *WT1* may confer genitourinary defects. *WT1* is a classic tumor suppressor gene, with loss of both copies required for the development of Wilms' tumor.

WT2 gene at chromosome 11p15: In a subset of Wilms' tumor, there is loss of heterozygosity at 11p15. This second putative Wilms' tumor gene has not yet been isolated but has been designated *WT2*. The 11p15 Wilms' tumor locus is also associated with BWS. Several candidate loci for Wilms' tumor and BWS have been proposed, including H19/IGF2 loci and p57Kip2.

Familial Wilms' tumor genes *FWT1* and *FWT2*: Familial Wilms' tumor represents 1–2% of cases. Analysis of families with Wilms' tumor has indicated that the predisposition is an autosomal dominant trait with incomplete penetrance. Linkage analysis has excluded both *WT1* and *WT2* as the loci for familial Wilms' tumor. Linkage analysis has mapped one familial Wilms' tumor gene, designated *FWT1*, to 17q12-21. A second locus, *FWT2*, has been mapped to 19q.

6. Give the recommendations for screening children who are at increased risk for developing Wilms' tumor.

Children with sporadic aniridia, WAGR syndrome, hemihypertrophy and BWS have an increased risk of developing Wilms' tumor. These children should have an abdominal ultrasound and urine analysis for microscopic hematuria every 3–4 months until at least age 7 yr and yearly until full growth is reached.

7. What are the histologic features that distinguish favorable histology (FH) Wilms' tumor from anaplastic Wilms' tumor?

Classic nephroblastoma is composed of varying proportions of three cell types: blastemal, the cellular component, stromal and epithelial tubules. Not all Wilms' tumors are triphasic, with biphasic blastemal and stromal patterns frequently seen. When anaplastic nuclear changes are not present, the tumor is classified as being an FH Wilms' tumor, due to the generally excellent prognosis. Anaplasia with extreme nuclear atypia is present in approximately 4% of cases of Wilms' tumor. Anaplasia is characterized by gigantic polyploid nuclei within the tumor specimen. The nuclei have diameters at least three times that of nearby cells, and the mitotic figures are multipolar or polyploid. Anaplastic cells are more resistant to chemotherapy. Patients require more intensive therapy and have a generally poorer prognosis than FH patients.

8. What is the importance of distinguishing focal from diffuse anaplasia?

Anaplastic changes may be either focal or diffuse in distribution. To meet the criteria of focal anaplasia, the anaplastic nuclear changes must be confined to a sharply restricted foci within the primary tumor and may not be present outside the kidney parenchyma. Diffuse anaplasia is diagnosed when anaplastic cells are present in more than one region of the primary tumor or in any extrarenal site, including the renal sinus, nodal or distant metastases. Patients with focal anaplasia Wilms' tumor have outcomes similar to those of favorable histology patients. Patients with diffuse anaplasia have high rates of relapse and death.

9. Describe the typical clinical presentation of a child with Wilms' tumor?

The most common presentation is an asymptomatic abdominal mass or swelling, often noted by a parent when bathing or dressing the child. Less common symptoms are fever, abdominal pain, gross or microscopic hematuria and hypertension. During the physical examination, special attention should be paid to signs of syndromes associated with Wilms' tumor, such as aniridia, hemihypertrophy and genitourinary anomalies.

10. Discuss the chief differential diagnosis of a child with an abdominal mass.

The most likely diagnoses in a child with an abdominal mass are neuroblastoma and Wilms' tumor. Clinically, children with advanced stage neuroblastoma appear ill, often having signs or symptoms of metastatic disease such as periorbital ecchymoses or pain from skeletal lesions. Computed tomography (CT) scan of the abdomen can usually distinguish between the two cancers, as neuroblastoma arises from the adrenal gland and compresses and displays the kidney, while Wilms' tumor is intrarenal and distorts the kidney.

11. What are the most common sites for metastatic spread of Wilms' tumor?

The most common sites of metastases in Wilms' tumor are the lungs, regional lymph nodes and liver. In patients with stage IV disease, the lungs are the only site of metastases in 80% of cases. Metastases to the liver, with or without lung metastases, is diagnosed in 15% of cases. Other sites of metastases in Wilms' tumor are uncommon. Metastases to the brain can occur in rhabdoid tumors and clear cell sarcoma of the kidney. Bone lesions can be found in clear cell sarcoma of the kidney.

12. Describe the work-up for a child with suspected Wilms' tumor.

Laboratory evaluation should include a complete blood count, a platelet count, liver function tests, renal function tests, serum calcium and urinalysis. Prothrombin time, partial thromboplastin time and fibrinogen should be obtained due to the risk of acquired von Willebrand's disease. If abnormal, factor VIII levels, von Willebrand's factor antigen level, and factor VIII ristocetin cofactor activity should be obtained.

Diagnostic imaging should include an abdominal ultrasound and CT scan to identify the intrarenal origin of the mass and to evaluate the contralateral kidney for its presence and function and for synchronous Wilms' tumors. The inferior vena cava should be carefully examined for the presence and extent of tumor. Echocardiogram is useful for detecting the presence of tumor in the right atrium. The liver should be evaluated for metastases. A chest x-ray, anterior, posterior and two obliques should be obtained, along with a chest CT scan to check for pulmonary metastases. It is currently recommended that patients be treated for pulmonary metastases, stage IV disease, based on the presence of pulmonary nodules appreciated on a chest x-ray. CT scan may be too sensitive, resulting in overtreatment of patients. A magnetic resonance imaging or CT scan of the brain should be done in the cases of rhabdoid tumors and clear cell sarcoma of the kidney, because both tumors are associated with intracranial metastases. A bone scan should be done in cases of clear cell sarcoma of the kidney.

13. Describe how Wilms' tumor is staged.

- Stage I: The tumor is limited to the kidney and was completely resected.
- Stage II: The tumor extends beyond the kidney but is completely resected. There is regional extension of tumor with penetration of the renal capsule. The blood vessels outside the renal parenchyma, including those of the renal sinus, contain tumor. The tumor is biopsied only or there is spillage of tumor before or during surgery that is confined to the flank.
- Stage III: Residual nonhematogenous tumor is present and confined to the abdomen. Any one of the following may occur:
  1. Lymph nodes within the abdomen or pelvis are found to be involved by tumor.
  2. The tumor has penetrated through the peritoneal surface.
  3. Tumor implants are found on the peritoneal surface.
  4. Gross or microscopic tumor remains postoperatively.
  5. The tumor is not completely resected because of local infiltration into vital structures.
  6. Tumor spill not confined to the flank occurred either before or during surgery
- Stage IV: Hematogenous metastases to the lung, liver, bone, brain, or other organ, or lymph node metastases outside the abdominal-pelvic region are present.
- Stage V: Bilateral renal involvement is present at diagnosis. An attempt should be made to stage each side according to the above criteria on the basis of the extent of disease prior to biopsy.

14. What is the general surgical approach for Wilms' tumor in North America?

The treatment of Wilms' tumor in North America has been guided for the past 30 years by the National Wilms' Tumor Study Group (NWTSG). The cornerstone of therapy is surgical removal of the primary tumor at diagnosis. The surgeon is responsible not only for removing the primary tumor intact but also for accurately accessing tumor spread. A transabdominal, transperitoneal, large incision is recommended for adequate exposure. Complete exploration of the abdomen should be done. The contralateral kidney should be palpated and visualized to rule out bilateral involvement. This should be done prior to nephrectomy to exclude bilateral Wilms' tumor. The surgeon should assign a "local-regional stage" to the tumor based solely on the operative findings. The presence or absence of disease in hilar and regional lymph nodes is an extremely important factor in accurate staging. Involved or suspicious lymph nodes should be excised. The renal vein and inferior vena cava should be palpated carefully before ligation to rule out extension of the tumor into the wall or the lumen of the vein. A tumor biopsy should not be taken prior to removal of the tumor. A radical nephrectomy should be performed, and care should be taken to avoid rupture of the tumor capsule with spillage of tumor cells. Partial nephrectomy is not indicated in the routine patient with Wilms' tumor. Exceptions include children with synchronous or metachronous bilateral disease or solitary kidneys. The recommended treatment approach for these patients is initial biopsy followed by combination chemotherapy before definitive surgical resection.

The NWTSG approach differs from the approach taken in Europe by the International Society of Pediatric Oncology (SIOP), where preoperative chemotherapy is advocated prior to primary resection. According to current SIOP recommendations, no biopsy is needed, with the diagnostic work-up based on radiologic findings, blood and urine tests and I-meta-iodobenzyl-guanidine scan, to evaluate for possible neuroblastoma. Using the SIOP protocol, there is a risk that chemotherapy will be given to a benign tumor, such as mesoblastic nephroma or that less-intensive therapy will be given to unfavorable tumors (i.e., rhabdoid tumor and clear cell sarcoma of the kidney).

15. Describe the role of radiation therapy in the treatment of Wilms' tumor.

Radiation therapy has been used to treat Wilms' tumor since 1915. Survival rates rose from 10–20% after nephrectomy alone to 25–35% when postoperative radiation was added. With the development of effective chemotherapy and to reduce late effects, the use of radiation therapy has been tailored for the stage and histology of the patient. Radiation therapy to the abdomen is no longer used for treatment of stage I patients. Currently, abdominal radiation is given to stage III favorable histology patients and to stage II–IV diffuse anaplasia patients. Lung radiation is reserved for patients with stage IV pulmonary metastases.

16. Which chemotherapy drugs are used for the treatment of Wilms' tumor and what are the current therapeutic regimens recommended by the NWTSG?

Between 1969 and 2001, there have been five studies conducted by the NWTSG. The first two studies, NWTS-I (1969–1973) and NWTS-II (1974–1978) demonstrated that postoperative local radiation was unnecessary for stage I patients, that the combination of vincristine and actinomycin D was more effective than either drug alone, and that the addition of doxorubicin improved survival in higher-stage patients. NWTS-III (1979–1986) and NWTS-IV (1986–1994), demonstrated that the addition of cyclophosphamide to the three-drug treatment regimen improved the 4-yr relapse-free survival rate of children with stage II–IV diffuse anaplasia. NWTS-V (1995–2001) is a single-arm therapeutic trial. Patients with stage I and II favorable histology and stage I anaplastic histology receive 18 weeks of vincristine and actinomycin D, but no irradiation. Patients with stage III favorable histology and stage II–III focal anaplasia receive 10.8 Gy abdominal irradiation and 24 weeks of vincristine, actinomycin D and doxorubicin. Patients with stage IV favorable histology receive abdominal irradiation according to the local tumor stage and 12 Gy to both lungs. Patients with stage II–IV diffuse anaplasia and I–IV clear cell sarcoma of the kidney receive irradiation to the tumor bed and chemotherapy with vincristine, doxorubicin, cyclophosphamide and etoposide. Due to the poor outcome on the previous NWTS studies, children with stages I–IV of rhabdoid tumor of the kidney receive the combination of carboplatin, cyclophosphamide and etoposide.

Therapeutic Recommendations of NWTS-V

STAGE	RADIOTHERAPY	CHEMOTHERAPY
Stage I and II, favorable histology Stage I, focal or diffuse anaplasia	None	Regimen EE-4A (18 weeks); vincristine, actinomycin D
Stage III and IV, favorable histology Stage II–IV, focal anaplasia	Yes	Regimen DD-4A (24 weeks); vincristine, actinomycin D, doxorubicin
Stage II–IV, diffuse anaplasia Stage I–IV, clear cell sarcoma of the kidney	Yes	Regimen I (24 weeks); vincristine, actinomycin D, doxorubicin, cyclophosphamide, etoposide
Stage I–IV, rhabdoid tumor of the kidney	Yes	Regimen RTK (24 weeks); carboplatin, cyclophosphamide, etoposide

17. What is the prognosis of patients with Wilms' tumor?

The overall prognosis for patients with FH Wilms' tumor is excellent. In NWTS-IV, FH patients had a 4-year relapse-free survival of about 90% for stages I–III and 80% for stage IV. Patients with bilateral stage V disease treated with an initial biopsy followed by postoperative chemotherapy had an 83% survival. The outcome for patients with localized stage I focal or diffuse anaplasia is also excellent, with an 88% survival. The 4-year relapse-free suvival for patients with stages II–IV focal anaplasia was 92%. In contrast, patients with stages II–IV diffuse anaplasia, given more intensive treatment with cyclophosphamide, had a 55% 4-yr relapse-free suvival. Patients with clear cell sarcoma of the kidney, regardless of stage, had a 4-yr relapse-free survival of 71%. Patients with rhabdoid tumor of the kidney had the worst outcome, with a a 4-yr relapse free survival of 27%.

BIBLIOGRAPHY

1. Argani P, Perlman EJ, Breslow NE, et al: Clear cell sarcoma of the kidney: a review of 351 cases from the National Wilms' Tumor Study Group Pathology Center. Am J Surg Pathol 24: 4–18, 2000.
2. Bernstein L, Linet M, Smith MA, Olshan AF: Renal tumors. In Ries L, Smith M, Gurney et al (eds): Cancer Incidence and Survival Among Children and Adolescents: United States SEER Program 1975–1995. National Cancer Institute, SEER Program, Vol. Pub. No. 99-4649, Bethesda, MD, NIH, 1999, pp. 79-90.
3. Choyke PL, Siegel MJ, Craft, W, et al: Screening for Wilms tumor in children with Beckwith-Wiedemann syndrome or idiopathic hemihypertrophy. Med Pediatr Oncol 32: 196–200, 1999.
4. Coppes MJ, Pritchard-Jones K: Principles of Wilms' tumor biology. Urol Clin North Am 27: 423–433, viii, 2000.
5. D'Angio GJ, Breslow N, Beckwith JB, et al: Treatment of Wilms' tumor. Results of the Third National Wilms' Tumor Study. Cancer 64: 349–360, 1989.
6. Faria P, Beckwith JB, Mishra K, et al: Focal versus diffuse anaplasia in Wilms tumor—new definitions with prognostic significance: A report from the National Wilms Tumor Study Group. Am J Surg Pathol 20: 909–920, 1996.
7. Green DM, Beckwith JB, Breslow NE, et al: Treatment of children with stages II to IV anaplastic Wilms' tumor: a report from the National Wilms' Tumor Study Group. J Clin Oncol 12: 2126–1231, 1994.
8. Neville HL, Ritchey ML: Wilms' tumor. Overview of National Wilms' Tumor Study Group results. Urol Clin North Am 27: 435–442, 2000.

35. NEUROBLASTOMA

Darrell Yamashiro, M.D., Ph.D.

1. What is neuroblastoma?

Neuroblastoma is a malignant tumor of infants and children originating from neural crest cells that normally give rise to the adrenal gland and the sympathetic ganglia. It can have widely varying outcomes: tumors can spontaneously regress, differentiate into benign ganglioneuromas or metastasize with a high mortality rate.

2. What is the incidence of neuroblastoma in the United States?

In the United States, approximately 650 infants, children and adolescents are diagnosed with neuroblastoma annually. Neuroblastoma accounts for 7.6% of all cancers in children younger than 15 yr, with an average age-adjusted incidence rate of 9.1 per million children. There is a marked age dependence in the incidence rate, with an incidence rate for infants (younger than 1 yr) of 64 per million, dropping to 29 per million during the second year of life. Ninety percent of all cases occur before age 10 yr. The figure shows incidence rates of neuroblastomas by year of age at diagnosis for the periods 1976–84 versus 1986–94. Among infants, the rate in the earlier time period was 53 per million compared with 74 per million in the later time period. The increased incidence rate among infants may be the result of the identification of previously undetected tumors in minimally symptomatic infants by noninvasive diagnostic tests and the routine use of prenatal ultrasound.

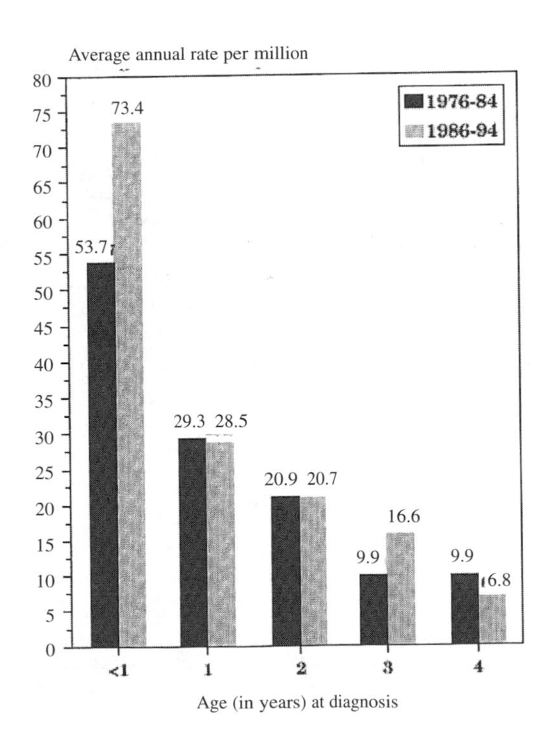

Neuroblastoma age-specific incidence rates by by age, all races, both sexes, SEER, 1976–84 and 1986–1994. From Ries et al: Cancer Incidence and Survival Among Children and Adolescents: United States SEER Program 1975–1995. Bethesda, MD, NIH, Pub. No. 99-4649.

3. Discuss the most common cancer occurring in the first year of life.

Neuroblastoma is the most common cancer occurring in the first year of life, with an incidence rate almost double that of leukemia, the next most common malignancy occurring in infants. Sixteen percent of infant neuroblastomas are diagnosed during the first month following birth, and 41% are diagnosed during the first 3 months of life.

4. In neuroblastoma, what is the utility of screening for urinary catecholamines?

About 90–95% of patients with neuroblastoma secrete one or both of the urinary catecholamine metabolites, homovanillic acid (HVA) or vanillymandelic acid (VMA). Screening of urinary VMA/HVA was conducted with the hope that earlier detection would lead to more localized disease and increase the possibility of cure. However, although screening of infants at 6 months of age or earlier leads to a marked increase in overall incidence of neuroblastoma, it does not reduce the incidence of advanced-stage patients with poor prognosis. Screening results in the overdiagnosis of tumors that would otherwise have spontaneously regressed.

5. What are the most common cytogenetic and molecular abnormalities found in neuroblastoma?

- Increased DNA index: Tumors of infants often demonstrate a hyperdiploid content (DNA index > 1). These infants are more likely to have lower stages of disease, improved response to chemotherapy and an overall improved outcome. Cytogenetically, the hyperdiploid tumors have whole-chromosome gains with few structural rearrangements.
- MYCN amplification: Genomic amplification of the proto-oncogene *MYCN* (also known as *N-myc*) occurs in about 25% of patients with neuroblastoma. Amplification may result in 30–400 copies of MYCN per cell. Amplification of MYCN (defined as >10 copies) is a powerful predictor of advanced stage, rapidly progressing disease, and poor prognosis.
- Loss at 1p: Deletion of the short arm of chromosome 1 is a common cytogenetic feature of neuroblastoma, occurring in 30–50% of tumors. The common region of loss is at the distal end in the area of 1p36 and is thought to contain a tumor suppressor gene(s) for neuroblastoma.
- Gain at 17q: Gain of genetic material on chromosome 17 is the most common genetic abnormality in neuroblastoma, occurring in 54–72% of cases. Gain at 17q is characteristic of tumors in children older than 1 yr and advanced-stage tumors, and is strongly associated with deletion of 1p and amplification of *MYCN*. The finding of recurring gains on chromosome 17 suggests the presence of one or more oncogenes that may contribute to neuroblastoma pathogenesis.

6. What are the most common sites at which neuroblastoma originates and metastasizes?

Neuroblastoma can originate from any site in the sympathetic nervous system. Most primary tumors arise in the abdomen (65%), with the primary site the adrenal gland occurring more frequently in children older than 1 yr (40%) than in infants younger than 1 yr (25%). Cervical and thoracic tumors occur more commonly in infants (33%) than in older children (15%). At presentation, about half of the patients will have metastatic disease. The most common sites of metastases include

- Bone marrow: 70%
- Bone: 56%
- Lymph node: 31%
- Liver: 30%
- Intracranial/orbit:18%

Infants are much more likely to have liver metastases than children older than 1 yr.

7. Describe the signs and symptoms of a child with neuroblastoma.

The signs and symptoms of neuroblastoma depend on the location and extent of the primary tumor, as well as the presence of metastases. Large abdominal masses can cause discomfort, vomiting and anorexia. High thoracic or cervical masses can present with Horner's syndrome (unilateral ptosis, miosis and anhidrosis). Epidural or intradural extension occurs in 5–16% of cases and can cause symptoms of spinal cord compression: pain, bladder and bowel dysfunction, paraparesis or paraplegia.

Metastatic neuroblastoma classically presents with proptosis and periorbital ecchymoses, as well as bone pain, resulting in irritability, limp or refusal to walk. Infants can have rapidly enlarging liver metastases that can cause respiratory compromise and renal and hepatic failure. Infants may have "blueberry muffin" lesions due to neuroblastoma metastasizing to the skin.

Patients may also have paraneoplastic syndromes due to neuroblastoma. Excessive secretion of catecholamines may rarely lead to attacks of sweating, flushing, pallor, headaches, palpitation and hypertension. Excretion of vasoactive intestinal polypeptide can cause intractable watery diarrhea. Infrequently, patients may have opsomyoclonus syndrome, with bursts of rapid chaotic eye movements along with frequent, irregular, jerking movements of muscles. Patients with opsomyoclonus have a favorable outcome with respect to survival. However, even when no tumor is present, many patients remain symptomatic, with long-term neurological deficits that include learning disabilities, motor and language delay and behavioral abnormalities.

8. Discuss the work-up for a child with suspected neuroblastoma.

Laboratory evaluation should include a complete blood count, platelet count, liver function tests, renal function tests, serum calcium and urinalysis. Serum ferritin and lactate dehyrogenase (LDH) should be measured, because elevated levels have been associated with a poorer prognosis. Prothrombin time, partial thromboplastin time and fibrinogen should be obtained due to the increased risk of disseminated intravascular coagulation in patients with metastatic disease. Urine should be tested for urinary catecholamine metabolites, HVA and VMA.

Diagnostic imaging should include a computed tomography scan and/or an magnetic resonance imaging to evaluate the primary tumor and liver and lymph node metastases. Bilateral bone marrow aspirates and biopsies are required to determine the presence of bone marrow metastases. For cortical bone involvment a metaiodobenzylguanidine scintigraphy or a ^{99}technetium (^{99}Tc) bone scan should be done. In infants, a skeletal survey should be performed, as it is generally a more reliable indicator of bone disease than a ^{99}Tc bone scan.

9. How is neuroblastoma staged?

To facilitate the comparison of clinical trials and biological studies, an international consensus regarding the criteria for the diagnosis of neuroblastoma, staging system and response criteria was published in 1988 and revised in 1993. The staging system is termed the International Neuroblastoma Staging System (INSS) and is described in the following table. Prior to implementation of the INSS, the two staging systems that were in use in the United States were those described by Evans and the St. Jude-Pediatric Oncology Group. The INSS takes into account the extent of tumor resection and also retains the "special" category of 4S for infants younger than 1 yr with a localized primary tumor who have metastases to the liver and skin and minimal amount in bone marrow: < 10%.

International Neuroblastoma Staging System

Stage	Definition
1	Localized tumor with complete gross excision, with or without microscopic residual disease; representative ipsilateral lymph nodes negative for tumor microscopically
2A	Localized tumor with incomplete gross excision; representative ipsilateral lymph nodes negative for tumor microscopically
2B	Localized tumor with or without complete gross excision, with ipsilateral lymph nodes positive for tumor; enlarged contralateral lymph nodes must be negative microscopically
3	Unresectable unilateral tumor infiltrating across the midline, with or without regional lymph node involvement, localized unilateral tumor with contralateral regional lymph node involvement or midline tumor with bilateral extension by infiltration (unresectable) or by lymph node involvement
4	Any primary tumor with dissemination to distant lymph nodes, bone, bone marrow, liver and other organs (except as defined for stage 4S)
4S	Localized primary tumor (as defined for stage 1, 2A or 2B), in a patient < 1 yr, with dissemination limited to skin, liver and/or bone marrow (marrow involvement should be minimal, with malignant cells < 10% of total nucleated cells)

10. Discuss the criteria necessary to make the diagnosis of neuroblastoma.

According to the INSS criteria, a diagnosis of neuroblastoma is established by one of the following:

- Unequivocal tumor histopathology
- Unequivocal tumor cells by bone marrow aspirate or biopsy and increased urinary catecholamines (VMA and/or HVA)
- If tumor histology is equivocal, then genetic features such as *MYCN* amplification or 1p LOH can be used to support the diagnosis of neuroblastoma

11. Describe the pathological classification of neuroblastoma.

The histopathologic appearance of neuroblastoma ranges from undifferentiated neuroblasts to more mature ganglioneuroblastoma to fully differentiated and benign ganglioneuroma. Currently, the morphologic system proposed by Shimada is used to classify tumors into favorable histology or unfavorable histology. The classification is dependent on age, the degree of neuronal differentiation, the mitotic rate and the presence or absence of Schwannian stromal development.

12. What prognostic factors are used to stratify patients into different risk groups?

Numerous prognostic factors have been described in neuroblastoma. Poor prognosis has been associated with the following parameters:

- Advanced stage
- Unfavorable histology
- Elevated serum ferritin
- Elevated LDH
- VMA/HVA ratio of < 1
- Diploid (DNA index = 1) tumors in infants
- Amplification of *MYCN*
- Loss at chromosome 1p
- Gain at chromosome 17q
- Low expression of nerve growth factor receptor TrkA
- Age > 1 year

The factors that are consistently independently prognostic have been age, stage, *MYCN* amplification, tumor histology and DNA ploidy in infants. These factors are used to stratify patients into low-, intermediate- and high-risk groups.

INSS	*Age (days)*	*MYCN*	*Histology*	*Ploidy*	*Risk*
1	Any	Any	Any	Any	Low
2A/2B	< 365	Any	Any	Any	Low
	≥ 365	Nonamplified	Any	—	Low
	≥ 365	Amplified	FH	—	Low
	≥ 365	Amplified	UH	—	High
3	< 365	Nonamplified	Any	Any	Intermediate
	< 365	Amplified	Any	Any	High
	≥ 365	Nonamplified	FH	—	Intermediate
	≥ 365	Nonamplified	UH	—	High
	≥ 365	Nonamplified	Any	—	High
4	< 365	Nonamplified	Any	Any	Intermediate
	< 365	Amplified	Any	Any	High
	≥ 365	Any	Any	—	High
4S	< 365	Nonamplified	FH	DI > 1	Low
	< 365	Nonamplified	FH	DI = 1	Intermediate
	< 365	Nonamplified	UH	Any	Intermediate
	< 365	Amplified	Any	Any	High

FH, favorable histology; UH, unfavorable histology; DI, DNA Index.

13. What is the treatment and prognosis for patients with low-risk neuroblastoma?

Low-risk patients are those with localized tumors and stage-1 disease, most patients with stage-2 disease and infants with stage-4S disease and favorable tumor biology. These patients have an excellent survival when treated primarily with surgery and supportive care.

Children with stage-1 and -2 disease treated primarily with surgery have a 5-yr survival of > 95%. Chemotherapy is reserved for the few patients with symptomatic disease due to paraspinal tumors resulting in spinal cord compression. Patients who do have a local recurrence of tumor after surgery are usually easily treated with either further surgery or with moderate chemotherapy or local radiation.

Infants with stage-4S disease and favorable biological features given minimal therapy also have an excellent survival: 85–90%. Treatment has ranged from supportive care only to modest chemotherapy regimens given over 4–5 months. Adverse prognostic factors for stage-4S patients include age younger than 2 months at diagnosis, *MYCN* amplification, unfavorable Shimada histopathology and diploid tumors. Infants with stage-4S disease who have a poor outcome are generally those with very extensive hepatic infiltration, causing respiratory compromise and occasionally renal and venous obstruction. These infants, despite receivingemergency abdominal decompression, mechanical ventilation, chemotherapy and hepatic radiotherapy, often die of sepsis or respiratory, renal or hepatic failure.

14. Describe the treatment and prognosis for patients with intermediate-risk neuroblastoma.

The intermediate risk group comprises patients who have an excellent prognosis: 80–90% survival. These patients include those with stage-3 diseasewith favorable tumor biology, those with stage-4 disease without tumor *MYCN* amplification and those with stage-4S disease whose tumors are diploid or have unfavorable histology. Treatment has consisted of surgery, moderately intensive combination chemotherapy and local radiation therapy for residual unresectable tumor. This group includes the patients of any age with biologically favorable stage-3 tumors, defined by the nonamplified *MYCN* and favorable histology. Infants with stage-3 disease and nonamplified *MYCN*, regardless of other biologic features, also have a favorable outcome. Infants with stage-4 disease whose tumors have a single copy of *MYCN* have a disease-free survival in excess of 85% with conventional chemotherapy, regardless of other prognostic features. The other group of intermediate-risk patients are infants with stage-4S disease who have either diploid DNA index or unfavorable histology. Currently, the Children's Oncology Group is treating intermediate-risk patients with favorable biology, with four cycles of chemotherapy given over 12 weeks, using a combination of carboplatin, etoposide, doxorubicin and cyclophosphamide. Patients with less-favorable biology, including infants with either unfavorable histology or diploid tumors, receive eight cycles of therapy.

15. Describe the treatment and prognosis for patients with high-risk neuroblastoma.

The high-risk group of patients with neuroblastoma consists primarily of patients with stage 4 disease older than 1 yr at diagnosis. Also included in the high-risk group are stage-3 patients with either *MYCN* amplification or who are older than 1 yr with unfavorable Shimada, stage-2 patients older than 1 yr with *MYCN* amplification and stage-3, -4 and -4s infants with *MYCN* amplification. Despite the use of increasingly aggressive combined modality treatments, which have increased remission rate and duration, the long-term survival for INSS stage-4 disease in children who are older than 1 yr at diagnosis has remained, until recently, < 15%. More recently, the introduction of platinum-based therapy, the use of increasingly dose-intensive chemotherapy combinations and the incorporation of myeloablative therapy followed by treatment for minimal residual disease has resulted in improvement in rates of progression-free survival and overall survival, with 3-yr estimates at 30%. The 4-yr survival for all stage 4 patients older than 1 yr at diagnosis in the Children's Cancer Group studies from 1978-1985 was 9%, compared with 30% for patients treated from 1991–1995. Current optimal therapy includes a chemotherapy induction phase, incorporation of local control with surgery and radiotherapy for bulky disease and myeloablative conditioning supported by hematopoietic stem cell reconstitution, finally followed by therapy for minimal residual disease. The most effective induction regimens are combination platinum-based regimens including a combination of other active drugs, such as cyclophosphamide, doxorubicin, etoposide, vincristine and ifosfamide. Consolidation therapy consists of myeloablative chemotherapy containing melphalan or thiotepa, with or without total body irradiation, followed by autologous bone marrow or peripheral blood stem cell transplant. Therapy for minimal residual disease includes cis-retinoic acid and antibody therapy against neuroblastoma specific antigens.

BIBLIOGRAPHY

1. Brodeur GM, Pritchard J, Berthold F, et a: Revisions of the international criteria for neuroblastoma diagnosis, staging, and response to treatment [see comments]. J Clin Oncol 11: 1466–1477, 1993.
2. Brodeur GM, SeegerRC, Barrett A, et al: International criteria for diagnosis, staging and response to treatment in patients with neuroblastoma. Prog Clin Biol Res 271: 509–524, 1988.
3. Goodman MT, Gurney JG, Smith MA, Olshan AF: Sympathetic nervous system tumors. In Ries LAG, Smith MA, Gurney JG, et al (eds). Cancer Incidence and Survival Among Children and Adolescents: United States SEER Program 1975–1995. NIH Pub. No. 99-4649. Bethesda, MD, National Cancer Institute, SEER Program, 1999, pp 65–72.
4. Maris JM, Matthay KK: Molecular biology of neuroblastoma. J Clin Oncol 17: 2264, 1999.
5. Matthay KK, Villablanca JG, Seeger RC, et al: Treatment of high-risk neuroblastoma with intensive chemotherapy, radiotherapy, autologous bone marrow transplantation, and 13-cis- retinoic acid. Children's Cancer Group. N Engl J Med 341: 1165–1173, 1999.
6. Matthay KK, YamashiroDJ: Neuroblastoma. In Holland JF, Frei E, Bast RC, et al (eds). Cancer Medicine, 5th ed. Hamilton, Ontario, B.C. Decker, 2000, pp. 2185–2195.
7. Shimada H, Ambros IM, Dehner LP, et al: The International Neuroblastoma Pathology Classification (the Shimada system). Cancer 86: 364–872, 1999.

36. RHABDOMYOSARCOMA AND OTHER SOFT TISSUE SARCOMAS

Julia Glade Bender, M.D.

1. What are soft tissue sarcomas?

Sarcomas are malignant tumors, which derive from the primitive mesenchyme. During the course of normal development, the primitive mesenchyme differentiates into the various structural tissues of the body, including bone, muscle, connective tissue, supportive tissue, and vascular and peripheral nerve tissue. Excluding bone sarcomas, which form a separate entity, soft tissue sarcomas represent the neoplastic counterpart of these tissue types and take their name from the normal tissue they most resemble.

SARCOMA TYPE	NORMAL TISSUE SARCOMA RESEMBLES
Rhabdomyosarcoma (RMS)	Skeletal muscle
Non-Rhabdomyosarcoma Soft Tissue Sarcomas (NRSTS)	
Leiomyosarcoma	Smooth muscle
Fibrosarcoma	Connective tissue
Malignant fibrous histiocytoma	Connective tissue
Liposarcoma	Adipose tissue
Synovial sarcoma	Synovium
Angiosarcoma	Blood vessel
Endothelial hemangiopericytoma	Pericyte
Neurofibrosarcoma/malignant peripheral nerve sheath tumors	Nerve sheath
Other	
Peripheral neural ectodermal tumor (PNET)	
Extraosseus Ewing's sarcoma	
Alveolar soft part sarcoma	
Undifferentiated sarcomas	

2. How common are pediatric soft tissue sarcomas?

While soft tissue sarcomas are relatively common in adults, they are less so in children, representing 7% of all pediatric malignancies, with an incidence of less than 500 cases per year. Of these, RMS is by far the most common, representing 50–60% of the group, or approximately 250 new cases each year. This makes RMS the third most common extracranial solid tumor after neuroblastoma and Wilms' tumor.

3. Discuss the most common associations predisposing a child to the development of RMS or one of the other soft tissue sarcomas.

The vast majority of soft tissue sarcomas are sporadic. However, there are several well-described predisposing factors:

- The familial cancer predisposition syndrome known as the *Li-Fraumeni syndrome*, characterized by a germ line mutation of the tumor suppressor gene *p53* on chromosome 17 and an autosomal dominant inheritance. The syndrome includes an increased incidence of soft and bony tissue sarcomas, leukemia, brain tumors, adrenocortical carcinomas and early-onset breast carcinoma in female relatives.

- *Neurofibromatosis type I (NF1, von Recklinghausen's disease)*, a relatively common autosomal dominant genetic disorder, characterized by mutation of the *NF1* gene mapped to 17q11.2. This disorder is associated with an increased risk of RMS and NRSTS, particularly malignant peripheral nerve sheath tumors/neurofibrosarcomas, as well as leukemias, Wilms' tumor and brain tumors.
- *Beckwith-Wiedemann syndrome*, a fetal overgrowth syndrome mapped to 11p15, the location of the insulin-like growth factor II gene, and characterized by hemihypertrophy, macroglossia, hypoglycemia, omphalocele and a predisposition most commonly to Wilms' tumor but also to hepatoblastoma, RMS and other tumors of embryonal origin.
- *Previous radiation or alkylator exposure*, particularly in the setting of a familial cancer syndrome such as Li-Fraumeni, NF1 or hereditary retinoblastoma (RB1 germ line mutation).
- Certain *congenital anomalies* of the genitourinary system and central nervous system are more frequent than expected in children with RMS.
- RMS in children with *other hereditary syndromes* including Rubenstein-Taybi syndrome, Gorlin's nevus basal cell carcinoma and trisomy 21 have been described.
- Leiomyosarcoma has been seen in children in the context of *immunosuppression* by human immunodeficiency virus (HIV), Epstein-Barr virus (EBV) and leukemia and following solid organ transplantation.

4. What is the most common clinical presentation of soft tissue sarcoma?

RMS or NRSTS most commonly presents as a painless, non-tender mass without antecedent history of trauma that may or may not cause interference of normal body functions depending on site of origin. Systemic symptoms are unusual.

5. Discuss the appropriate work-up for a soft tissue sarcoma.

As with any suspected malignancy, the corner stone of the initial work-up is an excellent history and physical examination with special attention to the draining lymph nodes. High-quality presurgical imaging studies are necessary to determine extent and surgical resectability of the local lesion, initial tumor volume (both prognostic and critical for radiation therapy planning) and evidence of metastatic spread. Whereas computer tomography (CT) with or without contrast has long been considered standard, many now favor magnetic resonance imaging (MRI) in the assessment of soft tissue tumors because of the superior resolution between tissue layers. Positron emission tomography (PET), which exploits the enhanced metabolic rate of malignant cells, has also found utility in the assessment of high-grade sarcomas. If positive at diagnosis, PET can be a particularly powerful tool in follow-up. CT of the chest and a radionucleotide scan with technetium-99m diphosphonate (bone scan) should also be obtained. If the lesion proves to be RMS or undifferentiated sarcoma, bone marrow aspirates and biopsies will be required in at least two sites to complete the metastatic work-up. Patients with parameningeal RMS should also undergo lumbar puncture to document negative cerebrospinal cytology. While there are no serologic markers for this family of tumors, routine laboratory studies should be obtained in anticipation of surgery and possible chemotherapy.

6. How should tissue be obtained for diagnosis?

A well-planned biopsy is absolutely essential for accurate diagnosis, subsequent definitive surgery, long-term survival and quality of life. The surgeon must be experienced and maintain awareness of future surgical options (e.g., limb or vital organ sparing) should the diagnosis of sarcoma be confirmed. For small tumors, wide excisional biopsy may be considered if complete removal with adequate margins and without major functional or cosmetic damage is anticipated. For larger tumors, incisional biopsy is usually preferable to core needle biopsy, although the latter is acceptable in some circumstances. Care should be taken to position the biopsy incision such that it can be re-excised at the time of definitive surgery and such that minimal dissection is required across tissue planes to reach tumor. Most commonly, this means avoiding a transverse incision on the extremity. The tissue obtained should be from an area felt to be most representative of the lesion and should be delivered to the pathology department fresh, so that cytogenetic and molecular testing can be performed, in addition to routine histologic evaluation.

7. What are the primary sites of origin for RMS, their relative frequency and predilection for age, sex and metastasis?

PRIMARY SITE	RELATIVE FREQUENCY (%)	PREDILECTIONS
Head and Neck	40	Female > male (slightly)
Orbit or eyelid	10 (25)	40% of RMS age 5–9 yr; Usually localized
Parameningeal (nasopharynx, middle ear, mastoid, paranasal sinuses, and pterygoid-infratemporal fossae)	20 (50)	Relatively high risk of metastasis to bone, brain, meninges and lung
Other (larynx, oropharynx, scalp, face, cheek, parotid and neck)	10 (25)	Metastasis to lung
Genitourinary tract	20	Male >> female
Bladder, prostate	12	75% < 5yr: Metastasis to lung, bone marrow
Paratesticular	6	Adolescents: Metastasis to retro-peritoneal nodes (30%), lung, bone
Vagina, uterus	2	Infant: Sarcoma Botryoides Older: Metastasis to retroperitoneal nodes
Extremities	20	Female > males (slightly); School age and adolescents: Metastasis to nodes (20%), lung, bone marrow, bone
Trunk	10	Spread to nodes unusual; metastasis to lung, bone
Other (intrathoracic, retroperitoneal, perineal-perianal, biliary tract, etc.)	10	Spread to nodes unusual; metastasis to lung, bone

8. Discuss the two major variants of RMS, their characteristic presentation, histologic appearance, clinical behavior and molecular alterations.

Embryonal (70–80%)

- Seen more commonly in young patients with head and neck or genitourinary primaries.
- Histologically, characterized by a mix of small, round and elongated cells in a stroma-rich environment, without open areas. A spindle cell (leiomyomatous) subvariant can be seen commonly in the paratesticular area, and a botryoid subvariant (5%) ("cluster of grapes" gross appearance) can be found in mucosa-lined organs, most often involving the vagina.
- Prior to the advent of more intensive chemotherapy regimens, this type had an improved prognosis over alveolar RMS, independent of stage at diagnosis. Leiomyomatous and sarcoma botryoids have a particularly favorable outcome.
- No pathognemonic molecular alterations. Nonetheless, embryonal tumors have consistently shown a loss of heterozygosity (LOH) at 11p15, perhaps involving the *IGFII* gene, which is believed to play a pathogenic role in RMS. Also has a 35% incidence of NRAS or KRAS proto-oncogene mutation.

Alveolar (20–30%)

- Seen more often in older patients and in lesions involving the extremities.
- Histologically characterized by small, round, dense-appearing cells with abundant eosinophilic cytoplasm surrounding open areas resembling the alveoli of normal lung tissue. There is also a solid variant.
- The more aggressive of the two variants, often with metastatic disease at the time of diagnosis. Requires intensive chemotherapy even in the setting of localized disease.
- The classic associated molecular abnormality is a chromosomal rearrangement of chromosomes 2 and 13 [t(2;13)(q35;q13)] leading to the *PAX3-FKHR* fusion gene. The novel chimeric protein encoded is presumed to exert its transforming potential via activation of inappropriate transcription and subsequent dysregulation of cell growth. A similar fusion gene PAX7-FKHR [t(1;13)] is seen in a minority of tumors; these are usually in younger patients with extremity primaries and lung or node metastasis but a slightly better clinical outcome.

9. Describe the staging system utilized for RMS and undifferentiated sarcomas.

Since 1972, RMS has been staged by the Intergroup Rhabdomyosarcoma Studies (IRS) using the Clinical Group system. This system relies on extent of tumor, but is post-surgical and therefore may reflect the skill or aggressiveness of the surgeon, rather than inherent tumor biology. From 1991-1997, during the fourth IRS study (IRS-IV), preoperative, clinical staging using a "tumor, nodes and metastasis" (TNM) system modified for site of origin was evaluated and found to be helpful in the up-front stratification of patients into risk-based treatment arms. Nonetheless, Clinical Group staging remained the most predictive of eventual disease-free/failure free survival. The current trials (IRS-V) stratify patients into high-, intermediate- and low-risk therapies based on an algorithm that takes both systems, as well as age and histology, into consideration. The use and dosage of radiotherapy is largely based on the Clinical Group staging system.

IRS Clinical Group

I	Localized disease, completely resected
II	Microscopic residual disease (regional nodes grossly resected)
III	Incomplete resection (or biopsy) with gross residual disease
IV	Metastatic disease at presentation

IRS TNM Pre-treatment Staging

STAGE	SITE	SIZE	NODES	METASTASIS
1	Orbit, other head/neck (excluding parameningeal), genitourinary (excluding bladder /prostate)	Any	Any	Absent
2	Bladder/prostate, extremity, parameningeal, other	≤5cm	N0, Nx	Absent
3	Bladder /prostate, extremity, parameningeal, other	≤5cm	N1	Absent
		>5cm	Any	
4	Any	Any	Any	Present

N0=Nodes not clinically involved, N1=nodes clinically involved, Nx=nodes unknown.

10. Discuss the treatment strategy in RMS and in undifferentiated sarcoma.

The two basic tenets of therapy for RMS and undifferentiated sarcomas are loco-regional control and eradication of micrometastasis. This is accomplished using three modalities: surgery, radiation therapy and chemotherapy. This timing of this multi-modality approach is tailored to the site and extent of the primary lesion.

All patients require systemic chemotherapy, usually lasting just under a year. Before treatment, wide, complete resection with an adequate margin of normal tissue is preferred in localized tumors if technically feasible. This is generally more applicable to primaries of the extremities and trunk than the head and neck and is not recommended in tumors arising from the orbit or genitourinary system. For parameningeal tumors with any evidence of having reached the dura (intracranial extension), upfront emergent radiotherapy is warranted. The most common approach for initially unresectable tumors is to begin combination chemotherapy, then undergo local control using radiation with or without additional surgery. The hope is that by shrinking the initial tumor with chemotherapy, the dose of radiotherapy and/or extent of surgical re-excision might be reduced. Whether radiation can be totally eliminated in low-risk, embryonal/botryoidal, Clinical Group I tumors is under evaluation in IRS-V.

11. Which chemotherapy agents are currently used in the treatment of RMS and undifferentiated sarcoma?

The standard regimen used to treat newly diagnosed RMS and undifferentiated sarcoma is vincristine, dactinomycin, and cyclophosphamide (VAC). While ifosfamide, etoposide, doxorubicin and cisplatin have all been show to have clinical efficacy in these diseases, both as single agents and in combination, as yet, no phase III randomized trial incorporating these agents has shown to be superior to VAC after dose intensification of the cyclophosphamide. The current IRS-V trials seek to evaluate the camptothecin derevatives, topotecan and irinotecan, topoisomerase I inhibitors, which have also shown clear anti-RMS activity in pilot and phase I/II clinical studies, to determine whether they offer any additional benefit to VAC. Other effective agents include melphalan and carboplatin.

12. According to the most recent IRS trials, what is the approximate failure-free survival (FFS) and survival by risk group for patients with RMS or undifferentiated sarcoma?

RISK	FFS (%)	SURVIVAL (%)
Low:		
Embryonal histology, Clinical Groups I, II (any site) or III (favorable sites only)	>80 (3 yr)	>90 (3 yr)
Intermediate		
Embryonal,Clinical Group III, unfavorable site	75 (3 yr)	>80 (3 yr)
Alveolar/undifferentiated, Clinical Group I–III	60 (5 yr)	65-80 (3 yr)
Embryonal, Clinical Group IV, age <10	55 (5 yr)	60 (3 yr)
High		
Clinical Group IV, embryonal (age ≥10) or alveolar/ undifferentiated	20 (5 yr)	25 (5 yr)

13. What is the treatment strategy in NRSTS?

Because of the small numbers and varying histologic diagnoses in this family of tumors, there have been very few prospective randomized trials to evaluate treatment strategies in children. The general principles are those extrapolated from single-institution case series and the adult literature.

The traditional approach is wide, surgical resection with the goal of obtaining an adequate margin of normal tissue. The general surgical principles applicable to RMS also apply to NRSTS. Neoadjuvant chemotherapy or preoperative radiation therapy has been utilized with some success in high-grade sarcomas for purposes of less morbid or limb-sparing surgery. External beam radiation is the treatment of choice for residual tumor at the surgical margin. The role of adjuvant chemotherapy in the treatment of NRSTS has yet to be established. In advanced disease, vincristine dactinomycin, cyclophosphamide, ifosfamide, adriamycin and etoposide are clearly active, but the optimal regimen and dose intensity have not been determined.

14. What are the common types of NRSTS, their characteristic presentations, molecular alterations and clinical outcome?

TUMOR TYPE	COMMON PRESENTATION	MOLECULAR CHARACTERISTICS	OUTCOME/SURVIVAL
Fibrosarcoma			
Congenital/infantile	<2yr old; Extremity (70%), trunk (30%) Adolescent; Extremity	t(12;15)(p13;q25) ETV6-NTRK3	Excellent, Surgery 84% (5 yr); 34–60% (5 yr)
Neurofibrosarcoma/ malignant peripheral nerve sheath tumor	Younger in NFI; Extremity (40%), retroperitoneum (25%), trunk (20%)	LOH at 17q11.2	Stage dependent Without NFI, 53%; with NFI, 16%
Synovial sarcoma	Adolescent, young adult: Extremity (lower > upper)	t(X;18)(p11;q11) SYT-SSX1(2)	Stage I or II, 70% Stage III or IV, poor
Malignant fibrous histiocytoma	Rare, 2nd decade of life: Extremity	loss of RB1	27–53% (5 yr)
Angiomatoid form	Young; Extremity		Excellent, Surgery
Hemangiopericytoma	Extremity, head/ neck, retroperitoneum		With adjuvant medication: Stage I, II (30–70%); stage III, IV poor
Adult	Rare: 2nd decade of life		
Congenital	<1 yr old		Excellent; surgery
Alveolar soft part sarcoma	Adolescent, young adult: Extremity (lower > upper), head/ neck	non-reciprocal t(X;17)(p1.2;q25) ASPL-TFE3	27–59% (5 yr) Short-term: good; long-term: poor
Leiomyosarcoma	Immunodeficiency, any age: Gastrointestinal tract, vessels, retroperitoneum		33%; site specific (non-gastrointestinal better; gastrointestinal with frequent metastasis)
Epithelioid form	Stomach: Young girls		Excellent; surgery
Liposarcoma	Two peaks (0-2yr/2nd decade): Extremity, retroperitoneum	t(12;16)(q13;p11) FUS/CHOP (myxoid type)	Very good, rarely metastasize; complete excision

15. What are some possible future directions for the treatment of RMS and NRSTS?

- *Sentinel lymph node mapping*: The injection of radiolabeled tracer and blue dye at the time of surgery to locate and excise nodes potentially involved by lymphatic spread.
- *Brachytherapy*: Catheters placed intra-operatively in the case of positive or questionable surgical margins, which can be "loaded" post-operatively with radioactive isotope for directed local control with reduced toxicity to surrounding tissue.
- *Intraoperative radiation therapy and intensity-modulated radiation therapy*: Novel technology in radiation oncology that may improve local control and minimize damage to normal tissue.
- *High-dose therapy with stem cell rescue*: Of possible utility in metastatic and relapsed RMS, although efficacy and optimal regimen (usually melphalan based) remain highly controversial.
- *Immunotherapy*: Vaccination with fusion-gene peptide products and/or immunomodulators such as interleukin-2 and granulocyte-macrophage colony-stimulating factor.

BIBLIOGRAPHY

1. Baker KS, Anderson JR, Link MP, et al: Benefit of intensified therapy for patients with local or regional embryonal rhabdomyosarcoma: results from the Intergroup Rhabdomyosarcoma Study IV. J Clin Oncol 12:2427–2434, 2000.
2. Crist W, Gehan EA, Ragab AH, et al: The Third Intergroup Rhabdomyosarcoma Study. J Clin Oncol 3:610–630, 1995.
3. Lanzkowsky P: Rhabdomyosarcoma and other soft tissue sarcomas. In Manual of Pediatric Hematology and Oncology, 3rd ed. San Diego, Academic Press, 2000, pp. 527–553.
4. Miser JS, Triche, TJ, Kinsella TJ, Pritchard DJ: Other soft tissue sarcomas of childhood. In Pizzo PA, Poplack DG (eds.). Principles and Practice of Pediatric Oncology, 3rd ed. Philadelphia, Lippincott-Raven, 1997, pp. 865–888.
5. Neville HL, Raney RB, Andrassy RJ, Cooley DA: Multidisciplinary management of pediatric soft-tissue sarcoma. Oncology 10:1471–1481; discussion, 1482–1490, 2000.
6. Pappo AS, Shapiro DN, Christ WM: Rhabdomyosarcoma: Biology and treatment. Pediatr Clin North Am 44:953- 972, 1997.
7. Ruymann FB, Grovas AC: Progress in the diagnosis and treatment of rhabdomyosarcoma and related soft tissue sarcomas. Cancer Invest 3:223–224, 2000.
8. Wexler LH, Helman LJ: Rhabdomyosarcoma and the undifferentiated sarcomas. In Pizzo PA, Poplack DG (eds.). Principles and Practice of Pediatric Oncology, 3rd ed. Philadelphia, Lippincott-Raven, 1997, pp. 799–829.

37. MALIGNANT BONE SARCOMAS: OSTEOSARCOMA AND EWING'S SARCOMA

Linda Granowetter, M.D.

1. What are the most common malignant bone tumors in children, adolescents and young adults?

Osteosarcoma (OS) is the most common bone cancer of children and adolescents. Among patients younger than 16 yr, the incidence of OS is about 3.3 per million per year, and the incidence of Ewing's sarcoma (ES) is about 1.5 per million per year.

Bone cancers comprise about 5% of all malignancies in children and adolescents younger than 16 yr. However, in adolescents as a group, bone cancers are the third most common malignancy, exceeded only by leukemias and lymphomas in incidence.

2. Discuss the most common age of presentation of OS and ES. Are there other important epidemiological factors?

OS is most common during the second decade of life, particularly around the time of the adolescent growth spurt. The median age for female patients is seventeen and for male patients, 20. The incidence rate of OS is 15% higher in U.S. patients of African heritage, compared with white Americans.

ES of bone is also most often a disease of the second decade, but the age range is wider, occurring in patients from about 5–30 yr of age. The female-to-male ratio is slightly increased in preadolescents and is equal in older patients. ES is rare in people of African and Asian heritage.

3. Describe the factors associated with the development of osteosarcoma.

The majority of patients with OS are not known to have any predisposition. However, there are known associations and risk factors:

- OS may occur as a secondary malignancy in irradiated bone.
- OS is one of the tumors seen in the Li-Faumeni familial cancer syndrome. In a retrospective study of pediatric osteosarcoma patients, 3% of the patients were found to carry germline p53 mutations consistent with Li-Fraumeni syndrome.
- Patients with bilateral retinoblastoma have a 10% risk of developing OS during their lifetime.
- Adults with Paget's disease have an increased incidence of OS.

4. Are certain factors associated with an increased risk of developing ES?

ES is very rare in people of African or Asian descent. This epidemiological fact has lead some investigators to wonder if there are specific genetic factors that predispose to, or protect against the development of ES that might be determined by investigating genetic polymorphisms. As we know that almost all ES tumor cells have a translocation involving chromosomes 11 and 22, there may be some constitutional predisposition to the occurrence of this translocation, although studies to date show no overt changes in the germline cells of patients with ES tumors.

5. How do OS and ES present?

Two thirds of OS occur around the knee, the distal femur and the proximal tibia are the most common sites. The proximal femur and lesions of the humerus follow in incidence. Axial lesions are uncommon. The typical presentation is pain, increasing over time and ultimately interfering with normal activities. A mass is often present. The patient is most often without systemic complaints.

In contrast, one third of ES of bone occurs in axial sites; about 20% is in the pelvis. The primary symptom is pain, with or without a visible or palpable mass. Systemic symptoms such as fever, fatigue and weight loss are common. The onset of symptoms may be 3–6 months prior to diagnosis. The axial lesions may present with one of the following constellations of signs and symptoms, often presenting as emergencies:

- Tumors of the rib and chest wall may present with pleural effusion and significant respiratory distress.
- Tumors of the pelvis may present with symptoms such as back pain and pain down the back of the leg or even bowel and bladder dysfunction. These symptoms may be due to sciatic nerve, spinal cord or cauda equina involvement.
- Tumors of the vertebrae and paraspinal tumors may present with clinical signs and symptoms of spinal cord compression such as dysesthesias, extremity weakness and bowel and/or bladder dysfuntion.

6. Describe the natural history of osteosarcoma.

When the primary treatment for osteosarcoma was limited to surgery, usually amputation, 50% of the patients presenting without known metastases would go on to develop pulmonary metastases within 6 months of diagnosis. An additional 30% would later develop metastatic disease in the lungs, bones or, less commonly, the brain. Most patients who developed or presented with metastases succumbed to the disease, although there were reports of patients with resectable pulmonary metastases surviving after aggressive surgery. In the pre-chemotherapy era, the overall survival rate with aggressive surgery of the primary and metastases resulted in survival rate reports of 20–40%.

7. Is it common for osteosarcoma patients to present with metastases?

Approximately 15% of OS patients present with pulmonary metastases and/or bone metastases. Rarely, patients present with multifocal OS, defined as multiple bone lesions in the absence of pulmonary metastases. "Skip" lesions are non-contiguous bone lesions in a single bone. Patients with multifocal OS skip lesions or metastases at diagnosis have a poor prognosis.

8. What is the natural history of ES?

Less than 10% of patient with ES treated in the pre-chemotherapy era survived and it was recognized that metastasis to lung, bone and/or bone marrow occurred rapidly, despite early amputation or irradiation of the involved site. In fact, when James Ewing identified the tumor in 1921, one of the important points in his initial report was that ES could be controlled with radium, unlike OS, which was relatively radiosensitive. The importance of this distinction at that time was that patients with a generally fatal disease—ES—could be spared amputation. Although radiation may still be used to treat the primary tumor, ES is now curable with combined modality therapy.

As many as 20% of ES patients present with metastases to bone, lung and /or bone marrow. The outlook for patients with metastases at diagnosis is extremely poor.

9. What is the current probability of cure for patients with OS and ES?

Multidisciplinary management of bone tumors, particularly the use of neoadjuvant chemotherapy, has resulted in markedly increased survival compared with historical data. At least 75% of patients with nonmetastatic OS are cured. OS patients presenting with metastases are cured less than 20% of the time; however, if fewer than five pulmonary metastases are resected, as many as 40% may be cured with aggressive surgery and chemotherapy. The outlook for patients with bone metastases remains poor.

Two thirds of patients with nonmetastatic ES of bone will be disease-free at 5 yr from diagnosis. Late metastases may occur with ES, so survival rates drop to about 50% at 10 yr. Patients who present with metastases have a disease free survival rate of <20%, despite aggressive therapy.

10. Name the clinical features that predict survival.

For both OS and ES, large-volume tumors and central axis tumors have a less sanguine prognosis. Children younger than10 yr with ES do better than older patients. At one time it was believed that younger patients with OS fared poorly; however, this is now not thought to be true. For both tumors, the extent of tumor necrosis in the primary tumor after initial chemotherapy is predictive of survival.

Currently, there is intensive investigation of molecular markers of these tumors, and there is preliminary evidence that the molecular phenotype of ES may help predict survival. There is extensive study of the molecular aberrations associated with OS as well. This will be further discussed later.

11. How does one make the diagnosis of a malignant bone tumor?

If the clinical presentation suggests a bone tumor, the first step is a radiograph of the affected bone. OS of long bones is most often involves the metaphysis, and the radiograph will show osteoblastic activity, as well as new bone formation. Commonly, one sees diffuse lines of calcification emanating from the periosteum called a sunburst, or a Codman's triangle, a lifting of the cortex. ES of the long bones involves the diaphysis, the bone most often appears moth-eaten, and there may be an onion skin appearance of the periosteum.

If the plain radiographs are suggestive of a malignant bone tumor, magnetic resonance imaging of the involved bone and a radionuclide (technetium) bone scan are indicated to better define the primary lesion and rule out skip lesions or distant bone metastases. The diagnosis must always be determined with a biopsy of the lesion.

12. What must be taken into consideration when planning a biopsy of a suspected bone malignancy?

State-of-the-art orthopedic surgery for malignant bone lesions generally involves a form of limb preserving surgery. Thus, it is essential that the biopsy be performed by an orthopedic surgeon able to perform limb preservation surgery so that the incision is placed in a site that will be excised at the time of definitive surgery. A horizontal incision that crosses fascial planes may spread tumor and may limit the patient's options for limb preservation.

It is also essential that the oncologist and pathologist coordinate plans with the surgeon prior to the biopsy to ensure that the tissue is handled appropriately. In addition to standard light microscopy studies and immunohistochemistry, it is essential to procure fresh tissue for cytogenetic studies and perform polymerase chain reaction or fluorescent in situ hybridization (FISH) reaction examination for molecular markers. Tissue may be required for an evolving set of biological investigations.

Occasionally, the diagnosis of a bone tumor is possible through the use of multiple needle biopsy specimens; however, it is often not possible to obtain sufficient tumor for all required studies. Most institutions do not rely solely on molecular diagnosis and require tissue for the full battery of immunohistochemical studies in addition to standard light microscopy. Further, the molecular diagnosis and evaluation of these tumors is in evolution. Thus, it is most often necessary to perform an open biopsy to procure adequate study for complete biologic studies.

If there is a very high probability of documenting malignancy, consideration should be given to placing a central venous catheter at the time of the biopsy to facilitate therapy. If ES is suspected, the staging bone marrow aspirate and biopsy may be done at the time of the biopsy as well.

13. Discuss the studies for molecular markers and biologic studies that are done on the fresh tissue.

Virtually all ES tumors have an 11;22(q24;q12) translocation or a related variant. The breakpoints identified join the *EWS* gene found on chromosome 22 to the *FLI* gene on chromosome 11, a known transcription factor. Further study has demonstrated that there are differing specific breakpoints, involving differing introns and exons. Preliminary data indicate that the specific site of the breakpoint may result in tumors with differing prognoses. Although these data are not currently mature enough to translate into the delineation of different treatments based on the molecular phenotype, the future of treatment may be tied more directly to molecular diagnosis.

OSs do not have a unifying genetic aberration. OS cells are often aneuploid, or have a variety of chromosomal aberrations. The specific chromosomal loci thought to be involved in the genesis of OS has not been worked out completely, but it is known that nonrandom changes may be seen at chromosome 13q14 and 17p13, sites that contain the retinoblastoma and p53 tumor suppressor genes.

14. What is the ES family of tumors?

Although the subject of this chapter is bone tumors, it should be noted that 20% of Ewing tumors occur in soft tissue. In addition, tumors called peripheral primitive neuroectodermal (PNET) tumors are related to Ewing tumors. PNET tumors also demonstrate the 11;22 translocation or a variant. They are Ewing-like tumors with some degree of neural differentiation. Thus, the ES family of tumors comprise ES and PNET tumors of bone or soft tissue. The derivation of this family of tumors appears to be neuroectodermal. The treatment of ES and PNET of bone and soft tissue is the same.

15. How are the bone tumors staged?

Staging is a reflection of natural history and known sites of metastases. Therefore, patients with OS should have a chest computed tomograph (contrast is not required due to the radio-opaque quality of the tumor) and a technetium bone scan to complete staging. ES patients require chest computed tomography, bone scan and bone marrow aspirate and biopsy. For both tumors, the patients are generally classified as metastatic versus nonmetastatic. Position emission tomography and thallium scanning are used at some centers at the time of diagnosis, so that they may be repeated after initial chemotherapy to help evaluate the response to initial therapy.

16. Discuss any blood tests essential in the evaluation of OS and ES.

The alkaline phosphatase is often elevated in OS, and when elevated the decline after therapy is indicative of the response to therapy. In both OS and ES, the lactate dehydrogenase may be elevated. Patients with ES and bone marrow involvement may have anemia but rarely present with other hematological abnormalities.

The renal and hepatic chemical profiles are generally normal in patients with OS and ES; however, as chemotherapeutic agents may affect renal and liver function, these examinations are required prior to beginning therapy.

17. Describe neoadjuvant chemotherapy.

Neoadjuvant chemotherapy is therapy given prior to resection of the primary tumor.

Neoadjuvant therapy allows treatment of micrometastases to begin immediately, generally facilitates surgery and allows the oncologist to determine the in vivo sensitivity of the tumor to the chemotherapeutic agents employed. For OS and ES, the duration of neoadjuvant therapy is generally 2–3 months

18. What is local control?

Local control is the eradication of the primary tumor. For OS, the preferred method of local control is always surgery, as the tumor is relatively radioinsensitive. For ES, local control may be surgery, radiation therapy or both. Although there is a trend toward better survival when surgery is employed for local control for ES, this seems to reflect the fact that smaller, more accessible tumors are most often treated surgically. Surgery is often considered preferable, because radiotherapy has adverse effects on bone and soft tissue growth and incurs the risk of a radiation-induced malignancy. For each patient, a decision on the best way to eradicate the tumor must be made based on the tumor's location, size, response to treatment, the patient's age and growth potential and potential functional and cosmetic results.

There are many options for limb preservation, including replacement of the bone with a titanium rod, expandable internal prosthesis, bone allografts from bone banks, or autografts. It is imperative that the patient and family are aware of choices, but the patient, family and physicians must always remember that the eradication of tumor is paramount. If amputation is required, it should be remembered that functional outcomes with external prostheses are generally very good and for some patients are better than one would expect after limb-preserving surgery.

19. What chemotherapy is used to treat ES and OS?

A high-dose regimen of methotrexate, cisplatin and doxorubicin has been the backbone of treatment of osteosarcoma. Recently, a national trial to determine if ifosfamide and/or MTP-PE, a monocyte activator that works as a biologic response modifier, added to the standard three drugs improves survival. The data are too new for complete analysis at this time.

Vincristine, cyclophosphamide and doxorubicin, alternating with ifosfamide and etoposide, are considered the agents of choice for ES tumors. A national study comparing these agents given in standard doses to the same agents given in a dose-intensified plan is closed to accrual, and results will be available in the near future.

For both OS and ES, neoadjuvant therapy is followed by local control measures. After local control has been accomplished, chemotherapy continues, depending on the regimen employed, for 4–10 months

20. What about very–high-dose therapy with stem cell or bone marrow transplantation?

There have been multiple reports of high dose chemotherapy followed by autologous transplant for the treatment for either metastatic, relapsed or high-risk (bulky, pelvic tumors) ES. Although some reports have seemed promising, the overall data from the European Transplant Consortium show no better overall survival with transplant than with other multimodality programs. Research in the area continues, and there is some interest in autotranplant programs combined with regimens to induce autologous anti-tumor cells. For OS, there is no significant evidence favoring transplantation over standard chemotherapy programs.

21. Discuss the late effects or complications of therapy for OS and ES.

The chemotherapeutic agents most often employed in the treatment of these tumors may result in the following late effects:

- Ifosfamide and less commonly, cisplatin may result in infertility in male patients and early menopause and decreased fertility in women. Men are advised to bank sperm prior to the initiation of therapy.

- Doxorubicin may affect myocardial function. Echocardiograms are examined during and after therapy with doxorubicin. Some treatment centers offer therapy with dexrazoxane, a cardioprotectant. Most limit the total cumulative dose of the doxorubicin.
- Cisplatin may cause renal dysfunction, including magnesium wasting.
- Cisplatin may cause hearing loss, particularly in the high frequencies.
- Methotrexate may affect kidney or liver function; however, significant permanent effects due to methotrexate are uncommon.
- Second malignancies, including brain tumors and leukemias, have been reported in survivors of OS about 2–3% of the time. These secondary cancers may be due to the treatment or, more likely, an interaction between the treatment and predisposing factors. Second malignancies outside of radiation fields occur in ES survivors as well. OS as a second cancer in ES patients treated with radiation has been reported in 4–30% of survivors, depending on the series reported.

The most important late effect to be considered is cure: Despite the risk of the significant late effects listed here, the majority of ES and OS survivors go on to enjoy normal lives.

38. GERM CELL TUMORS

Gustavo del Toro, M.D.

1. Describe the classification of Germ Cell Tumors (GCT).

- Teratoma
  - Mature teratoma
  - Immature teratoma
  - Malignant teratoma
- Germinoma
  - Seminoma: testicular germinoma
  - Dysgerminoma: ovarian germinoma
  - Germinoma
- Embryonal carcinoma
- Yolk sac tumor: endodermal sinus tumor
- Choriocarcinoma
- Gonadoblastoma
- Polyembryoma

2. Where are germ cell tumors usually located?

Germ cell tumors (GCTs)can be divided into two main categories: gonadal (ovary/testicle) and extragonadal. The most common extragonadal locations are the anterior mediastinum, the brain, and the sacrococcygeal area. Fifty percent of GCTs are gonadal, 25% are sacrococcygeal, and 20% are found in the central nervous system.

3. Describe the tumor markers that are secreted by GCTs.

The most common serum tumor markers secreted by GCTs are alpha-fetoprotein (AFP), beta-human chorionic gonadotropin (bhCG), lactic dehydrogenase-1 (LDH1), and placental alkaline phosphatase (PLAP). The level of the tumor maker in the serum correlates with tumor burden.

Yolk Sac Tumor	AFP
Embryonal Carcinoma	AFP
Choriocarcinoma	bhCG
Germinoma	bhCG
Polyembryoma	AFP
	bhCG
Dysgerminoma	LDH1
Seminoma	PLAP

4. Describe the clinical presentation of GCTs.

The clinical presentation of GCTs depends on the site of origin and the size of the primary tumor:

- Ovarian tumors: The most frequent presenting signs and symptoms of ovarian GCTs include an abdominal or pelvic mass, abdominal distention, and acute or chronic abdominal pain. Less commonly, patients may present with precocious puberty, constipation, enuresis, amenorrhea, vaginal bleeding, and torsion of the affected ovary.
- Testicular tumors: Testicular tumors usually present as painless scrotal masses.

Twenty percent of testicular GCTs are accompanied by testicular hydroceles or inguinal hernias.

- Sacrococcygeal tumors: Sacrococcygeal tumors present as a presacral mass that may extend into the abdomen or buttocks. Urinary frequency, constipation, and leg weakness are other possible signs.
- Mediastinal tumors: Mediastinal GCTs are usually asymptomatic in adolescents. However, in infants, severe cough, dyspnea, and hemoptysis are the common presenting symptoms. The usual location is the anterior mediastinum.
- Intracranial tumors: GCTs of the central nervous system may present with visual disturbances, nystagmus, Parinaud's syndrome, diabetes insipidus, anorexia, precocious puberty, and signs of increased intracranial pressure, such as headaches, nausea, and vomiting.

5. What is the relationship between cryptorchidism in male infants and children and GCTs?

Patients with cryptorchidism have a 30-fold increased risk of developing testicular cancer. The testicular cancer is most likely to develop between the ages of 30 and 50 yr. These tumors are usually GCTs—seminomas or embryonal carcinomas.

6. Describe the surgical management of sacrococcygeal GCTs.

The surgical management of sacrococcygeal GCTs must incorporate total excision of the coccyx. The risk of recurrence is 40% in patients in whom the coccyx is not removed.

7. GCTs in infants are different than GCTs in adolescents. Describe the major age-dependent differences.

GERM CELL TUMOR	INFANT	ADOLESCENT
Yolk-sac tumor	Common	Rare
Seminoma	Rare	Common
Extragonadal location	Common	Rare
Isochromosome 12p	Absent	Common

8. What is the most common ovarian GCT in pediatric and adolescent patients?

Mature cystic teratoma of the ovary is the most frequent GCT diagnosed. It is often cystic, it occurs at a median age of 13 yr, and approximately 10% of the cases are bilateral. Most patients present without significant symptoms, and 90% of mature ovarian teratomas have neither cytogenetic nor molecular abnormalities.

9. What is the most common testicular tumor in pediatrics?

Yolk sac or endodermal sinus tumor of the testis is the most frequently diagnosed testicular tumor. It occurs at a median age of 2 yr, is highly malignant, and is often metastatic to retroperitoneal lymph nodes. AFP is elevated in the majority of cases and serves as a serum marker of disease activity. An abnormality of chromosome 1 is appreciated in approximately 90% of cases. Treatment is surgical extirpation from an inguinal approach and must include a lymph node dissection; postoperative chemotherapy is often necessary.

10. Which characteristics define high-risk GCTs?

In general, GCTs of childhood have a relatively high cure rate; however, certain characteristics exist at the time of diagnosis that may correlate directly with an unfavorable outcome. The factors that may predict a poor prognosis include

- Bulky tumors that are unresectable at the time of initial surgery
- Tumors of extragonadal origin
- Tumors that histologically have a high mitotic rate and contain neuroepithelial elements
- GCTs with elevated serum tumor markers that do not decline to normal levels after surgery and chemotherapy
- The presence of lymph node involvement and distant parenchymal involvement at diagnosis

11. Why must one use caution when using AFP as a serum tumor marker?

Normal, healthy infants may have elevated serum AFP levels until 8–9 months of life. Thus, the use of AFP as a marker of disease status in this age group may be confusing. In addition, AFP has a serum half-life of approximately 8-10 days; this has to be taken into consideration when assessing the effectiveness of surgical tumor removal or chemotherapy—a persistently elevated AFP after surgery may just be due to the expected, slow drop in the AFP.

12. Does radiation therapy have a role in the management of GCTs?

Radiation therapy is the treatment of choice for central nervous system germinomas. However, although other gonadal and extragonadal GCTs may respond to high-dose radiation therapy, this treatment is not part of the initial therapeutic plan. Thus, radiation therapy is not used as first-line management.

13. Name the GCT most likely to be misdiagnosed as an ectopic pregnancy.

Choriocarcinoma. Choriocarcinomas secrete large amounts of bhCG. An ovarian choriocarcinoma can present as a pelvic / abdominal mass with a high serum level of hCG.

14. What are the most effective chemotherapy agents in the treatment of GCTs?

Cisplatin, bleomycin, and etoposide are the three standard drugs used to treat malignant GCTs. Carboplatin is effective in GCTs of the central nervous system. The standard treatment for non-central nervous system malignant GCTs involves four to six cycles of bleomycin, etoposide, and cisplatin. This combination is commonly known as "BEP" (**B**leo., **E**topo., cis**P**lat.).

CONTROVERSY

15. It is well established that mature teratomas are benign tumors and that malignant teratomas require full use of chemotherapy. However, immature teratomas present a dilemma. These tumors do not express any truly malignant tissues, but do express immature and neuroectodermal elements that are thought to warrant chemotherapy by some experts.

BIBLIOGRAPHY

1. Castleberry RP,. et al. Germ cell tumors. In PizzoPA, Poplack DG (eds): Principles and Practice of Pediatric Oncology. Philadelphia, Lippincott-Raven, 1997, pp 921– 946.
2. Pinkerton CR. Malignant germ cell tumours. In Pinkerton CR, Michalski AJ, Veys PA (eds): Cinical Challenges in Paediatric Oncology. Oxford, Isis Medical Media, 1999, pp 163–172.
3. Pinkerton CR. Malignant germ cell tumours. In Pinkerton CR, PlowmanPN: Paediatric Oncology Clinical Practice and Controversies. London, Chapman & Hall, 1997, pp 507–522.

39. CLINICAL EMERGENCIES IN CHILDREN WITH CANCER

Kara M. Kelly, M.D.

1. What organs are most affected by leukemia-associated hyperleukocytosis?

The intracerebral and pulmonary circulations. Patients may be asymptomatic or present with frontal headaches, seizures, mental status changes, weakness, papilledema or retinal venous distension. Long-term sequelae of cerebral vascular infarction are potential risks. Pulmonary leukocytosis may be associated with shortness of breath, hypoxemia and failure of the right side of the heart. Life-threatening cardiorespiratory failure may result, analogous to the situation seen with acute chest syndrome in sickle cell anemia.

2. Tumor lysis syndrome may develop with which tumors?

Most often in Burkitt's lymphoma and T-cell acute lymphoblastic leukemia, both of which are associated with a large tumor burden and high sensitivity to chemotherapy. Risk factors include bulky abdominal disease, elevated pretreatment serum uric acid and lactate dehydrogenase levels and poor urine output. The risk of renal failure is exacerbated in the setting of renal parenchymal tumor infiltration or tumor-induced ureteral or venous compression. More rarely, tumor lysis syndrome may be seen with hepatoblastoma or stage-IVS neuroblastoma. Tumor lysis syndrome typically occurs before initiation of therapy or up to 5 days after the start of cytotoxic therapy.

3. What is the management of tumor lysis syndrome?

Treatment is largely preventative. Laboratory evaluation involves frequent assessment of serum sodium, potassium, chloride, bicarbonate, calcium, phosphorus, uric acid, blood urea nitrogen and creatinine. Complete blood counts are useful as a marker of tumor burden. Ultrasonography of the kidneys may aid in revealing tumor infiltration of the kidneys or hydronephrosis. An electrocardiogram (ECG) should be ordered if the serum potassium is > 7.0 mEq/L. Vigorous hydration is essential. The addition of sodium bicarbonate to the intravenous fluids enhances excretion of uric acid, although overalkalinization may aggravate symptoms of hypocalcemia by shifting calcium to its nonionized form. Allopurinol or urate oxidase is employed to enhance uric acid excretion. Phosphate binders help to aid phosphate excretion. However, when conservative measures are ineffective in correcting electrolyte disturbances and improving urinary flow, short-term hemodialysis may be necessary.

4. What are the signs and symptoms of spinal cord compression?

Back pain is the most common symptom, occurring in 80% of children with spinal cord compression. Back pain may occur at any level of the spine, and movement, straight-leg raising, neck flexion or the Valsalva maneuver may worsen it. Weakness that may lead to partial or complete paralysis and incontinence tend to develop later in the course if the symptoms persist and continue to elude diagnosis. Sensory deficits may also occur but are difficult to elicit, especially in younger children.

5. Describe the signs and symptoms of the superior vena cava (SVC) syndrome.

The SVC syndrome is a clinical phenomenon that develops when a mass lesion obstructs the blood flow through the SVC. Collateral veins of the thorax, neck and head engorge and produce the classic symptoms that include the following:

- Dyspnea
- Fullness and plethora of the face, head and upper extremities
- Periorbital edema
- Dysphagia
- Chest pain

Frequently in children with a mediastinal mass lesion respiratory symptoms and compromise predominate; in fact, the term *superior mediastinal syndrome* has been used to describe the entity in pediatric and adolescent patients.

The severity of the symptoms is directly proportional to the rapidity of the SVC obstruction. The more acute the onset of the SVC obstruction, the more significant the signs and symptoms present and the more imperative it is to initiate lifesaving therapy. The patient should be treated empirically with high-dose glucocorticoids and/or radiotherapy, and the biopsy to confirm the diagnosis should be delayed until it can be performed safely.

6. What are the most common causes of the SVC syndrome?

Malignant tumors. The “terrible Ts”—T-cell non-Hodgkin’s lymphoma (lymphoblastic lymphoma or large cell lymphoma), T-cell acute lymphoblastic leukemia, malignant teratoma, thyroid cancer and thymoma—may all cause this syndrome. Hodgkin’s disease is not infrequently associated with SVC syndrome, whereas neuroblastoma, rhabdomyosarcoma and Ewing’s sarcoma are rare causes. Occlusion of a central venous catheter in a child with cancer may cause a secondary form of SVC syndrome.

7. What is the most appropriate diagnostic work-up of a patient presenting with a mediastinal mass?

The diagnostic work-up should begin with the least-invasive procedure, as children with anterior mediastinal masses are at particular risk for respiratory failure or circulatory collapse during general anesthesia. Bone marrow aspiration, pleurocentesis, pericardiocentesis or lymph node biopsy with local anesthesia may be diagnostic. Fine needle cytologic aspiration under computerized tomography (CT) or fluoroscopic guidance also may be of benefit. Measurement of the serum markers, beta human chorionic gonadotrophin or alpha-fetoprotein may lead to the diagnosis of a germ cell tumor. If these measures are not possible, the risk associated with induction of anesthesia should be assessed with pulmonary function tests, CT scan, ECG and echocardiogram. If, for example, pulmonary function tests show the tracheal area and peak expiratory flow rates to be < 50% predicted or the echocardiogram shows impaired venous return, general anesthesia should not be given.

8. Discuss the leading diagnosis and management of right lower quadrant abdominal pain in a neutropenic child.

Typhlitis, or necrotizing colitis of the cecum, is a major concern in a child with prolonged, severe neutropenia (absolute neutrophil count < 200) who presents with localized right lower-quadrant abdominal pain. Bacterial invasion of the mucosa may progress from inflammation to infarction and perforation. *Clostridium septicum* and *Pseudomonas aeruginosa* are most often involved. Children with acute myeloid leukemia are most at risk because of the prolonged neutropenic phase and the common use of chemotherapeutic regimens that are toxic to the gastrointestinal tract. CT scan may reveal thickening of the cecal wall or in advanced cases, pneumatosis intestinalis. Treatment is primarily supportive with antibiotic coverage for gram-negative and anaerobic organisms; however, a surgical consult should be requested as some patients may require surgical intervention.

9. Which chemotherapeutic agents are associated with a risk of acute cerebral infarctions?

L-asparaginase can cause either cerebral vascular hemorrhage or thrombosis as a result of its inhibition of synthesis of coagulation factors. Cisplatin can lead to cerebral ischemia from renal wasting of solutes with subsequent hypomagnesemic arterial spasm or direct thrombotic endothelial injury. Methotrexate, after either high dose intravenous or intrathecal administration, may also lead to cerebral infarction, either from direct vascular injury or from an embolic effect. In a series of pediatric patients with acute cerebral infarctions, 30% were directly related to chemotherapy.

10. Hypercalcemia may be encountered with which pediatric malignancies?

Hypercalcemia of malignancy (HCM) is the most common paraneoplastic syndrome in adult patients with cancer; however, it is quite rare in children with cancer, with an incidence of only 0.4–0.7%. When seen, it is most often observed in children with acute lymphoblastic leukemia or the alveolar subtype of rhabdomyosarcoma. It has also been associated with rhabdoid tumor, hepatoblastoma, Hodgkin's disease, non-Hodgkin's lymphoma, acute myeloid leukemia, brain tumors, neuroblastoma, angiosarcoma and malignant tumor of unknown origin.

HCM is diagnosed when the serum calcium levels exceed normal parameters. In the past, the etiology of HCM was thought to be related to the release of calcium by bone osteoclasts after its invasion and destruction by cancer cells. Recently, however, parathyroid hormone-related protein (PTH-rP), a substance secreted or mediated by cancer cells, has been identified. PTH-rP regulates calcium levels, but it is not regulated by the normal feedback mechanisms that suppress parathyroid hormone in the face of hypercalcemia. Additional factors that may play a role in HCM are osteoclast-activating factors, transforming growth factors and prostaglandins. Other conditions that contribute to the development of HCM include immobilization, thiazide diuretics, androgens and estrogens.

11. Describe the signs and symptoms of hypercalcemia associated with malignancy.

Calcium is essential in the formation of bones and teeth, contractility of muscle cells, nerve conduction, hemostasis, granulocyte chemotaxis and cardiac automaticity. Thus, the symptoms of HCM are varied and may involve multiple organ systems. The most common signs and symptoms include

- Psycho-emotional: lethargy, confusion, somnolence, depression
- Neurological: weakness, visual disturbance, hyporeflexia
- Cardiovascular: hypertension, bradycardia, arrhythmias, cardiac arrest
- Musculoskeletal: bone pain, pathologic fractures
- Metabolic: polyuria, nocturia, dehydration, azotemia, alkalosis, renal failure
- Gastrointestinal: anorexia, nausea, vomiting, constipation, ileus
- Miscellaneous: ectopic calcification, pruritus, hypercoagulopathy

12. What are the causes of shock in the child with cancer?

Shock is often related to hypovolemia. The most common etiologies include sepsis and hemorrhage. With respect to the latter, hemorrhage may be secondary to either gastrointestinal problems from *Clostridium difficile* infection or typhlitis, or pulmonary problems from *Aspergillus* infection or direct tumor invasion. Distributive shock results when there is abnormal distribution of blood volume and is most often seen with anaphylaxis or sepsis. Cardiogenic shock is less frequent but may be observed in children who have received high dose anthracycline therapy with or without cardiac irradiation or following high-dose cyclophosphamide therapy, especially in the setting of stem cell transplantation. The following outline (modified with permission from Pizzo PA, Poplack DG: Principles and Practice of Pediatric Oncology, 3rd ed. Philadelphia, Lippincott-Raven Publishers, 1997, p 1045) describes the common causes of shock in children with cancer:

1. Hypovolemic
   - Sepsis
   - Hemorrhage: bladder, (drug, adenovirus), intestinal (typhlitis, *Clostridium difficile*), hemoptysis (infection, tumor)
   - Intractable emesis
   - Pancreatitis: L-asparaginase, glucocorticoids
   - Addisonian crisis
   - Diabetes mellitus
   - Hypercalcemia
2. Distributive
   - Anaphylaxis: etoposide, teniposide, carboplatin, L-asparaginase, cytosine arabinoside, amphotericin B, blood products, gammaglobulin, interleukin-2, tumor necrosis factor
   - Sepsis
   - Veno-occlusive disease
   - Syndrome of inappropriate antidiuretic hormone
3. Cardiogenic
   - Treatment-related: anthracyclines, cyclophosphamide, radiation therapy
   - Cardiac tamponade: intracardiac tumor, intracardiac thrombus, pericardial effusion, pericarditis
   - Myocarditis: bacterial, viral, fungal
   - Metabolic: hyperkalemia, hypokalemia, hypocalcemia

BIBLIOGRAPHY

1. Kelly KM, Lange B: Oncologic emergencies. Pediatr Clin North Am 44:809–830, 1997.
2. Lange B, O'Neill JA Jr, Goldwein JW, et al: Oncologic emergencies. In Pizzo PA, Poplack DG: Principles and Practice of Pediatric Oncology, 3rd ed. Philadelphia, Lippincott-Raven Publishers, 1997, pp 1025–1049.

40. PERIPHERAL BLOOD AND BONE MARROW TRANSPLANTS

M. *Brigid Bradley*, M.D.

1. When are autologous and allogeneic stem cell transplants performed?

Autologous transplants are used to restore bone marrow function in patients receiving myeloablative doses of therapy for malignancies. Autografts are used mainly in the treatment of solid tumors where increasing dose intensity is the major aim. Some investigators are using autologous transplants for the treatment of autoimmune disorders.

Allogeneic transplants are used to replace abnormal or malignant hematopoiesis or immune systems with normal hematological and immune cells from a healthy donor. Allogeneic transplant is favored in diseases where graft-versus-tumor reactions is desirable. Allografts may also benefit patients with hematological malignancies, aplastic anemia, congenital bone marrow disorders, hemoglobinopathies, immune deficiency states and some inborn errors of metabolism.

2. Why is human leukocyte antigen (HLA) typing done and what is its importance when choosing an allogeneic stem cell donor?

The immunologic relationship between the donor and recipient influences the outcome of a hematopoietic stem cell transplant. The major histocompatability complex (MHC) molecules are the HLAs. There are two classes of MHC molecules: the HLA class I and class II antigens. HLA typing is an important variable when choosing a donor for transplant.

The HLA antigens are encoded by genes located on chromosome six. Three loci are classically screened when the donor and recipient are typed. These loci have been identified to be important in stimulating immune reactions in hematopoietic stem cell transplantation. They are HLA class IA and B and HLA class II DRB1. There is evidence to show that matching at the HLA class IC locus is also important.

HLA matching benefits all allogeneic transplants. Graft rejection and risk of graft versus-host-disease (GVHD) correlate with the degree of HLA matching. The ideal donor is an HLA-identical sibling. If one is not available, alternative donors can be used. One antigen–mismatched family member, one antigen–mismatched unrelated donor or one or two antigen–mismatch cord blood donor sources are also used with success. If the disparity of typing is more than this, graft manipulation with T cell depletion is often employed to decrease the risk of rejection and GVHD.

3. What are the sources of stem cells used in hematopoietic stem cell transplantation?

Stem cells can be isolated from the bone marrow, mobilized peripheral blood products or cord blood.

4. What is the advantage of using mobilized peripheral blood stem cells rather than bone marrow as a source for hematopoietic reconstitution?

Mobilized peripheral blood stem cells (PBSCs) have essentially replaced bone marrow as a source of autologous stem cells. PBSCs are also being used more frequently for allogeneic stem cell transplants. The use of mobilized PBSCs has resulted in a decreased duration of neutropenia, more rapid immune reconstitution and decreased duration of platelet transfusion dependence. A PBSC transplant typically results in myeloid engraftment (absolute neutrophil count [ANC] > .5 x 109/L) by day 11–14. With a standard bone marrow transplant, myeloid engraftment is typically not seen until day 20–24.

Although PBSCs have been used in allogeneic transplantation for a shorter duration, studies to date show, despite a higher T cell number in the PBSC graft, there is no increased incidence of acute GVHD. There are reports of an increased incidence of chronic GVHD when mobilized PBSC are used, but further investigation is needed. There is belief that the higher T cell number in the PBSC graft may also result in an increased graft-versus-tumor effect, resulting in a decreased relapse rate.

5. Describe the methods used to mobilize peripheral blood progenitor cells (PBPCs).

Hematopoietic progenitor cells and stem cells reside in the bone marrow under steady-state conditions. The frequency of these cells is 2/100,000 peripheral blood mononuclear cells. Mobilization of the progenitor cells from the marrow into the peripheral circulation can be approached in three ways:

- Collection of PBPC during the recovery phase after myelosuppressive chemotherapy
- Collection of PBPC after the administration of hematopoietic growth factors such as granulocyte colony–stimulating factor (G-CSF) or granulocyte-macrophage colony–stimulating factor (GM-CSF)
- Collection of PBPC after the combination of chemotherapy followed by growth factors

The combined use of myelosuppressive chemotherapy with G-CSF or GM-CSF enhances the mobilization of CD34+ PBPC up to 1000-fold when compared with mobilization with growth factors alone.

Cyclophosphamide has been used most frequently in combination with G-CSF or GM-CSF for PBPC mobilization. However, a large number of mobilizing chemotherapy regimens have been developed, most are disease specific and none has been found to be superior to the other regimens.

6. What is the goal of the preparative regimen for stem cell transplantation?

Treatment regimens must accomplish two goals, depending on the patient's disease and the source of stem cells. First, for transplants performed for the treatment of a malignant disease, the regimen must provide tumor cytoreduction and disease eradication. Second, for allogeneic transplants, the regimen also must be sufficiently immunosuppressive to overcome host rejection of the donor stem cells.

7. What is veno-occlusive disease (VOD) of the liver? How is it diagnosed and how is it managed?

A complication related to the chemotherapy and radiotherapy utilized in both autologous and allogeneic transplants. It develops in 10–60% of patients during the first few weeks after transplant. Predisposing conditions that place a patient at increased risk of developing VOD include inflammatory hepatitis, bacterial or viral infection prior to transplant, previous radiation therapy to the liver and a previous history of stem cell transplant.

Pathophysiologically, occlusions develop in the small hepatic venules and the small endothelium-lined pores that connect the sinusoids to the hepatic venules. Subsequently, obliteration of the venules and fibrosis of the sinusoids occurs. A diagnostic hepatic ultrasound may show a reversal of portal venous flow in advanced disease. A liver biopsy is diagnostic but poses a risk when performed in a severely thrombocytopenic patient.

VOD is a clinical diagnosis of jaundice, weight gain, ascites and painful hepatomegaly. Clinical features vary according to the severity of disease. Mild VOD may be clinically detected but resolves completely without treatment. Moderate disease involves signs and symptoms that require supportive care measures, such as diuretics and pain management, but resolves completely. Severe VOD is observed in patients with poor prognostic signs, such as refractoriness to platelet transfusions and serum transaminases greater than five times normal; despite therapeutic intervention, severe VOD has significant morbidity and mortality. Overall, 70% of patients with VOD recover spontaneously; the treatment is primarily supportive. Therapeutic interventions such as anticoagulation and thrombolytic therapies have been investigated, but to date these interventions do not provide therapeutic benefit.

8. What is GVHD? How is it prevented? How is it treated? Describe the long-term complications that can result from GVHD.

GVHD is a major risk in allogeneic stem cell transplantation and contributes significantly to its morbidity and mortality. GVHD occurs when immunocompetant cells from the donor graft recognize antigenic differences expressed by tissues and cells of the recipient. The HLA antigens are primarily involved in triggering this response. Both acute and chronic forms of this disorder exist. There are three requirements for acute GVHD to occur:

- The graft must contain immunologically competent cells
- The recipient must express tissue antigens not present in the donor
- The host must be incapable of mounting an effective immunological reaction against the donor cells

The target organs of acute GVHD are classically the skin, liver and gastrointestinal tract, although other organs can be involved. GVHD of the skin manifests as a fine maculopapular rash that can progress to generalized erythroderma with bullae formation in more severe cases. Liver involvement is manifested by a rise in the bilirubin and transaminases and painless hepatomegaly. Gastrointestinal tract symptoms include diarrhea, gastrointestinal bleeding, crampy abdominal pain and ileus.

Eliminating or blocking donor T-cell function can prevent acute GVHD. T cell depleting the donor graft by various methods reduces the risk of GVHD; however, manipulating the graft in this manner increases the risk of graft rejection and relapse of malignant disease. Another approach is the use of immunosuppressive drugs such as methotrexate, cyclosporin, cyclophosphamide, steroids, total lymphoid irradiation, anti-thymocyte globulin (ATG), FK506 and mycophenolate mofetil alone or in combination to help prevent acute GVHD. Effective supportive care, protective isolation and the administration of intravenous immunoglobulin can also contribute to a lower incidence of GVHD. The treatment of acute GVHD includes high-dose steroids. In steroid refractory disease, ATG and monoclonal antibodies may be effective in the treatment of steroid-refractory AGVHD.

Chronic GVHD classically presents beyond 100 days after allogeneic transplant. There is no standard classification for this disorder. It can evolve in a patient with acute GVHD or in patients with no history of acute GVHD. It can be limited to only the skin or be extensive, affecting multiple organ systems. Skin involvement shows sclerodermatous changes resulting in contractures. Hair loss keratoconjunctivitis and xerostomia can develop. Patients can develop chronic obstructive pulmonary disease with bronchiolitis obliterans that may be associated with an increased risk of chronic pulmonary infections. Chronic cholestasis and decreased gastrointestinal motility and absorption are also seen. Profound immune deficiency and pancytopenia can also occur. All of these symptoms can significantly affect a patient's quality of life after transplant. Imuran and thalidomide have both been used in the treatment of chronic GVHD.

9. What is a placental cord blood transplant?

Placental cord blood has become a widely accepted source of hematopoietic stem cells. Initially, placental cord blood was obtained from siblings, but now unrelated donor transplants are done using placental hematopoietic stem cells. Allogeneic stem cell transplants using cord blood stem cells have been performed, and results confirm that stable engraftment can be achieved. There is a decreased risk of acute and chronic GVHI, allowing for increased HLA disparity between the donor and recipient. Despite the decreased incidence of GVHD, reports show there is no increased incidence of relapse in patients with leukemia and lymphoma who underwent transplant using cord blood stem cells.

10. Describe viral and bacterial complications of stem cell transplant.

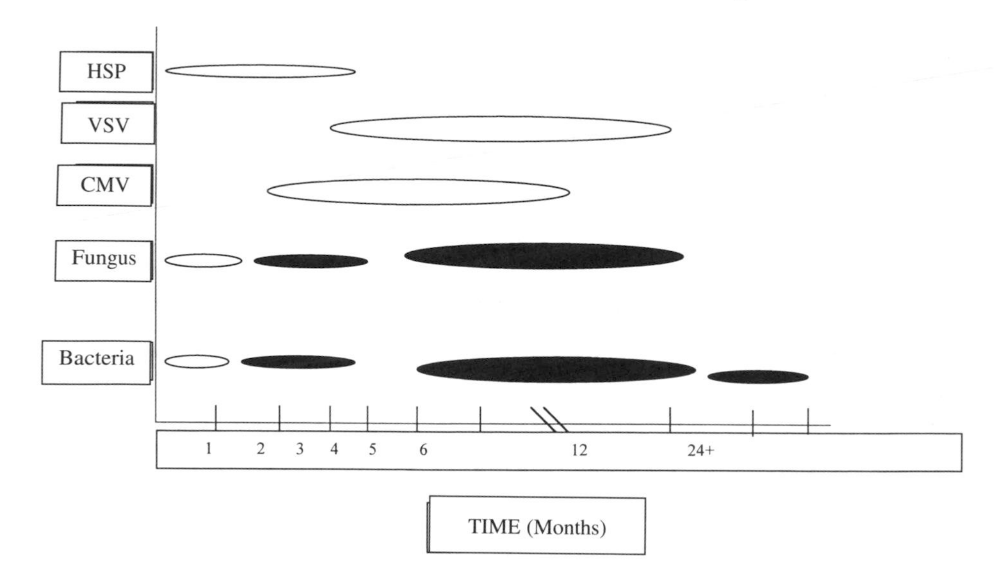

This time course shows when viral and bacterial complications typically occur in transplant patients. Bacterial infection risk is during the neutropenic phases and when the course is complicated by acute and chronic GVHD (filled circles). HSV = herpes simplex virus; CMV = cytomegalovirus; VZV = varicella zoster virus.

11. Describe the grading system for acute GVHD.

Skin		*Liver*		*Gut (Diarrhea)*	
0	No rash	0	T bili < 2mg/dL	0	< 5mL/kg/day
1	Rash < 25%	1	T bili 2–3 mg/dL	1	5-10 mL/kg/day
2	Rash 25–50%	2	T bili 3–6mg/dL	2	10-15 mL/kg/day
3	Rash 50–100%	3	T bili 6-15 mg/dL	3	> 15 mL/kg/day
4	desquamation/bullae	4	T bili > 15mg/dL	4	Severe abdominal pain +/- ileus

Overall Grade of Acute GVHD

GRADE	SKIN	LIVER	GUT
I	Stage 1–2	Stage 0	Stage 0
II	Stage 3	Stage 1	Stage 1
III	Stage 3	Stage 2–3	Stage 2–4
IV	Stage 4	Stage 4	

12. What is the graft-versus-leukemia (GVL) effect?

A mechanism where donor immunocompetent cells such as T cells and natural killer (NK) cells induce a strong immune-mediated reaction against recipient leukemia cells to prevent relapse. It has been demonstrated that there is a reduced relapse rate in patients with acute and chronic GVHD. Conversely, there is an increased risk of relapse in syngeneic transplants and T cell–depleted transplants. Most importantly one can induce a durable remission with donor lymphocyte infusions in patients who relapse after allogeneic stem cell transplant.

MHC-restricted CD4+ and CD8+ T lymphocytes and NK cells are the cells proposed to induce the GVL response, but the mechanism of action and the target antigens remain under investigation.

13. Describe the time course of immune system reconstitution after allogeneic stem cell transplant.

Immune reconstitution is delayed after hematopoietic stem cell transplantation, resulting in a prolonged period of immune suppression and an increased risk of infectious complications. The barriers to immune recovery are age at the time of transplant, the presence of acute and chronic GVHD, immune-suppressive medications, the stem cell source and the manipulation of stem cell product. In general, recovery is shorter utilizing mobilized PBSC than bone marrow cells, which in turn is more rapid than cord blood stem cells. The following table summarizes the time recovery of the components of the immune system:

Component	*Time to Recovery*
Myeloid: ANC > 500/μL	12–24 days
NK cells	1–2 months
Lymphoid: ALC > 500/μL	24–30 days
CD3+ T cells	3 months
CD8+ T cells	4 months
CD4+ T cells	6–9 months
T cell function	4–6 months
B cells: antibody production	4–6 months
IgM	4–6 months
IgG	6–9 months

ALC = absolute lymphocyte count; Ig = immunoglobulin.

14. What immunizations that should be given to a child after transplant?

Patients undergoing allogeneic transplant will lose immunity to the common childhood diseases and should be reimmunized after transplant.

	Time after HSCT		
VACCINE	12 MONTHS	14 MONTHS	24 MONTHS
Diphtheria, tetanus, pertussis			
< 7 years	DTP or DT	DTP or DT	DTP or DT
> 7 years	Td	Td	Td
Haemophilus influenzae type B (H1b) conjugate	Hib conjugate	Hib conjugate	Hib conjugate
Hepatitis (Hep B) Only at 12 months ×1 for patients previously immunized	Hep B	Hep B	Hep B
Pneumoccoccal polysaccharide (PPV23)	PPV23		PPV23
Influenza	Lifelong before transplant and resume > 6 months after HSCT		
Inactivated polio (IPV)	IPV	IPV	IPV
Live-attenuated vaccine measles-mumps-rubella (MMR)			MMR only if off all immunosuppression no evidence of GVHD

15. Describe some of the strategies used to prevent infection in stem cell transplantation.

Factors that increase the risk of infection after bone marrow transplant are neutropenia, impaired cell-mediated immunity, impaired humoral immunity, disrupted anatomical barriers and hyposplenism. Some methods used to reduce infection include

- Suppressing endogenous flora
- Reducing exposure to exogenous flora
- Suppressing latent infection
- Augmenting the host's immune function
- Administrating of growth factors such as G-CSF and GM-CSF

During the pre-engraftment period, the combination of neutropenia and altered barriers place the patient at increased risk for infection from endogenous flora. Attempts to reduce the microbial load are made by diligent oral hygiene and bathing. Decreasing exposure to exogenous flora is achieved by placing the patient in a protective environment of reverse isolation during the neutropenic phase; effective air filtration, such as hepa filtration, helps to remove all bacteria and fungi from the environment. Good handwashing by staff and visitors and passive immunotherapy in the form of intravenous immunoglobulins are also used to prevent infection. Empiric antibiotics are administered. Fluconazole prophylaxis is routinely given during the neutropenic period and has helped to eliminate *Candida albicans* infection. However, fungal infections not susceptible to fluconazole, such as those caused by *C. krusei, C. glabrata*, and aspergillus still occur.

Transplant patients are *also* at increased risk of reactivating latent infections such as herpes simplex when they are seropositive. Prophylactic acyclovir given during the neutropenic period may suppress reactivation. Antiviral prophylaxis with ganciclovir has reduced the frequency of cytomegalovirus (CMV) reactivation. For CMV-positive patients, weekly CMV surveillance cultures and prompt initiation of therapy are essential. Screened CMV-negative blood products and filtered blood products for CMV-negative patients have been shown to be effective in preventing transfusion-acquired CMV infections. During the postengraftment period, prophylaxis against *Pneumocystis carinii* pneumonia is required for the duration of immunosuppression.

BIBLIOGRAPHY

1. Baron F, Beguin Y: Adoptive immunotherapy with donor lymphocyte infusions after allogeneic HPC transplantation [see comments]. Transfusion 40:468–476, 2000.
2. Champlin R, Khouri I, Kornblau S, et al: Allogeneic hematopoietic transplantation as adoptive immunotherapy. Induction of graft-versus-malignancy as primary therapy. Hematol Oncol Clin North Am13:1041–1057, 1999.
3. Thomas ED, Blume KG, Forman SJ (eds): Hematopoietic Cell Transplantation, 2nd ed. Malden, MA, Blackwell Science Inc. 1999
4. Foot AB, Potter MN, Donaldson C, et al. Immune reconstitution after BMT in children. Bone Marrow Transplant 11:7–13, 1993.
5. Heitger A, Neu N, Kern H, et al: Essential role of the thymus to reconstitute naive (CD45RA+) T-helper cells after human allogeneic bone marrow transplantation. Blood 90:850–857, 1997.
6. Mackall CL, Granger L, Sheard MA, et al: T-cell regeneration after bone marrow transplantation: Differential CD45 isoform expression on thymic-derived versus thymic-independent progeny. Blood 82:2585–2594, 1993.
7. Small TN: Immunologic reconstitution following stem cell transplantation. Curr Opin Hematol 3:461–465, 1996.
8. Small TN, Papadopoulos EB, Boulad F, et al: Comparison of immune reconstitution after unrelated and related T-cell–depleted bone marrow transplantation: effect of patient age and donor leukocyte infusions. Blood 93:467–480, 1999.
9. Treleaven JG, Barrett J (ed): The Clinical Practice of Stem-Cell Transplantation, 1st ed. Vols. I and II. Oxford, United Kingdom, Isis Medical Media Ltd., 1998.
10. van Burik JA, Weisdorf DJ: Infections in recipients of blood and marrow transplantation. Hematol Oncol Clin North Am 13:1065–1089, 1999.

41. EXPERIMENTAL THERAPEUTICS IN PEDIATRIC HEMATOLOGY-ONCOLOGY

Kiery A. *Braithwaite,* M.D., *and Mitchell* S. *Cairo,* M.D.

CYTOKINES, GROWTH FACTORS, AND COLONY-STIMULATING FACTORS

1. Briefly describe hematopoiesis.

Hematopoiesis is a complex process involving the production, differentiation and maturation of all erythroid, myeloid, thrombopoietic and lymphoid cells. This process begins with uncommitted stem cells within the bone marrow that are the earliest known pluripotent hematopoietic stem cells. Colony-stimulating factors (CSFs) facilitate the production and differentiation of these early cells by stimulating stem cells to mature into progenitor cells. Early progenitor cells are referred to as colony-forming units (CFUs) and are named for the cells they become, such as CFU-GM, which give rise to granulocytes and macrophages. Progenitor cells subsequently differentiate further into various lineages depending on their exposure to growth factors, or cytokines. As the cells develop, they become more committed and ultimately become mature, lineage-restricted functioning cells within the peripheral circulation.

2. Discuss the role of endogenous granulocyte colony–stimulating factor (G-CSF).

Granulocyte colony–stimulating factor is a hematopoietic growth factor involved in the regulation of neutrophils by its ability to stimulate the proliferation and maturation of granulocytes and their precursors. The function of G-CSF in normal hematopoiesis is unclear; however, it has been demonstrated that during stressed states, such as sepsis, the endogenous level of G-CSF rises in inverse relation to the circulating absolute neutrophil count (ANC). G-CSF is produced principally by mature macrophages, as well as by other cells such as fibroblasts, endothelial cells and mesothelial cells. A rise in endogenous G-CSF levels results in the proliferation and maturation of committed progenitor cells in the bone marrow, a decrease in the neutrophil storage pool and a more rapid release of neutrophils into the blood. This translates into a dramatic increase in the peripheral neutrophil count. Furthermore, G-CSF additionally enhances mature neutrophil function by stimulating chemotaxis, phagocytosis and the production of superoxide radicals.

3. Explain the use of G-CSF in pediatric patients undergoing chemotherapy for malignancies.

The overall prognosis for children diagnosed with malignancies has greatly improved over the past few decades secondary to better drugs, intensified regimens of induction, maintenance therapy and improvements in supportive care. However, infectious complications remain a major cause of morbidity during chemotherapy and may cause delays in treatment cycles. The risk of infection in patients receiving myelosuppressive chemotherapy correlates directly with the severity and duration of neutropenia. Studies have examined the ability of G-CSF to alleviate the immunosuppression associated with the hematological toxicity of chemotherapy. It has been demonstrated that cancer patients treated with prophylactic G-CSF following chemotherapy had a significant reduction in the duration and severity of their neutropenia, translating into a decrease in infections, hospital days and antibiotic use.

Prophylactic use of G-CSF in children receiving myelosuppressive therapy for acute lymphoblastic leukemia (ALL) accelerates recovery from neutropenia and significantly decreases the median hospital stay for febrile neutropenia; however, it does not decrease the number of severe infections. If G-CSF prophylactically administered between chemotherapy cycles reduces the incidence of febrile neutropenia, culture-confirmed infections and the duration of parenteral antibiotics, it will allow a tighter adherence to planned treatment schedules.

4. Does G-CSF promote leukemogenesis in leukemic patients?

The concern that G-CSF may encourage the proliferation of abnormal leukemic cells originated with the observation that leukemic cells may express G-CSF receptors. However, patients treated with G-CSF versus placebo have similar remission rates as well as long-term event-free survival rates, suggesting that G-CSF does not promote or stimulate leukomogenesis. Longer follow-up studies in larger patient populations are required to definitively answer this question.

5. Discuss the use of G-CSF in the setting of bone marrow transplants (BMTs) for children with malignancies.

Administration of G-CSF decreases the duration of neutropenia following myeloablative regimens for both autologous and allogeneic BMT, and it promotes engraftment as well. Moreover, there is no evidence that G-CSF is able to stimulate malignant cells that survive the conditioning regimen for BMT. G-CSF is also commonly used to mobilize donor stem cells in anticipation of peripheral blood stem cell collection for transplantation. Peripheral blood primed with G-CSF is superior to unprimed bone marrow and/or unprimed peripheral blood and leads to a more rapid engraftment in the recipient.

6. What is the role of G-CSF in treating neutropenia of the newborn?

Newborns have an increased susceptibility to infection due to an immaturity in their immune system, both quantitatively and qualitatively. Compared with older children and adults, they have fewer bone marrow progenitor cells, a smaller neutrophil storage pool and increased neutrophil consumption during infection. Premature neonates are especially susceptible to this immaturity during bacterial sepsis or other periods of stress. However, except in cases of severe neonatal neutropenia, the use of G-CSF during the newborn period remains controversial.

Granulocyte colony–stimulating factor has proven to be efficacious in cases of congenital neutropenia. Kostmann's syndrome (familial severe neutropenia) is associated with impairment in neutrophil maturation within the bone marrow, resulting in a severely depressed ANC. G-CSF significantly increases the peripheral neutrophil count in these children, resulting in dramatic clinical improvement. Children with cyclic neutropenia and autoimmune neutropenia have also responded to treatment with G-CSF.

7. Discuss the role of endogenous granulocyte-macrophage colony-stimulating factor (GM-CSF).

Endogenous GM-CSF is similar to G-CSF in its ability to stimulate the production, differentiation and maturation of myeloid precursor cells; however, it is an earlier-acting cytokine than G-CSF, and it stimulates early hematopoietic progenitors of multiple cell lineages. Many cell types, including activated T cells, mast cells and fibroblasts, produce GM-CSF. GM-CSF also enhances the function of mature circulating neutrophils, eosinophils and monocytes/macrophages. Effects of GM-CSF on peripheral myeloid cells include enhanced neutrophil oxidative metabolism, improved chemotaxis and phagocytosis, increased leukotriene release, augmented intracellular killing and antigen procession by macrophages and increased eosinophilic protozoal killing.

8. Discuss the clinical role of GM-CSF.

The clinical role of GM-CSF is similar to that of G-CSF. It decreases the duration and severity of neutropenia, as well as the incidence of infections in children undergoing chemotherapy for solid tumors. It enhances neutrophil recovery and decreases the number of infections following both autologous and allogeneic BMT. When used for mobilization of peripheral blood progenitor cells (PBPCs) for transplantation, treatment with GM-CSF results in more efficient apheresis in the donor, as well as enhanced granulocyte recovery in the recipient. Furthermore, recipients of GM-CSF–mobilized PBPC demonstrated earlier platelet and erythrocyte transfusion independence than those patients who received non-mobilized PBPC. The use of GM-CSF also has potential efficacy in treating children with severe aplastic anemia, neutropenic newborns, and patients with AIDS.

9. What are the most common side effects of G-CSF and GM-CSF?

Bone pain is the most common side effect during treatment with either G-CSF or GM-CSF. The bone pain likely reflects the proliferation of progenitor cells and stem cells within the bone marrow. Long-term administration may be associated with osteopenia or osteoporosis. Additional side effects include rash, fever, myalgias and increased serum lactate dehydrogenase, uric acid and/or alkaline phosphatase. Occasionally, patients may experience flushing, hypotension, tachycardia and dyspnea during initial administration of GM-CSF. Fluid retention leading to generalized edema and pleural and pericardial effusions has been noted with higher doses of GM-CSF.

10. Discuss the role of endogenous erythropoietin (Epo).

The glycoprotein hormone Epo is the primary regulator of red blood cell production, or erythropoiesis. The liver initially produces Epo during fetal life, but this process shifts to the kidneys around the time of birth. Epo levels are regulated in a classic negative feedback mechanism that is stimulated by hypoxia and/or anemia. Normally, there is a linear inverse relationship between red blood cell mass and the serum Epo level. During episodes of hypoxia and/or anemia, a rapid rise in Epo levels occurs through an exponential increase in the number of Epo-producing cells in the kidney. Epo subsequently stimulates erythropoiesis by binding to specific cell surface receptors on erythroid progenitor cells within the bone marrow. The colony-forming unit erythroid is the primary target cell for Epo, and with further maturity of the erythroid cell, receptor expression decreases to undetectable levels in circulating reticulocytes. Epo additionally interacts with other growth factors to stimulate myeloid, monocyte and megakaryocyte cell maturation.

11. What is the clinical role of recombinant human erythropoietin (rhEpo)?

Since rhEpo was first introduced in 1985, it has been utilized in a variety of clinical settings. It is generally very well-tolerated in children and adults, with hypertension as the most common adverse effect. Its utilization in the pediatric hematology/oncology population is summarized below.

- Anemia of end-stage renal disease: RhEpo causes a significant rise in hemoglobin levels, thus decreasing transfusion requirements and even allowing some dialysis patients to become transfusion-independent. It was further shown to improve the quality of life in these patients.
- Anemia of cancer: Anemia associated with cancer is often multifactorial, and patients are often anemic even prior to the initiation of cytotoxic therapy. Endogenous Epo levels are inappropriately low in solid tumor patients for any given degree of anemia when compared with control patients with anemia secondary to iron deficiency or hemolysis. The normal Epo response in the cancer patient is blunted, and there is an absence of the normal inverse relationship between endogenous Epo and hemoglobin.

Moreover, the Epo response to anemia is further dulled once chemotherapy is initiated. Nevertheless, the ability of rhEpo to improve the anemia associated with cancer has been well documented and significantly reduces the number of PRBC transfusions. Furthermore, a decrease in the number of platelet transfusions was additionally noted with rhEpo.

12. Discuss the function and regulation of endogenous thrombopoietin in hematopoiesis.

Thrombopoietin is the primary hematopoietic factor responsible for the growth and maturation of megakaryocytes. It increases the size and number of megakaryocytes, increases ploidy and stimulates the expression of platelet-specific markers. Other thrombopoietic cytokines, such as interleukin (IL)-3, IL-6 and IL-11, act in conjunction with thrombopoietin, and are thrombopoietin-dependent. Thrombopoietin functions synergistically with other cytokines to stimulate the growth of erythroid progenitor cells.

The platelet mass regulates endogenous levels of thrombopoietin by an inverse relationship. Mature circulating platelets express thrombopoietin receptors (c-mpl) that bind the growth factor, thus lowering its plasma level. Thrombopoietin levels have been measured in patients with different forms of thrombocytopenia. Patients with thrombocytopenia due to bone marrow hypoplasia secondary to myelosuppressive chemotherapy or aplastic anemia have significantly increased levels of thrombopoietin. On the other hand, patients with idiopathic thrombocytopenic purpura had low levels of thrombopoietin. Because idiopathic thrombocytopenic purpura is characterized by peripheral destruction of platelets, these patients have increased production of megakaryocytes and platelets, which increases the binding of thrombopoietin, thus decreasing its plasma level.

The fact that platelet mass rather than megakaryocyte levels regulates thrombopoietin has significant clinical consequences. For example, when myelosuppressive chemotherapy and/or irradiation is initiated, it destroys the megakaryocytes and their progenitors but not the previously circulating platelets bound to thrombopoietin. Thus, the rise in thrombopoietin is delayed until thrombocytopenia occurs days later secondary to the bone marrow hypoplasia.

13. Describe the role of exogenous thrombopoietin in the clinical setting.

The Food and Drug Administration has yet to approve thrombopoietin, which is currently undergoing phase I evaluation in children. However, in adults, thrombopoietin accelerates platelet recovery after conventional doses of chemotherapy and may decrease the need for platelet transfusions following autologous BMT. Thrombopoietin may enhance the mobilization of peripheral blood progenitor cells. This may greatly improve both autologous and allogeneic peripheral stem cell transplantations by decreasing the number of aphereses required to harvest a sufficient number of stem cells. Similarly, the administration of thrombopoietin to healthy platelet donors during platelet pheresis boosts the count in the donated product and results in greater increments in the platelet count in the recipient following transfusion. However, the safety profile of thrombopoietin must be thoroughly considered before its use can be justified in healthy donors.

14. Discuss the use of IL-11 in treating thrombocytopenia.

Interleukin-11 is a hematopoietic growth factor that, in combination with other cytokines, such as IL-3, thrombopoietin and/or stem cell factor, increases peripheral platelet counts by stimulating megakaryocytopoiesis. IL-11 receptors have been detected on megakaryocytes but not on platelets. This suggests that IL-11 acts directly on megakaryocytes and their progenitors but has little or no effect on the mature circulating platelets. By accelerating platelet recovery, IL-11 decreases the need for platelet transfusions following chemotherapy for nonmyeloid malignancies. IL-11 also has potential efficacy in treating the thrombocytopenia associated with the Wiskott-Aldrich syndrome, an x-linked genetic disease characterized by the clinical triad of thrombocytopenia, eczema and immunodeficiency, prior to allogeneic stem cell transplant.

IMMUNOTHERAPY

15. What is a monoclonal antibody?

A purified antibody produced against a particular antigen expressed by a specific cell population. Monoclonal antibodies are being investigated to both diagnose and treat malignancies. Monoclonal antibodies may be used alone, or they may be conjugated to toxins, radioisotopes or drugs. For monoclonal antibodies to be effective in the treatment of malignancies, several criteria must be met:

- The target antigen must be expressed on tumor cells.
- The antigen should be unique to the targeted malignant cells and not expressed by other normal cells.
- The monoclonal antibody must be able to be delivered to the antigen and induce a cytotoxic response.
- The unconjugated antibody binds to the antigen and induces cell death by complement-dependent cytotoxicity, antibody-dependent cellular cytotoxicity (ADCC) and apoptosis.
- Conjugated antibodies must be internalized so that the cytotoxic drug or toxin can exert its effect.

16. Discuss the challenges in using monoclonal antibodies to treat malignancies.

Monoclonal antibodies theoretically combat malignancies by effectively targeting and destroying tumor cells that express specific tumor antigens. However, theory does not always correlate with practice, and since the introduction of monoclonal antibodies, several challenges have arisen. Potential problems include

- The inability of the monoclonal antibody to reach target tumor cells
- The expression of tumor antigens on normal cells
- Cross-reactivity
- The inability to mediate ADCC and other effector mechanisms in the setting of large tumor burden
- The production of antibodies against the monoclonal antibodies themselves

Therefore, the efficacy of monoclonal antibodies for first-line, single-agent therapy for malignancies is limited. However, monoclonal antibodies may show efficacy in maintenance therapy or states of minimal residual disease.

17. Does the monoclonal antibody IDEC-C2B8 (rituximab) have efficacy in the treatment of B cell tumors?

IDEC-C2B8 (rituximab) is an anti-CD20 chimeric monoclonal antibody that targets and binds to the CD20 antigen. CD20 is a phosphoprotein that is expressed on the surface of normal, circulating B cells, as well as more than 90% of B cell tumors. It is not shed into the peripheral blood and when bound to antibody does not internalize. Rituximab has high specificity and affinity for CD20 and on binding to CD20, rituximab induces complement-dependent cytotoxicity, antibody-dependent cellular cytotoxicity and apoptosis; it has additionally been shown to increase sensitivity to chemotherapy. Rituximab has demonstrated efficacy in treating B cell lymphoma and leukemia in adults and has proven to safe and efficacious in children as well.

18. Discuss the side effects associated with rituximab.

The CD20 antigen is expressed on normal peripheral B cells as well as B cell tumor cells. Therefore, treatment with rituximab results in peripheral B cell lymphocytopenia. However, the depletion of normal B lymphocytes is only temporary, as bone marrow stem cells and progenitor cells are not affected. Furthermore, plasma cells do not express CD20, and thus antibody production continues during B lymphocytopenia. Other toxicities include low-grade fever, chills, headache, hypotension, rash and rarely, respiratory distress.

19. What is the role of the monoclonal antibody CMA-676 (gemtuzumab) in the treatment of acute myeloid leukemia (AML)?

CMA-676 (gemtuzumab) has recently been approved by the Food and Drug Administration to treat adult patients (> 60 years old) with relapsed CD33-positive AML. This novel drug comprises the monoclonal antibody anti-CD33 conjugated to the cytotoxic drug calicheamicin, which promotes cell death by inducing the breaking of double-stranded DNA. CD33 is a hematopoietic surface antigen expressed by leukemic blast cells in 80–90% of patients with AML. It is ordinarily expressed on myeloid precursor cells and megakaryocytes but not on pluripotent hematopoietic stem cells. Gemtuzumab has shown promising results in patients with relapsed AML, with remission rates similar to those reported with conventional chemotherapy. The efficacy of gemtuzumab as first-line treatment of AML has yet to be proven.

20. Discuss the B43-PAP immunotoxin that is currently undergoing phase III trials for pediatric ALL.

The immunotoxin B43-PAP is currently undergoing phase III clinical trials in children with B lineage ALL. This immunotoxin is prepared by convalently linking the murine immunoglobulin G1 anti-CD19 monoclonal antibody B43 to the plant toxin PAP (pokewood antiviral protein). PAP is an enzyme isolated from the leaves and seeds of the pokewood plant (*Phytolacca americana*) that inactivates ribosomes, resulting in an irreversible shutdown of protein synthesis. The monoclonal antibody B43 binds the antigen CD19, which is expressed on virtually all B lineage ALL clonogenic blasts and when bound to the antibody B34, induces internalization of antibody. CD19 is unique and not expressed in nonlymphohematopoietic tissue. Preliminary trials with B43-PAP have demonstrated significant antileukemic activity.

21. Explain the theory behind using anti-idiotypic antibodies as tumor vaccines.

A tumor or cancer vaccine introduces tumor antigens that stimulate T cells and other immune system responses to create anti-tumor antibodies. These antibodies subsequently recognize and attack malignant cells. However, attempts to use tumor antigens as vaccines have been mostly unsuccessful because the tumor antigens have been found to be poor antigens, or poor stimulators of the immune system. Therefore, efforts have been made to convert these weak antigens into stronger antigens that are able to overcome the immune tolerance of the host. The network hypothesis utilizes anti-idiotypic antibodies that are designed against anti-tumor antigen antibody. Thus, by creating an antibody to the antibody of the original tumor antigen, one produces a more potent antigen that has similar three-dimensional structure to the original antigen.

22. What anti-idiotypic (anti-Id) tumor vaccine is currently being investigated in children?

The anti-Id antibody 1A7 is currently being investigated in children with advanced neuroblastoma. This monoclonal antibody is an antibody to the anti-GD2 monoclonal antibody. GD2 ganglioside is highly expressed in neuroblastomas, as well as in melanoma, small cell lung carcinoma, sarcomas and some brain tumors. GD2 is poorly immunogenic; therefore, anti-Id antibodies have been developed as potential tumor vaccines. The anti-Id antibody 1A7 shows promise as a vaccine for neuroblastoma patients with microscopic residual disease, or for maintenance therapy.

NOVEL THERAPY

23. Discuss the role of all-trans-retinoic acid (ATRA) in the treatment of acute promyelocytic leukemia (APL).

Acute promyelocytic leukemia is characterized by hypergranular blast cells, coagulopathy and the t(15;17)(q22;q21) translocation that results in the fusion of the promyelocytic leukemia gene with the retinoic acid receptor alpha gene. Although 65–80% of patients with newly diagnosed APL achieve complete remission with standard chemotherapy, relapse rates are very high, resulting in an overall poor 3-year survival rate. Furthermore, 10–20% patients die either prior to or during initiation of chemotherapy secondary to bleeding complications.

Physicians in Shanghai first reported the clinical efficacy of ATRA in the treatment of APL in 1987. Since then, it has been shown that ATRA improves disease-free and overall survival rates when used as induction and/or maintenance treatment, compared to chemotherapy alone. ATRA works by its ability to differentiate leukemic promyelocytes into mature granulocytes. It has several advantages over standard chemotherapy, including more rapid correction of coagulopathies, induction of clinical remission without bone marrow aplasia and earlier attainment of normal peripheral blood counts. It is also administered orally and is inexpensive compared with chemotherapy. However, the duration of remission with ATRA alone is usually brief, and thus the early addition of chemotherapy to ATRA and maintenance therapy with both chemotherapy and ATRA are necessary to decrease the likelihood of relapse and improve overall survival.

24. What is the retinoic acid syndrome?

Retinoic acid syndrome is the major toxicity associated with ATRA, occurring in 40–50% of patients with APL. It is characterized by fever, respiratory distress with pulmonary infiltrates, pleural effusions, pericarditis and weight gain secondary to fluid retention. It usually occurs within the first 3 weeks of ATRA treatment. Although it can be fatal, most patients do well without discontinuation of therapy. Treatment with dexamethasone is standard and should be initiated at the earliest suggestion of symptoms.

25. Discuss the utilization of 13-cis-retinoic acid in the treatment of pediatric neuroblastoma.

Neuroblastoma, a malignancy arising from the adrenal medulla or other sympathetic nervous system ganglia, is the most common extracranial solid tumor of childhood. It is generally associated with a poor prognosis. 13-cis-retinoic acid has been demonstrated to decrease proliferation and induce differentiation in neuroblastoma cell lines. Children with high-risk neuroblastomas treated with high-dose 13-cis-retinoic acid after completing treatment regimens including chemotherapy, irradiation, surgery and/or transplantation had a significant improvement in event-free survival rates, regardless of the type of prior therapy.

26. Briefly describe the significance of tyrosine kinase inhibitors as a potential therapy for malignancies.

Patients with chronic myeloid leukemia characteristically express the t(9;22)(q34;q11) translocation, otherwise known as the Philadelphia chromosome. In this translocation, the proto-oncogene c-abl is juxtaposed to the *bcr* gene, and the resulting *bcr-abl* gene is an abnormal tyrosine kinase that suppresses apoptosis while promoting cell growth. In vitro studies have demonstrated that the tyrosine kinase inhibitor CGP 57148 is a potent inhibitor of the change to abelson leukemia protein tyrosine kinase; in vivo animal studies have further suggested that this tyrosine kinase inhibitor is selectively toxic to cells expressing the fused bcr-abl protein and thus displays antitumor activity.

Although chronic myeloid leukemia is not a childhood malignancy, therapy with tyrosine kinase inhibitors may show promise for many malignancies, both pediatric and adult. For example, the Philadelphia chromosome is also expressed in some patients with ALL. The ability to design compounds that target the binding sites of abnormal, malignancy-promoting proteins opens the door to novel therapies with increased potency and specificity.

BIBLIOGRAPHY

1. Abu-Ghosh A, Bracho F, Kirov I, Cairo MS: Hematopoietic colony-stimulating factors. In Grenvik A, Ayers SM, Holbrook PR, Shoemaker WC (eds): Textbook of Critical Care, 4th ed. Philadelphia, W.B. Saunders, 2000, pp 542–561.
2. Bracho F, Krailo M, Blazar B, et al: Clinical and hematological recovery in children with recurrent/refractory solid tumors treated with ifosfamide, carboplatin, & etoposide (ICE) followed by sequential trials of IL-11/G-CSF, IL-6/G-CSF, PIXY321, or G-CSF: Children's Cancer Group (CCG) and Genetics Institute experience [abstract]. Proc Am Soc Clin Oncol 18:43a, 1999.
3. Druker B: Status of BCR-ABL tyrosine kinase inhibitors in CML. The ASH Education Program Book, 1999. The American Society of Hematology, Washington, DC.
4. Fenaux P, Chastang C, Chevret S, et al: A randomized comparison of all transretinoic acid (ATRA) followed by chemotherapy and ATRA plus chemotherapy and the role of maintenance therapy in newly diagnosed acute promyelocytic leukemia. The European APL Group [see comments]. Blood 94:1192–1200, 1999.
5. Kaushansky K. Thrombopoietin. N Engl J Med 339:746–754, 1998.
6. Matthay KK, Villablanca JG, Seeger RC, et al: Treatment of high-risk neuroblastoma with intensive chemotherapy, radiotherapy, autologous bone marrow transplantation, and 13-cis- retinoic acid. Children's Cancer Group. N Engl J Med 341:1165–1173, 1999.
7. Sen G, Chakraborty M, Foon KA, et al. Preclinical evaluation in nonhuman primates of murine monoclonal anti-idiotype antibody that mimics the disialoganglioside GD2. Clin Cancer Res 3:1969–1976, 1997.
8. Sievers EL, Larson RA, Estey E, et al: Efficacy and safety of CMA-676 in patients with AML in first relapse [abstract]. Blood 94:3079, 1999.
9. Tallman MS, Andersen JW, Schiffer CA, et al: All-trans-retinoic acid in acute promyelocytic leukemia [see comments]. [Published erratum appears in N Engl J Med 337(22):1639, 1997.] N Engl J Med 337:1021–1028, 1997.
10. Tepler I, Elias L, Smith, JW, et al: A randomized placebo-controlled trial of recombinant human inte leukin-11 in cancer patients with severe thrombocytopenia due to chemotherapy. Blood 87:3607–3614, 1996.

42. SUPPORTIVE CARE

Judith R. Marcus, M.D.

1. Describe supportive care for children with cancer.

Because cancer treatment is generally immunosuppressive as well as myelosuppressive, prevention of infection and quick intervention if infection is suspected are key supportive measures. Prevention and control of hemorrhage, thrombosis and drug and radiation toxicities are extremely important aspects of supportive care. Of course, nutritional support, prevention and treatment of nausea and vomiting, skin and mouth care, indications for and care of venous access devices and pain management all fall under the broad definition of supportive care. Other related topics, such as hospice and home care, psychosocial support and alternative medicine will be dealt with in other chapters of this book.

2. How can we prevent infection in children with cancer?

Although we cannot prevent many infections and rely on timely assessment of symptoms and signs followed by rapid institution of therapeutic measures, reduction of certain known infective agents can be accomplished.

***Pneumocystis carinii* pneumonia prophylaxis:** Trimethoprim-sulfamethoxazole given orally or intravenously at 2.5 mg/kg of trimethoprim every 12 hr three days a week. Other agents that can be given to accomplish the same end are pentamidine, which can be administered intravenously at 4 mg/kg over 60 minutes every month or by inhalation at 8 mg/kg in children younger than 5 yr and 300 mg for those older than 5 by Respirgard II nebulizer every month, or dapsone 2 mg/kg orally as a single dose daily. These measures should be instituted at diagnosis and continued for 2–6 months after chemotherapy is stopped.

***Candida* prophylaxis:** Nystatin, 5–10 ml of the 100,000 U/mL suspension, swish and swallow twice to four times a day, depending on risk for mouth ulcers and esophageal candidiasis. Clotrimazole troche, one twice a day to be sucked on for 20 minutes is an alternative.

Herpes simplex prophylaxis: In patients with past history of recurrent Herpes simplex who are on intensive chemotherapy protocols or are bone marrow transplant recipients acyclovir, 200–600 mg/m^2 per day orally in three to six doses or 250 mg/m^2 intravenously every 8 hr during periods of severe neutropenia.

Granulocyte stimulating factor: Although current data do not show a reduction of actual number of septic episodes in neutropenic patients in controlled studies, filgrastim (rhG-CSF, Neupogen®) at 5 μg/kg per day subcutaneously can reduce the length of time of neutropenia. It is indicated and part of many protocols where the period of anticipated neutropenia is 7 days or more. Use of filgrastim may reduce the frequency and duration of fever and neutropenia admissions.

3. Discuss the toxic side effects of chemotherapy that can be prevented with supportive care.

Several drugs have been very useful in preventing the unpleasant nauseating effects of highly emetogenic chemotherapies such as high dose cyclophosphamide, ifosfamide, cisplatin, melphalan, high dose cytosine arabinoside, high-dose methotrexate, anthracyclines such as doxorubicin, daunorubicin, idarubicin, mitoxantrone, and more. Most effective have been the serotonin antagonists which work on both the chemoreceptor trigger zone in the medulla of the brain stem and peripherally on the vagal nerve terminal. These drugs are often given in combination with corticosteroids and antihistamines for optimal effect. Possible drug regimens include the following:

- Serotonin antagonists:
  Ondansetron (Zofran®) given at 0.15 mg/kg orally or intravenously 30 minutes prior to chemotherapy and 4 and 8 hr thereafter daily or every 8 hr for a 5-day course of chemotherapy or 0.45 mg/kg as a one-time daily dose 30 minutes prior to chemotherapy. A single dose at 0.15 mg/kg may be given prior to less nausea-provoking chemotherapy such as low-dose cytosine arabinoside, low-dose methotrexate and others.
  Granisetron (Kytril®) is given at 10 μg/kg intravenously or orally as a single daily dose 30 minutes prior to chemotherapy. Individual patients may respond better to one serotonin antagonist than another. Cost factors at institutional pharmacies may influence pharmacopiae.
- Corticosteroids: Dexamethasone (Decadron®), used in conjunction with serotonin antagonist for highly emetogenic chemotherapeutic agents. Dosage is 0.2 mg/kg, with a maximum dose of 10 mg given 30 minutes prior to chemotherapy.
- Antihistamines: Hydroxyzine (Atarax®, Vistaril®) may be added if the serotonin antagonist and dexamethasone do not provide relief. Dosage is 1 mg/kg per dose, 50 mg maximum per dose intravenously or orally every 6 hr.
- Several drugs that are effective anti-emetics have a high incidence of extrapyramidal effects in children and have been used less since the advent of serotonin antagonists. They should always be administered with diphenhydramine (Benadryl®) at 1 mg/kg per dose, maximum 50 mg per dose every 6 hr concurrently to prevent the extrapyramidal effects. These drugs include the phenothiazines prochlorperazine (Compazine®), promethazine (Phenergan®) and chlorpromazine (Thorazine®). Also, metoclopramide (Reglan®) and droperidol (Inapsine®) are effective anti-emetics with frequent extrapyramidal reactions.
- Although not antiemetics per se, benzodiazepines are often prescribed for their amnesic effect. They should always be used in conjunction with an antiemetic. Lorazepam (Ativan®) at 0.04 mg/kg, maximum dose 2 mg, orally or intravenously every 6 hr or diazepam (Valium®) at 0.2 mg/kg IV or orally every 6–8 hr, maximum dose 0.6 mg/kg per day.

Cardiotoxicity is anticipated with anthracyclines such as daunorubicin (Daunomycin®), doxorubicin (Adriamycin®), idarubicin (Idamycin®) and mitoxantrone (Novantrone®), especially as the cumulative dosages in a patient increase to more than 450 mg/m^2 for daunorubicin and doxorubicin and more than 125 mg/m^2 for idarubicin. The cardiotoxicity is increased when the heart receives more than 1000 cGy of radiation therapy, such as in mantle radiotherapy for Hodgkin's disease. Baseline echocardiograms and/or MUGA scans prior to chemotherapy and regularly during chemotherapy in anthracycline-containing regimens can benefit the individual patient by identifying those whose cardiac function begins to deteriorate so that the anthracyclines can be eliminated from that patient's treatment protocol before he or she develops irreversible cardiac myopathy. As the cumulative dose of the anthracycline increases, the frequency of the cardiac studies also increases prior to each course of chemotherapy after a cumulative dose of 300 mg/m^2 for doxorubicin and daunorubicin. If there is an abnormality in either the echocardiogram or the radionuclide cineangiography, the other test should be performed to confirm the abnormality. A myocardial biopsy is sometimes necessary to confirm myocardial damage. A Holter monitor test will identify rhythm abnormalities which can also signify myocardial damage to the conducting system. Normal values for children are fractional shortening >28% and left ventricular ejection fraction >54%. Cardiotoxicity may be acute during therapy, or late effect may occur years after chemotherapy. If a patient shows no deterioration in cardiac function after 1 yr off chemotherapy, the risk for late-appearing cardiotoxicity is reduced.

Significant reduction in the cardiac toxicity seen after giving bolus doses of anthracycline has been shown with the administration of dextrazone (Zinecard®) 15 minutes prior to the anthracycline bolus, at a dose of 10 times the doxorubicin dose. The dextrazone does not work for continuous infusion or infusion over several hours doxorubicin.

Renal toxicity is seen after cis-platinin, ifosphamide, high-dose cyclophosphamide and methotrexate. Renal toxicity is increased when the baseline renal function is already reduced, such as after aminoglycoside or amphotericin B treatment for infection, from pretreatment with nephrotoxic chemotherapeutic agents, in patients with hydronephrosis, after radiation to the kidney and when the patient is dehydrated. Supportive care measures include measurement of renal function prior to each course of chemotherapy to determine if dose modification is necessary, hyperhydration during chemotherapy, careful measurement of intake and output during chemotherapy administration and at least daily weights during the chemotherapy. At the first sign of decreased urinary output, furosemide (Lasix®), 0.5–1 mg/kg, is administered. Fluid compensation for emesis and diarrhea during chemotherapy must be calculated at least daily. Urine output must be maintained at 70% fluid intake or better to minimize kidney damage. Renal tubular damage can cause aberrations in serum sodium, potassium, chloride, magnesium, phosphate, glucose, protein, alkaline phosphatase, bicarbonate and pH. These parameters must be followed and abnormalities corrected. Fanconi's syndrome with markedly decreased serum potassium, phosphate, and bicarbonate associated with glycosuria and aminoaciduria as a consequence of ifosphamide or high-dose cyclophosphamide can persist for years. Amifostine may protect against renal damage and is being tested in children in several protocols with nephrotoxic drugs.

Bladder toxicity in the form of hemorrhagic cystitis is seen after cyclophosphamide and ifosfamide chemotherapy. Prevention includes hyperhydration and administration of the bladder protectant Mesna® 360 mg/m^2 during and four doses after the chemotherapy during the 10 hr after completion of the cyclophosphamide or ifosfamide infusion. Years after completion of chemotherapy, bladder contraction leading to vesicoureteral reflux and hydronephrosis can later complicate prior episodes of hemorrhagic cystitis, particularly in those who received radiation therapy to the bladder.

Many chemotherapeutic drugs are detoxified or metabolized in the liver, and when the liver cannot perform that function, the effective doses of the drugs or drug levels are higher, leading to increased general toxicity of the drugs such as mucositis and bone marrow suppression. The specific drugs that have liver-dependent metabolism are vincristine, vinblastine, etoposide, daunorubicin, doxorubicin, idarubicin, actinomycin D, methotrexate, cyclophosphamide, CCNU, BCNU, 5-fluorouracil, cytosine arabinoside, DTIC and procarbazine 6-mercaptopurine, 6-thioguanine and L-asparaginase. Guidelines for dose modification depend on the extent of bilirubin and enzyme elevation. For grade three or higher toxicity, bilirubin and enzymes five times normal or higher, the chemotherapy drugs listed here are held until the bilirubin and enzymes have improved. A syndrome of venous occlusive disease has been described after 6-thioguanine and actinomycin D consisting of liver enlargement and ascites, with or without bilirubin or enzyme elevation, and thrombocytopenia caused by decreased flow or obstruction of the hepatic venules leading to passive congestion of the liver. In extreme cases, a Tips procedure connecting the hepatic circulation to the portal circulation may be necessary. Generally, supportive care and cessation of the therapeutic agent until recovery are all that is necessary.

Neurotoxicity can be subtle or profound. Vincristine and cisplatin in cumulative dose are associated with peripheral neuropathy, such as foot drop, lid lag, weakness, and paresthesias, which are increased with increased cumulative doses over a short period of time.

Acute encephalopathic changes may be seen after high-dose methotrexate, L-asparaginase, ifosfamide and intrathecal therapy. Vincristine can cause trigeminal pain, reflected as jaw pain, and also cause autonomic dysfunction leading to an ileus with constipation. Supportive care measures include oral laxatives to prevent constipation, appropriate pain medication and neurological workup to discount other causes of the symptom, such as infection or non-chemotherapy drug with neurological side effects. Learning disabilities are often seen after chemotherapy for leukemia, many of which are mild, but some are severe, especially in children younger than 2 yr who received cranial radiation.

Pulmonary toxicity is fortunately uncommon and is primarily seen after treatment with bleomycin and less frequently after methotrexate, busulfan and CCNU. Bleomycin toxicity is manifested by decreased inspiratory vital capacity and decreased pulmonary capillary blood volume. The chest x-ray shows an interstitial pneumonitis–type picture and when coupled with tachypnea and decreased oxygen saturation, pulmonary toxicity of chemotherapy should be considered as well as infectious etiologies. High-flow oxygen may initiate pulmonary toxicity. When bleomycin is given in combination with nephrotoxic drugs, the concentration of the bleomycin can rise if the renal function decreases, leading to more pulmonary toxicity, as described previously in the renal toxicity section.

4. What supportive measures can be taken during bone marrow suppression?

Red cell support: The reticulocyte count helps determine whether the child will recover soon from the anemia. Actual hemoglobin number to transfuse will depend on when it is likely the child will recover the hemoglobin spontaneously and on symptoms, the need for a higher hemoglobin for radiotherapy (must be >10 g/dL) or respiratory condition.

Transfusions: All blood products for children on chemotherapy should be irradiated to prevent graft-versus-host disease, and to prevent leukocyte reactions, use leukopoor filtered blood, which also removes cytomegalovirus. Both the patient and the donor blood should be screened for unusual antibodies and a cross-match done. Blood is transfused at 15 cc/kg over 3–4 hr. Premedication of acetaminophen, 10 mg/kg orally and benadryl, 1 mg/kg orally or intravenously, prevents most febrile and allergic reactions.

Recombinant erythropoietin, 150 IU/kg per dose subcutaneously three times a week, may help keep up the hemoglobin.

Children on chemotherapy are not generally iron deficient but may have low serum iron from anemia of chronic disease accompanied by high ferritin levels.

Platelet support is necessary to prevent hemorrhagic complications. All would agree to platelet transfusions for patients with platelets under 10K and for children who are bleeding with platelet counts under 20K. For simple surgery, 40K is acceptable, and for lumbar puncture, 50K is preferred. Premedication, irradiation, leukopoor filtration are the same as for red cells. The platelets should be transfused rapidly over approximately 30 minutes. 1 U of platelets per 7.5 kg will raise the platelet count by 40–50K 1 hr after the transfusion thoretically, but many patients are partially refractory and require more per transfusion or very frequent platelet transfusions. The variability in actual platelet counts achieved by a particular platelet transfusion is influenced by infection, hypersplenism, prior alloimmunization, damage to the platelets during collection, storage or transfusion. HLA-matched single-donor platelets can reduce the refractoriness in patients documented to have HLA platelet antibodies. Single-donor platelets have the equivalent of 8 U of platelets and can be used for older children. Sometimes they come in half packs equivalent to 4 U, which are more practical for children. The criteria for platelet transfusion vary from institution to institution:

Interleukin-11 (Neumega®) is an available cytokine that stimulates platelet production. It is given daily at 50 μg/kg subcutaneously.

Recombinant thrombopoietin is in final testing and will soon be commercially available. It will be given subcutaneously.

White cell support: Granulocyte transfusions are reserved for the seriously ill immunocompromised septic patient who is severely neutropenic and not likely to recover the white cell count in the next week. (See discussion of granulocyte-stimulating factor in response to the question about preventing infection in children with cancer.)

5. Describe how else we can prevent hemorrhage in the child with cancer.

Pediatric cancer patients are subject to several hemorrhagic mechanisms: disseminated intravascular coagulation (DIC) from infection or disseminated tumor (neuroblastoma, acute promyelocytic leukemia, any leukemia with white count over 100,000), vitamin K deficiency in severe malnutrition and after certain antibiotics, liver dysfunction and L-asparaginase–induced coagulopathy due to hypfibrinoginemia, decreased protein C and S and anti-thrombin III.

Common Coagulation Issues in Children with Cancer

COAGULATION ISSUE	ABNORMAL TESTS	COMMON PRESENTATION	MANAGEMENT
DIC	↑ PT, ↑PTT, ↓ PLTS, ↓ fibrinogen, ↑ D-dimer	Sepsis, APML, leukemia white blood cell count >100K, disseminated neuroblastoma	Correct underlying condition (antibiotics, chemotherapy), fresh frozen plasma, platelet infusions
Vitamin K deficiency	↑ PT, ↑ PTT, PLTS and fibrinogen normal	Malnutrition, prolonged antibiotic therapy with cephalosporins, unexplained bleeding diathesis	Vitamin K replacement, 1–5 mg orally or 2–20 mg subcutaneously Fresh frozen plasma Cryoprecipitate Prothrombin complex 50 U/kg for life-threatening hemorrhage
L-asparaginase coagulopathy	↑ PT, ↑ PTT, ↑ fibrinogen, ↑ anti-thrombin III, ↑ protein C & S	Large-vessel thrombosis or cerebrovascular accident; rarely, hemorrhage	Supportive care, fresh frozen plasma
Liver dysfunction	↑ PT, ↑ PTT, PLTS and fibrinogen normal or ↓, ↓ factor VII	Jaundice, hepatomegaly, gastrointestinal hemorrhage	Fresh frozen plasma

6. What are the common thromboses in children with cancer and what is their treatment?

Thrombosis has been associated with central venous access lines. Different centers report different incidence rates, but rates can be as high as 35% for some centers. The risk for venous thrombosis is higher in children who have underlying thrombophilic conditions such as factor V_{Leiden} (4–5% of caucasians), prothrombin-20210 (2%), anti-thrombin III deficiency (20–50 per 100,000) or protein C or S deficiency (200–500 per 100,000). In addition, thrombosis is associated with active cancer, total parenteral nutrition and immobility. The signs of thrombosis are venous dilatation of the chest or arm veins in a child with a central venous catheter or pain, erythema and swelling of a venous area in the lower extremity. Acute pleuritic pain accompanied by shortness of breath can be a sign of pulmonary embolism arising from a thrombosis. Focal neurological signs or focal seizures can be a sign of cerebrovascular thrombus.

Treatment of common thromboses in children with cancer

SITE	SIGNS & SYMPTOMS	DIAGNOSTIC STUDIES	THERAPY
Central venous catheter	No blood return, cannot flush line	Radio-opaque dye study	Tissue plasminogen activator, 1 mg for 1 hr, remove solution and flush
Upper extremity	Venous dilatation in chest wall or extremity	Bilateral arm venogram; doppler may not be accurate	Same as for lower extremity*
Lower extremity	Swollen, erythematous, tender, cords along veins	Duplex doppler study; MRI of pelvis and extremity; venogram	Same as for upper extremity*
Pulmonary embolism	Acute pleural pain, shortness of breath, decreased oxygen saturation	VQ scan, pulmonary angiogram	Respiratory support same as for extremity*
Cerebral venous thrombosis	Focal neurological signs, decreased level of consciousness, focal seizures	MRI-MRA	Neurological assessment, same as for extremity*

MRI = magnetic resonance imaging.

*In all cases, anticoagulation begins with heparinization using either traditional heparin (start with 75 U/kg loading dose followed by 20–28 U/kg/hr continuous infusion), or low-molecular-weight heparin (no loading dose, give 1–1.5 mg/kg/day subcutaneously). For the former, the activated PTT is used to monitor the effect, and for the latter antifactor Xa level can be used, but most do not monitor the low molecular weight heparin. The ideal level for enoxaparin-treated patients antifactor Xa level is 0.5–1.0 U/mL. Coumadin® (warfarin), 0.2 mg/kg loading dose is added on day 2–4 and the INR of the PT is followed. By day 4–6, as the INR rises to 2–3, the heparin is stopped. Weekly measurements of the INR are taken to ensure that anticoagulation is appropriate and the Coumadin® is continued for 3–6 months.

7. How can we provide nutritional support for children undergoing cancer treatment?

The data show that children with severe wasting in a catabolic state do not tolerate chemotherapy, radiotherapy and bone marrow transplants as well as those who are in positive nitrogen balance. Although perhaps some tumors—notably soft tissue sarcomas—may actually grow faster in some cases, the consensus is that enhancing nutrition benefits the patient more than the risk of fostering tumor growth.

The first approach to enhancing a child's nutrition is to do a 3-day calorie count. Next, one should ascertain what the child's likes and dislikes are and using that information, add high-calorie meals and snacks to provide more energy and protein. Intervention is necessary when the child has lost more than 5% of his or her baseline weight. When a child will not take in enough calories and the gastrointestinal mucosa is intact, then enteral feedings via nasogastric, nasoduodenal or nasojejunal tubes or traditional gastrostomy or percutaneous gastrostomy should be given. Feedings can be intermittent or continuous or a combination of continuous during the night and bolus during the day to simulate meals. There are many products on the market appropriate for children, including Pediasure®, Kindercal®, Peptamen Junior®, Vivonex Pediatric®, Portogen®. Starting at 1–2 mL/kg/hr, the volume is increased daily by 1 mg/kg/hr until the caloric and protein needs are met.

Daily Allowances for Calories and Protein in Children

AGE	CALORIES (kcal/kg/d)	PROTEIN (g/kg/day)
0–6 months	110	2.2
6 months–1 yr	100	1.6
1–3 yr	100	1.2

4–6 yr	90	1.2
7–10 yr	70	1.0
11–14 yr	50	1.0
15–18 yr	45	0.9

Children who cannot tolerate enteral feedings are placed on total parenteral nutrition (TPN) to meet their caloric and protein needs. Prior to placing a child on TPN, bloodwork is undertaken to evaluate the biochemical status. A full chemistry panel including electrolytes, kidney function, liver function, albumin, triglycerides, cholesterol, liver enzymes and calcium, magnesium and phosphorus is examined. Using the recommended daily allowances for protein, lipid (1-2 g/kg/day), carbohydrate (~5–8 mg/kg/minute), calories and electrolytes, a solution tailored to each child is administered intravenously over 24 hr. Start with a solution containing dextrose 10%, which can be given peripherally or via central line. The dextrose is increased gradually to 20% to meet the caloric needs, and when >10%, requires a central line. After stabilizing the patient on a 24-hr regimen, the TPN may be cycled to 10–12 hr a day. Close monitoring of daily weight, intake and output, glucose twice daily, electrolytes, minerals and liver function is mandatory. When the child can resume eating or enteral feedings are again possible, the TPN should be tapered and stopped and the alternative feeding restarted.

8. Discuss the types of venous access devices used in children.

Almost all of the children treated with chemotherapy have venous access devices placed to minimize the possibility of extravasation and to provide convenience of access to the patient and medical staff. External devices such as Broviac, Hickman, Groshong and plasmapheresis catheters are inserted surgically and tunneled through the skin so that they are semi-permanent until removed surgically. Their chief advantage is that they require no needles for access; however, they require frequent dressings, cap changes and heparinization. Showering and swimming require extra-special care and infection is a major complication. Internal devices include Mediport and Portacath, which are subcutaneously implanted. A non-coring needle called a Huber needle is required for access. Preparation of the skin with a topical anesthetic, EMLA cream, minimizes the trauma of needle access for young children. While the risk of infection is less with the internal device, infection is still a concern, and extravasation and bleeding from improper movement of the needle is at higher risk than with the external devices. Care requirements are much less, and showering and swimming is not an issue.

Children who become febrile with either internal or external devices require immediate attention. Blood cultures should be obtained from all ports, and intravenous antibiotics should be given until the 48-hr culture results are obtained. If the child has an absolute neutrophil count (ANC) of >1,000, the daily dose of ceftriaxone can be given daily until the cultures come back. If the ANC is <1,000, the child should be admitted and treated for fever and neutropenia, with the suspicion of line sepsis. Antibiotics will need to be continued in that case until the neutropenia resolves.

Care protocols for the external devices vary from institution to institution. Studies have shown that as long as the care is consistent, the complication rate is the same for all the variations in care. These devices require dressing changes three times a week to daily, heparinization three times a week with 250 units per port to daily with 25 units per port and weekly cap changes. Care for internal devices requires flushing with saline and 500 U of heparin after use.

In addition to systemic line infection, local infection at the exit site (the area where the device is tunneled under the skin) and reservoir infection can be troublesome and lead to systemic infection. Local and parenteral antibiotics and increased local care can usually control such infections, except for the reservoir infection which generally requires removal of the device.

Occlusion and partial occlusion of the line is a frequent occurrence and is managed with flushing with normal saline, heparin or instillation of TPA (1 mg) or urokinase (5,000 U), waiting 30 minutes to an hour, removing the TPA or urokinase, and then flushing with saline and heparin.

Many external venous access devices survive the entire chemotherapy protocol for periods greater than a year. Occasionally, after a long period of time the body starts to extrude the velcro cuff and the catheter falls out. Other lines need to be replaced because of occlusion or infection.

9. How is mucositis managed in children?

The best treatment is prevention, which cannot always be accomplished due to the damage caused to the mucosa by chemotherapeutic agents such as anthracyclines and methotrexate. Good oral hygiene, including daily toothbrushing with a soft-bristle brush, flossing and mouthwash with sodium bicarbonate (1/2 teaspoon in 1 cup of water) when the ANC is >1,000 and wiping the teeth with the bicarbonate mouthwash with a toothette or gauze pad, is necessary. If the white count or platelet count is low, brushing and flossing should be discontinued. Twice to three times daily nystatin, 5 mL swish and swallow or Mycelex troches help prevent and treat mucositis. At the earliest sign of esophagitis, fluconazole can be started.

Once mouth sores have developed, "magic mouthwash" is often helpful for reducing pain and allowing for some oral intake. The recipe for magic mouthwash varies from place to place, but equal parts of 2% viscous lidocaine, liquid Maalox® or Mylanta®, and liquid diphendydramine (Benadryl®) swish and spit provide some relief. Consider swishing and spitting Ulcerease® 5–10 mL every 2 hr. For the child with severe mucositis, patient-controlled analgesia with morphine may be required.

The child with severe lower mucositis should be placed on stool softeners, and "butt paste" may provide comfort. Butt paste recipes also vary from place to place, but most include nystatin cream, EMLA® cream, and Desitin®. The perianal area should be inspected carefully for signs of infection.

10. Describe how to prevent constipation in children with cancer.

Prevention of constipation is important, not only for the well being of the child but also to avoid infection and pain. Vincristine and opiate analgesics are particularly constipating and children receiving these frequently should be placed prophylactically on stool softeners such as Colace®, Pericolace® or Senokot S®. If the patient becomes constipated, lactulose or Miralax® (1 tablespoon in 8 ounces of water) is often effective. In a non-neutropenic, non-thrombocytopenic patient, Dulcolox® suppositories or a Children's Fleet enema with oil can be used. Prevention goes a long way to provide comfort and compliance should be monitored closely.

11. What can be done to minimize pain from disease and treatment?

Much progress has been made in assessing and treating pain in children. The theory is that pain can be managed with appropriate medication in just about all cases. Current management starts with oral medications that have both anti-inflammatory and analgesic effects and works up to oral oxycodone and morphine preparations. If oral treatment is not appropriate for the patient, then patient-controlled analgesic morphine or fentanyl patches can be prescribed. (Please see the chapter on palliative care for more detailed pain management.)

BIBLIOGRAPHY

1. Ablin A: Supportive Care of Children with Cancer. Baltimore, Johns Hopkins University Press, 1997.
2. Children's Cancer Group, Supportive Care Guidelines, private communication.
3. Pizzo P, Poplack D: Principle and Practice of Pediatric Oncology, Philadelphia, J.B. Lippincott, 1998.
4. http://www.oncolink.com/support

43. LATE EFFECTS OF CHILDHOOD CANCER

M. Brigid Bradley, M.D.

1. What is the risk of a cancer survivor developing a second malignancy?

Childhood cancer survivors are at an increased risk of developing second malignancies. Sixty to seventy percent of children diagnosed with cancer can be cured using combined regimens of chemotherapy, radiation therapy and surgery. The incidence of a second malignancy developing in a child who has been cured of a primary malignancy is 8–12% at 20 years. This is 10–15 times greater than that of age-matched controls. The bones and soft tissues of growing children whose cells are actively dividing are prone to developing second malignancies.

Not all patients have the same risk. The primary malignancies with the greatest risk of developing second malignancies include retinoblastoma, Hodgkin's disease, Ewing's sarcoma and acute leukemia. Patients with a history of the genetic form of retinoblastoma are predisposed to developing second malignancies before including the treatment-related variables. Hodgkin's disease survivors treated with nitrogen mustard, vincristine, prednisone and procarbazine (MOPP) have a high risk for the development of radiation-associated sarcomas and leukemia,

Some of the secondary malignancies, such as cancers of the skin, thyroid gland and central nervous system (CNS) meningiomas, are curable. Others, such as second cancers of the bone, soft tissue sarcomas, non-Hodgkin's lymphoma, and acute myelogenous leukemia are more serious, require intensive therapy, and often prove fatal.

Radiation treatment is a major risk factor for the development of a second malignancy. The dose, radiation source, age at which radiation was given and the addition of chemotherapy all influence a patient's risk of developing a second malignancy after radiation therapy. Patients with a history of bone and soft tissue sarcomas treated with doses greater than 30 Gy have a risk 100 times greater of developing secondary bone sarcomas.

Alkylating agents are well-known leukemogens. Nitrogen mustard, procarbazine, carmustine and cyclophosphamide are associated with the development of leukemia. The epipodophylotoxins, etoposide and teniposide, are also leukemogenic. The schedule of administration plays a major role—twice weekly and weekly schedules increase the risk of developing secondary acute myelogenous leukemia (AML). The latent period for the development of secondary leukemia is 3–10 years.

2. Describe the effects on the endocrine system after stem cell transplantation.

Both chemotherapy and radiation used in the preparative regimens for stem cell transplantation can have an effect on the endocrine function of patients after transplant. The only risk factor associated with the development of abnormal thyroid function after transplant is total body irradiation (TBI). Irradiation of the thyroid gland can result in hypothyroidism, thyroiditis and thyroid malignancies. After 12–15 Gy of fractionated TBI, 10–14% of patients will develop compensated hypothyroidism, and fewer than 5% will develop overt hypothyroidism.

Growth can also be affected. Irradiation to the CNS results in growth hormone deficiency. In addition, direct irradiation to the skeletal system may account for some of the growth inhibition. Retardation of growth is related to the child's age at the time of radiation and the dose received. All children who receive cranial radiation plus TBI are at risk of growth hormone deficiency. Decreased growth rates are also reported after chemotherapy-only regimens that include busulfan and cyclophosphamide.

Hormone production and germ cell viability are affected by high doses of alkylating agents and TBI. The patient's age and sex and type and dose of therapy all most be considered. Prepubertal children who receive cumulative doses of cyclophosphamide up to 200 mg/kg will not be at increased risk and will undergo puberty at a normal age. When a combination of busulfan and cyclophosphamide is the preparative regimen used gonadal failure develops in female patients; and impaired spermatogenesis develops in male patients. Following TBI, delayed development of puberty has been observed in more than 70% of girls and more than 78% of boys. Girls with delayed puberty have primary gonadal failure, and boys who receive additional testicular radiation have testicular failure.

3. What are the clinical signs of cardiac damage exhibited by patients after anthracycline therapy?

Clinical abnormalities seen after anthracycline therapy are usually dose related and can range from minor changes on an electrocardiogram (ECG) to congestive heart failure. The incidence of congestive heart failure increases logarithmically at a cumulative dose of 550 mg/m^2. Acute anthracycline-induced cardiotoxicity can be seen during or within 6 months of completing therapy. Symptoms include fatigue, exercise intolerance, dyspnea, tachycardia and tachypnea. Hepatomegaly, rales and altered heart sounds by auscultation may be noted on physical examination.

Late cardiac effects can be seen 10–15 years after treatment. The risk for late cardiac failure is greatest in those patients who show abnormal cardiac function on echocardiogram (ECHO) after completing therapy. There is a 12% risk if the ECHO is normal at the end of therapy, versus 70% risk if the ECHO is abnormal at the end of therapy. Late-onset anthracycline-induced cardiomyopathy may manifest with congestive heart failure or ventricular arrhythmias. A prolonged QTc interval on ECG can be seen in patients who have received higher doses of anthracyclines. This is a more sensitive indicator of cardiac injury than ECHO.

4. In long-term survivors of childhood cancer who have received cardiotoxic therapy, what annual cardiac evaluations should be performed?

Patients at risk are those who have received anthracyclines, high-dose cyclophosphamide and cardiac irradiation. The baseline for all patients should include a thorough history, physical examination, chest radiograph, 12-lead ECG, and an ECHO. Patients treated with anthracyclines should have as ECG and ECHO every 2–3 years. Those who have had an abnormal test result either at the end of therapy or at the time of initial long-term follow-up should have more frequent cardiac screening. Changes in exercise tolerance, dyspnea on exertion, palpitations and syncope should be evaluated. The manifestations of late anthracycline-related cardiotoxicity are congestive heart failure and arrhythmias. Echocardiogram and ECG exercise testing have been shown to reveal cardiac injury that is not evident on resting studies. Asymptomatic patients who will be subject to increased cardiac stress should undergo careful baseline evaluations and scheduled monitoring.

5. Describe the complications seen in children who have received cranial irradiation.

The delayed effects experienced by children who receive cranial irradiation are varied. Patients will commonly exhibit cognitive defects. They can also exhibit deficits in general intelligence, developmental skills, reading, arithmetic, language, visual and perceptual motor skills, memory and attention. The severity is determined by the age of the patient when radiation therapy is administered and the cumulative dose delivered. Children treated before 5 or 6 years of age and especially < 3 years are at greatest risk of developing cognitive impairments. The neuropsychological deficits in children treated with cranial radiation do not become manifest until 1 or 2 years after irradiation.

One rare but devastating effect of radiation therapy is radiation necrosis. It can be seen in 1–5% of patients treated with 5–6 Gy of radiation. Signs and symptoms include headache, nausea, seizures, hemiparesis, papilledema and focal deficits. They can be seen from 3 months to many years after radiation therapy is delivered.

6. What off-therapy screening evaluations should patients treated for acute lymphoblastic leukemia undergo to identify potential therapy related effects?

Patients with acute lymphoblastic leukemia (ALL) are often treated with a combination of radiation therapy and chemotherapy. If a patient has received cranial irradiation and chemotherapy with methotrexate and 6 mercaptopurine, an educational assessment should be done each year and a baseline neurocognitive evaluation should be done and repeated every 2–3 years. A dental examination should be performed by age 5 years. An eye examination should also be performed every year. Patients should be monitored for precocious puberty and growth curves should be followed.

If a patient received spinal radiation, a thyroid examination should be done every year for the first 10 years. Growth assessment with standing and sitting height should also be done. A patient who has received testicular radiation should have leutenizing hormone (LH), follicle stimulating hormone (FSH) and testosterone levels measured on an annual basis.

Patients who received methotrexate and 6 mercaptopurine should have liver function studies done once a year. If a patient received cyclophosphamide levels of LH, FSH, estradiol and testosterone should be followed after age 12 and a urine analysis should be done once a year. If an anthracycline was given, an ECG and ECHO should be done at least every 3 years. A neurologic examination and complete blood count should be done each year in patients who received etoposide, and a neurological examination is recommended after cytarabine therapy.

7. Which chemotherapeutic agents are clearly associated with an increased risk of developing a secondary leukemia?

The alkylating agents melphalan, nitrogen mustard and cyclophosphamide have all been identified as leukemogenic agents. The secondary leukemia that develops as a result of these therapies is usually AML, and typically abnormalities of chromosome 5 and 7 are appreciated. The epipodophylotoxins such as etoposide are also associated with secondary leukemias and often exhibit 11q23 abnormalities. Patients who have a history of receiving these therapies and present with pallor, bruising, fatigue or petechiae should be evaluated with a complete blood count and bone marrow to rule out secondary leukemia.

8. Describe the etiology of pulmonary complications and how patients with respiratory compromise should be evaluated.

Both radiation therapy and chemotherapy can acutely and chronically alter lung function. Late effects of the lung after radiation can lead to progressive fibrosis. The chemotherapeutic agents responsible for pulmonary toxicity are bleomycin, chlorambucil and nitrosureas. Patients who receive methotrexate, cyclophosphamide, procarbazine and bleomycin can also develop pneumonitis, which may be a precursor of chronic pulmonary fibrosis. Pulmonary venocclusive disease, with vasculitis and intimal fibrosis resulting in pulmonary hypertension, has been reported with bleomycin and mitomycin.

In a child, impairment of the proliferation and maturation of alveoli can lead to chronic respiratory insufficiency. Inhibition of growth of the thoracic cage can also limit chest wall compliance, resulting in restrictive problems. Therefore, younger children are at increased risk for developing chronic toxicity.

Patients can present with cough, fever and shortness of breath. Tachypnea and the presence of a pleural effusion are the principle signs of delayed radiation-induced pneumonitis. A pulmonary function test can be performed to determine the pattern of pulmonary disease.

Restrictive patterns are most often seen after radiation and chemotherapy; reductions in vital capacity, lung volumes and total lung capacity are appreciated. However, combined obstructive restrictive patterns also can be seen. The basic evaluation for patients who have had lung injury consists of measuring the maximum inspiratory and expiratory pressures, forced vital capacity (FVC) and the FEV, as well as FEV1/FVC%. This differentiates an obstructive from a restrictive pattern and to what degree the pulmonary function is impaired. The total lung capacity should also be examined; similarly, it is also necessary to perform a carbon monoxide diffusing test to measure the degree of alveolar capillary block.

9. What sort of therapy affects growth in children treated for malignancy?

Decreased linear growth is a common problem in children with cancer. Severe growth retardation has been observed in as many as 30–35% of survivors of childhood brain tumors and in 10–15% of patients treated for leukemia.

Whole-brain radiation therapy has been identified as the principal cause of short stature. The affects appear to be age related; children younger than 5 years are more susceptible. The effect is also dose related. Administration of 3000 cGy to the hypothalamus and pituitary results in severe growth retardation in more than 50% of the patients treated for brain tumors. Chronic growth retardation in children with a history of acute leukemia treated with 1800–2400 cGy cranial radiation is less frequent and is milder. The mechanism by which cranial radiation induces short stature is not clear. Growth hormone deficiency has been identified as the cause in some patients. Early onset of puberty in girls also may contribute to loss of final height. Direct inhibition of vertebral growth by spinal irradiation often contributes to short stature. This change is seen most commonly in brain tumor patients whose entire spinal column has received doses in excess of 3500 cGy.

Chemotherapy alone may also contribute to decreased linear growth. However, when chemotherapy is given alone without cranial radiation, the growth retardation is usually temporary.

10. Describe the effects on the reproductive system in long-term survivors of childhood cancer.

Both germ cell depletion and abnormalities of gonadal endocrine function have been seen in male survivors of cancer secondary to the radiation, surgery and chemotherapy they received during treatment. Testicular irradiation affects germ cell number. Reduced sperm production is seen in a dose-dependant manner. At doses of 400–600 cGy, azoospermia develops and may persist for 3–5 years. At doses above 600 cGy, germinal loss with resulting increases in FSH and decreases in testicular volume usually appears and are irreversible. Prepubertal germ cells also appear to be radiosensitive, although tubular damage may be difficult to assess until the patient has gone through puberty. Radiation therapy is also toxic to the Leydig cells, resulting in inadequate production of testosterone. Boys treated prepubertally with 2400 cGy for testicular leukemia show germ cell depletion, and are at a high risk of delayed sexual maturation associated with decreased testosterone levels.

Chemotherapy alone can also interfere with testicular function. Alkylating agents decrease spermatogenesis in long-term survivors of cancer. Cyclophosphamide, procarbazine and chlorambucil inhibit spermatogenesis. The effect is dose dependent and is reversible in 70% of the patients. Many studies suggest that prepubertal testes are resistant to chronic toxicity. The effects of chemotherapy on Leydig cell function is also age related, with normal puberty developing in patients treated at a prepubertal age and gynecomastia with low testosterone and increased LH levels in patients treated during adolescence. The alkylating agents and antimetabolites have not been reported to produce Leydig cell failure.

An evaluation of the effects of radiation or chemotherapy on hormonal and reproductive function in female survivors is more difficult. The effects of radiation therapy on the ovary are also age and dose dependent. Irreversible ovarian failure usually occurs after 400–700 cGy is delivered to both ovaries in woman older than 40 years. Total body irradiation has been associated with primary ammenorhea and absent secondary sexual characteristics in most patients treated as young girls and followed for 10 years. Premature menopause has also been reported. Ovarian failure has also been associated with chemotherapy. Alkylating agents such as cyclophosphamide, busulfan, nitrogen mustard and procarbazine have been the best-described agents. Toxicitiy also appears to be dose and age dependent.

BIBLIOGRAPHY

1. Blatt J. CD, Bleyer W. Late effects of childhood cancer and its treatment. In Pizzo PP (ed): Principles and Practice of Pediatric Oncology, 3rd ed. Vol. 1. Philiadelphia, Lippincott-Raven, 1997.
2. S. K. Paediatric problems. In Barrett JTJ(ed): The Clinical Practice of Stem-Cell Transplantation. Vol. 2. Oxford, U.K., Isis Medical Media Ltd, 1998.
3. S. S. Endocrine and reproductive dysfunction in adults. In Barrett JTJ (ed): The Clinical Practice of Stem-Cell Transplantation. Vol. 2. Oxford, UK, Isis Medical Media Ltd, 1998.
4. Schwartz CHW, Constine L, Ruccione K: Survivors of childhood cancer. In L C (ed): St. Louis, MO, Mosby, 1994.

44. PSYCHOSOCIAL ASPECTS OF CARE OF THE CHILD WITH CANCER

Kenneth S. Gorfinkle, Ph.D.

1. How can the oncologist ease a child's distress when administering painful or invasive treatments?

- Explain the purpose and nature of the procedure in language intelligible to the child. Offer help to parents on how to answer questions about the procedure.
- Use honest, informative and positive language when describing what is planned. Instead of telling the child how much pain he or she might feel, describe it in terms such as "how uncomfortable" it might be.
- Give some thought to an appropriate period for the child to prepare for a procedure. A good guideline for this is to consider how the child, parents and medical team can best use the time to prepare for the procedure. Too much time allows unnecessary worry, but too little time takes away a patient's perceived control over treatment. Younger children have limited understanding of time. Furthermore, they are less able to productively use long preparation time. For minor procedures that are not routine parts of treatment (i.e., not regularly scheduled), consider warning a child 6 to 18 hours beforehand. This might apply to subcutaneous, intramuscular or intravenous injections and Ifusaport access. For procedures requiring short-acting general anesthesia such as Broviac removal, LP and BMA, consider 24 to 48 hours or more, especially for children over 10 years of age.
- Rehearse the procedure, simulating the timing, location and, importantly, the physical position and movements required of the child. Communicate what will be expected of the child. For example, avoid phrases such as "be cooperative" or "be good." Instead, tell the child what part of the body must be held in what position and for how long.
- When feasible, allow the child to observe the procedure being performed on a child who has mastered his or her fears.
- During procedures, engage the child's attention without attempting to block the child's vision or awareness of the procedure. Let the child watch as closely as he or she wishes, using mirrors if requested, e.g., for LPs. An adult may want to tell stories, sing songs or even interact with imaginary playmates. Children are capable of maintaining simultaneous awareness of play and a needle.
- If requested, provide a verbal or visual signal when a procedure is to begin. Many children wish to count down from three to one before a needle is inserted. This works best if counting down does not prolong the procedure.
- When praising a child after a procedure, do so in proportion to the effort the child made. Too much praise can signal a patronizing attitude. Too little praise deprives the child of useful information on how well he or she fulfilled expectations.
- If painful procedures must be repeated throughout treatment, and the physician knows how many will be performed, the physician should count them in reverse order, giving the child information on how many more remain to be done. Never promise an end to treatment if there is a chance that it may need to be extended.
- Use physical restraint only when necessary and with the least amount of physical force needed to complete a procedure safely. Do not assume restraint will be needed

unless clearly indicated, even if it was needed previously. Avoid using punitive or threatening language when instituting physical restraint. For example, do not attempt to gain compliance by telling a child you will hold him down if he cannot hold still. Think of physical restraint as a way of supporting a child, making him or her feel safe, recognizing that holding an arm still for venipuncture is often not possible without help from an adult. Gradually decrease the amount of force used for subsequent procedures. Many children are capable of learning sufficient self-control to sit still for finger sticks, blood draws and other repeated procedures.

2. How should children be informed about a diagnosis of cancer, leukemia, or lymphoma?

The meaning of the word *cancer* is not the same for children as it is for their parents, who were born in an era when few cancers were treatable. Remember that the idea of cancer is unfamiliar to laypeople, many of whom associate cancer with the death of older people. Parents often postpone disclosure of diagnosis for fear that the child will interpret this as a death sentence. Children feel less anxious when they can ask questions, and see that adults are not afraid to respond with simple, candid answers. Children rarely ask deep existential questions about morality and risk unless they have been recently exposed to others with the disease. If a child does become preoccupied with concerns about death, open discussion goes a long way towards reassuring children about essential concerns.

3. What are children concerned with after receiving new medical information such as cancer diagnosis, suspicion of worsening disease, or relapse?

Top worries for children are:

- Pain and discomfort: How much will I feel it?
- Dislocation: When can I sleep in my own bed?
- Disorientation: Where will Mommy and Daddy be? When can I go home? Where is Child Life?
- Unfamiliar food, people and procedures: Why are there different doctors and nurses on different days?
- Missed school and interrupted social or travel plans.

Children gauge their reactions to news of diagnosis, recurrence, or treatment failure against those of the adults around them. Children under age 12 or 13 rarely ask broad existential questions about mortality and our fate on Earth unless directly prompted to do so. When a child asks, "Why me?" it is best to ascertain the child's intent before offering a response. Does he want to know if he did something to cause the illness such as eat bad food or disobey his elders? Does he expect a direct answer to such a question, or is the child asking for general reassurance? Make every effort to respond to children's questions at a level appropriate to their understanding and ability to cope. If you are unsure, parents are the best judges of a child's ability to respond to and understand difficult news.

4. What approaches are effective when a child becomes resistant to or unable to eat as a result of tumor impact, chemotherapy, radiation or surgical complications?

When a child is very ill and under the care of physicians and nurses in a hospital, feeding is often one of the few remaining functions a parent can fulfill in caring for the child. However, feeding is often profoundly impaired by disease or treatment side effects. When the nourishment function is taken away from parents, they may become understandably frustrated. A common response is to make Herculean efforts to induce the child to increase food and fluid intake. Often this is successful, and even life saving. Equally prevalent is a battle over eating and drinking between parent and child, and even between the child and the entire medical team. While oncologists understand the effect of treatment on taste, appetite, digestion and elimination, they may fall into placing higher expectations on some children than can be humanly met.

A few tips on responding to treatment-induced anorexia:

- Classic anorexia nervosa is very rare in patients undergoing cancer treatment. Once physiological causes are ruled out, food refusal is likely to be related to conditioned food aversions. These develop as a result of Pavlovian pairing of emetigenic treatments with food intake. Once conditioning occurs, food alone induces nausea in the absence of chemotherapy.
- Take a careful survey of all organic and chemical influences on reduced appetite. This may include central nervous system pathology; esophageal, gastric and bowel pathology; side effects of antibiotic and antifungal treatments; as well as radiation treatment when any portion of the gastrointestinal tract is in the treatment field. There may be significant individual differences in patients' ability to eat when not feeling well. Avoid basing expectations of one patient too closely on the performance of another patient.
- Research on nausea and vomiting has documented a relationship between a premorbid sensitive stomach and a higher vulnerability to nausea and vomiting during treatment. In short, if the child typically was motion sick in cars, he or she will be more vulnerable to GI side effects of chemotherapy.
- Anxiety lowers the vomiting threshold. For this reason, benzodiazepines are effective adjuvant antiemetic agents. Similarly, psychotherapeutic anxiety management is also an effective tool for controlling gastrointestinal treatment complications. Maintain modest expectations of children's food consumption while on treatment. When medically feasible, stimulate appetite by reducing tube or TPN feeds. At these times, offer a wide variety of foods at frequent time intervals. It is important (but challenging) to offer food in a calm, dispassionate way. Do not be offended by a patient's refusal to eat. Some parents may need significant support in this area. A child may refuse an item six times in 2 hours, and then eat it on the seventh offer. This is less likely if the offers are made while applying heavy emotional pressure to eat. Younger children are bewildered by being asked to eat food that tastes bad to them, especially when not hungry. It is advisable to rule out clinical depression in children who will not eat. Antidepressants in such cases can bring a return of appetite. A skilled diagnostician can make the difficult distinction between drug side effects and neurovegetative signs of depression.

BIBLIOGRAPHY

1. Gorfinkle KS, Redd WH: Behavioral control of anxiety, distress and learned aversions in pediatric oncology. In: Breitbart W, Holland JC (eds): Psychiatric Aspects of Symptom Management in Cancer Patients. American Psychiatric Press, 1993, pp 129-146.
2. Gorfinkle KS: Soothing Your Child's Pain: From Teething to Tummy Aches to Acute Illnesses and Injuries—How to Understand the Causes and Ease the Hurt. Contemporary Books, 1998.
3. Manne SL, Redd WH, Jacobsen PB, et al: Behavioral intervention to reduce child and parent distress during venipuncture. J Consult Clin Psychol 58(5):565-572, 1990.
4. Manne SL, Bakeman R, Jacobsen PB, et al: Adult-child interaction during invasive medical procedures. Health Psychol 11:241-249, 1992.
5. Manne SL, Bakeman R, Jacobsen PB, et al: An analysis of a behavioral intervention for children undergoing venipuncture. Health Psychol 13(6):556-566, 1994.

45. PALLIATIVE CARE AND END OF LIFE CARE

Linda Granowetter, M.D.

1. What is the difference between Palliative Care and End of Life Care?

The World Health Organization (WHO) defines palliative care as:

> Control of pain, of other symptoms, and of psychological, social and spiritual problems...The goal of palliative care is the achievement of the best quality of life for patients and their families. Many aspects of palliative care are applicable in the course of illness in conjunction with anticancer treatment. When one considers the goals of palliative care, it becomes obvious that the principles of palliation should be integrated into all patient care during all life stages. End of Life cares focuses on the care of patients with diseases that cannot be cured and are dying. The transition between medical care with the goal of cure and end of life care is most often a gradual development.

Palliative and end of life care involves the treatment of all possible physical and emotional symptoms. Obviously, due to the broad scope of the field, this chapter addresses only the most common issues.

2. Are pediatricians generally successful in treating pain?

Multiple studies have demonstrated that there is a gap between patients' and families' perceptions of distressing symptoms and physicians' perceptions. From the patients' perspective, pain and other symptoms are inadequately treated. As pain and suffering are, by definition, subjective, it is imperative that pediatricians incorporate symptom assessment and management techniques into their thinking about patient care.

3. What are four of the most common symptoms experienced by children with cancer?

- Pain due to tumor, treatment, or procedures
- Nausea and vomiting
- Constipation
- Fatigue

4. How does one evaluate pain in children and adolescents?

The history and physical should always incorporate the evaluation of pain:

History

- Speak with the patient; if possible, use validated pain scales.
- Verify the specific pain medications used in the last 24 hours and determine if they have been sufficient.
- Discuss the patient's course with the nurse and family members who have been by the bedside, particularly if the patient is unable to speak.
- Determine if the patient has been able to sleep.
- Review the chart notes to determine if problems were noted.

Physical

- Check vital signs—is there increased blood pressure or heart rate out of proportion to other medical factors?
- Check for signs of physical injury that could result in pain; for example, mucositis, erythema at an intravenous site, pressure sores.

- Monitor the patient's reactions during the examination, such as grimacing, stiffness, ease of movement.

5. What are "pain scales"?

Several validated "pain scales" may be used to attempt to quantitate pain. Scales may be visual analog scales, numerical scales (0 = no pain, 10 = worst possible pain), or a scale based on facial expressions. The primary use of the pain scale is to follow changes in the intensity of pain over time and in relation to analgesia employed.

6. What is the ladder?

The WHO has described a three-step approach to analgesia, based on the level of pain the patient reports, called a ladder. Pain is classified as mild, moderate, or severe.

- Step 1: non-opioid such as acetaminophen and or NSAIDs
- Step 2: addition of mild opioid such as codeine
- Step 3: increased strength opioid such as morphine

7. Should pain medications be prescribed as requested, prn (pro re nata)?

It has been demonstrated that when analgesic medications are given around the clock, on a schedule, the cumulative dose of analgesia required is less than that required when pain medications are given prn. The reason is that by the time a patient asks for the medication, a higher dose is required to alleviate the pain.

8. What are appropriate methods of analgesic administration?

The most common routes of delivering pain medication are oral and intravenous. In the absence of vomiting, mouth pain, nausea, and vomiting, the appropriate titration of oral medication can effectuate pain control as well as intravenous delivery. Unfortunately, for the reasons mentioned above, many patients cannot tolerate oral analgesia. Other effective routes of delivery are:

- **Transdermal**: fentanyl is currently available as a transdermal patch. Some pharmacies will make up a gel of morphine or other medications for transdermal absorption.
- **Subcutaneous** (sc): sc injection or infusion may be very effective when the drug dose may be concentrated. Infusions of up to 5 cc/hour are generally tolerated subcutaneously. Injections of less than 1 ml are well tolerated. EMLA or other absorbed local anesthetic for the skin may be used to minimize the pain of sc injection.
- **Sublingual**: small doses of liquid opioids such as concentrated morphine or hydromorphone may be rapidly absorbed sublingually for patients who cannot swallow
- **Epidural, intraspinal, or intraventricular** administration of opioids may be considered for patients who require high doses of opioids that are not tolerated systemically. Indwelling catheters may be placed for ongoing delivery. Patients who are not responding to other routes of administration may be referred to pain-control experts for consideration of these routes.
- **Rectal**: medications given per rectum are generally avoided in neutropenic and/or thrombocytopenic patients in order to avoid causing infection or bleeding. However, some patients receiving palliative care may not be myelosuppressed, and if necessary a per rectum (pr) route may be considered in the absence of other options. Several opioids are available in a pr form.

NOTE: Intramuscular administration of analgesia should be avoided due to erratic absorption and the pain of the injection.

9. What are the most important side effects of opioids, and how are they managed?

- **Constipation** is the most common and a potentially very painful complication of opioids. The key is **prevention**: any patient receiving opioid therapy should receive concomitant treatment to prevent constipation. Adequate fluid intake and the intake of fiber (bran) and bowel stimulants (prune juice) are advised when possible. Most patients will require a combination of stool softeners (docusate) and a senna laxative. The dose of docusate/senna should be titrated so that the patient has a soft bowel movement at least every other day. If a patient is constipated at the start of therapy or becomes constipated, lactulose or even enemas may be required if the constipation is severe.

- **Nausea and even vomiting** are common complications of opioids. Nausea, vomiting, and abdominal cramps are often related to untreated constipation. If there is no evidence of constipation, antiemetics such as promethazine, prochlorperazine, lorazepam, ondansetron, or granisetron may be effective. Many patients become accustomed to the opioid and the nausea passes, others may benefit from a change to an alternate opioid.
- **Pruritus** is a common complication of opioids. Some patients respond to a change of opioids. Antihistamines such as diphenhydramine and hydroxyzine may be useful.
- **Urinary retention** may occur infrequently. Usually the patient will respond to running water or bladder massage. If these measures are not sufficient, intermittent straight catheterization may be required; often after once or twice the patient will resume normal micturation. A decrease in dose or change of opioid may be required. If persistent urinary retention occurs, etiology other than the opioid should be considered.
- **Respiratory depression** is uncommon. Most health care providers have an exaggerated concern about respiratory depression, resulting in inadequate pain control for the patient. If a patient is easily arousable, significant respiratory depression is unlikely. If there is true respiratory depression—such as a respiratory rate of less than 8/minute for longer than 30 minutes that does not increase when the patient is stimulated—intervention may be considered. The best intervention is stimulation and a decrease of the dose of narcotic infusion or dose by two-thirds. If required, naloxone may be given, but it must be noted that naloxone can induce a severe withdrawal reaction and thus naloxone should only be used if absolutely necessary.
- **Confusion, hallucinations, and dizziness** may occur. Usually these effects are transient, and it may not be necessary to titrate the opioids to a lower dose. Electrolyte abnormalities, especially hypercalcemia, may cause confusion and should be ruled out.
- **Fatigue** due to the opioids is a common complaint. Very often, the cause of the fatigue is the illness as much as the pain medication. If a patient is anemic, transfusions may help and are appropriate for an ambulatory or still-active patient. Dehydration or electrolyte disturbance should be ruled out as a cause of fatigue. Some patients will benefit from the use of methylphenidate.

10. What is the usual starting dose of intravenous morphine sulfate? How are changes between opioids made?

Although one need not remember the dose of each medication, morphine is the gold standard, and is the one to remember. The starting IV dose of morphine for a narcotic-naïve patient is 0.1 mg/kg/dose. The duration of action of morphine is 2-4 hours, thus the interval between doses should not be more than every 4 hours. If a patient is in pain, and has been using an opioid, the starting dose should be 10% to 20% higher than the patient's usual dose.

Patients who have been receiving opioids and are being changed to an alternative IV opioid should start at a dose about 25% less than the equianalgesic dose, as cross-tolerance between opioids is incomplete.

Opioid medication doses must always be checked: memory is fine, but a decimal point error can be very dangerous, so always check doses with a published reference.

The following table lists some of the most commonly used pain medications and relative doses:

MEDICATION (BRAND NAME)	INTRAVENOUS DOSE	ORAL DOSE	DURATION OF ACTION IN HOURS
MORPHINE	**10**	**30**	**IV: 2–4** **PO: 3–4**
Controlled-release morphine (MSContin)			PO 8–12
Methadone	10	20	6–8
Hydromorphone (Dilaudid)	1.5		
Codeine	—	200	3–4
Oxycodone (available as Roxicodone, or as Percocet in fixed combination with acetaminophen)	—	15	3–5
Controlled-release oxycodone (available as Oxycontin)	—	15	8–12
Hydrocodone (available as Vicodin—in a fixed combination with acetaminophen)	—	30	3–5

11. How is an intravenous dose of an opioid converted into an oral form?

Each opioid is different in regard to conversion to oral from the parenteral form. The following table demonstrates the equianalgesic doses and conversion from parenteral to oral of the most common opioids. It is not necessary to try to memorize these conversions, provided that you know where to find the information. In fact, dose conversions should not be made without checking a standard reference, so that the chance of inadvertent errors is minimized. The PDR or Internet-based systems such as Micromedex are useful, as is the Internet-based Texas Pain Initiative handbook.

1. Determine the total amount of narcotic received in the last 24 hours.
2. Multiply by the conversion factor in the Table below
3. Divide the number of doses per day based on the duration of drug action, as noted below.

THE CONVERSION FROM IV TO ORAL MORPHINE IS 1:3
(10 MG IV morphine is equivalent to 30 mg po morphine)

FROM ORAL	TO ORAL MORPHINE	FROM IV	TO IV MORPHINE
Methadone	1.5	Methadone	1
Hydromorphone	4	Hydromorphone	6.7
Codeine	0.15		
Oxycodone	2		

FORMULATION	DURATION OF ACTION
Intravenous morphine	2–4 hours
Oral morphine intermediate release (IR)	3–4 hours
Morphine slow release (MS Contin)	8–12 hours
Oxycodone	4–6 hours
Oxycodone slow release (Oxycontin)	8–12 hours

For example, using the table above, a patient who has been receiving 5 mg of IV morphine every 3 hours has received 40 mg of IV morphine in 24 hours. This is equivalent to a total of 120 mg of oral morphine in 24 hours.

120 mg oral morphine = 20 mg of IR oral morphine every 4 hours.
20 mg of IR oral morphine every 4 hours = 60 mg of slow release morphine every 12 hours

12. What is PCA?

PCA means patient-controlled analgesia. This generally refers to intravenous administration of analgesia, using a programmed pump. The pump may be programmed to give continuous medication with the ability for the patient to self-administer "bolus" increases, or it may be programmed only for bolus administration. The pump is programmed to permit a maximum dose, so as not to cause oversedation. Most PCA pumps register not only the exact amount of medication given, but also the number of attempts at administration by the patient. By reviewing the patient's history of attempts and medication delivered, one may have an objective measure of the patient's use of analgesia. If the patient has many attempts registered above delivered, it would indicate that the current level of analgesia is insufficient, and the rate and or bolus amount should be increased.

PCA was developed for adults, with the concept that if one were awake enough to push the demand button oneself, one could not overdose and cause respiratory depression. PCA is employed for younger children as well; when used for children the parent must be instructed how and when to use the pump, and it must be set so as not to allow for overdose by the parent.

13. What opioid analgesic should never be used as a continuous infusion and why?

Meperidine has an unacceptable risk of seizures due to accumulation of neurotoxic metabolites when used by infusion. Thus, continuous infusion or long-term use of bolus meperidine is inappropriate.

14. What is a "ceiling" effect?

Non-opioid analgesics such as acetaminophen and NSAIDs have a maximum dose over which no additional benefit is seen. This is considered the "ceiling" effect for these medications. There is no ceiling effect for opioids.

15. What is the difference between dependence, addiction, and tolerance?

Dependence means that if the medication is abruptly stopped, the patient will develop a withdrawal syndrome. This is an expected physical response to prolonged narcotic usage, and can be avoided by a slow taper for patients who have been treated for a long time, Dependence is NOT synonymous with addiction, which is a form of psychological dependence. True psychological addiction rarely occurs among patients receiving therapy for pain.

Pseudoaddiction is the onset of apparent addiction and drug-seeking behavior in patients who have been inadequately treated for pain, for example receiving medication with a 4-hour duration of action every 6-8 hours, or being given insufficient pain medication. To the physician, this may appear as inappropriate drug seeking; however, if the patient is inappropriately medicated by the physician, the drug seeking is appropriate.

Tolerance means that a sustained stable dose of medication no longer controls the pain. In other words, higher doses are required to attain the same degree of pain relief over time. Tolerance to opioids generally develops gradually. A very rapid increase in opioid need is most often due to an increase in the underlying pain.

16. Name some adjuvant medications used with analgesics for pain control.

- Antidepressants may be used in combination with analgesics. Some have analgesic properties. Concomitant sleep disorders and/or depression may be alleviated by the adjuvant use of antidepressants. Neuropathic pain may respond to tricyclic antidepressants. However, the newer serotonin-specific uptake inhibitors have fewer side effects and should be considered before tricyclics.
- Anticonvulsants such as carbamazepine and gabapentin are useful in the treatment of neuropathic pain. Gabapentin appears to have few side effects except drowsiness at higher dose ranges. Anticonvulsants should not be stopped abruptly as seizures may be precipitated.
- Hydroxyzine and lorazepam may help alleviate sleeplessness and/or anxiety.

- Haloperidol in small doses may alleviate nausea, anxiety, and sleep disturbance. However, extrapyramidal reactions are a possible side effect.
- Dexamethasone may be useful for severe bone pain, and pain due to swelling near nerve roots.

17. What behavioral interventions have been shown to be useful in pain control?

The patient's feelings and anxieties should be acknowledged. Patients may respond to cognitive and behavioral therapy. Specific relaxation programs, hypnotherapy, self-hypnosis, and guided imagery may all be useful. Engagement in pleasurable activities such as child life programs, music, and computer activities may be very helpful for young children and adolescents.

18. What methods may be used to alleviate the pain of venipuncture?

The best method to alleviate the pain of venipuncture is the use of lidocaine-prilocaine creams (EMLA). Unfortunately, for the peak effect to occur, it is ideal to have the cream, covered with Tegaderm, in place for 45–60 minutes.

19. What methods of pain control may be used to decrease the pain of procedures such as lumbar punctures and bone marrow aspirates and biopsies?

Conscious sedation is used in many centers. It must be noted that conscious sedation must be monitored appropriately. Most centers now arrange for procedures to be done while the patient is receiving short-acting anesthesia such as propofol, under the direction of an anesthesiologist.

20. What are methods that may be used to treat anorexia and weight loss?

Megestrol is commonly used for the treatment of anorexia in adult patients. This agent is rarely used in pediatrics. Parenteral nutritional therapy, or enteral feeding via tube, may be considered on an individual basis based on the patient's and parent's desires. Weight loss and anorexia are often very distressing to a parent, but less so to the child who may not want tube or intravenous feeding. It is important that children and adolescents are not subjected to treatments for anorexia and weight loss during end of life care, unless it is truly beneficial to the patient's sense of well-being, and consistent with the patient's wishes.

21. Name some of the classes and medications are useful in alleviating nausea and vomiting.

- Phenothiazines such as prochlorperazine are helpful but sedating and in high doses may cause extrapyramidal side effects
- 5HT antagonists such as ondansetron and granisetron are useful because they do not cause drowsiness or extrapyramidal reactions. An occasional side effect is headache, which may be alleviated by switching from one 5HT antagonist or another.
- Benzodiazepines such as diazepam and lorazepam are useful, but are sedating. They are especially useful for treatment of anticipatory vomiting.
- Antihistamines such as diphenhydramine and hydroxyzine are mild antiemetic agents, and are useful as adjuncts to therapy with 5HT and/or antianxiolytics
- Corticosteroids have an antiemetic effect, and are particularly useful for the treatment of increased intracranial pressure.
- Cannabinoids are available as tablets, dronabinol. Some patients find cannabinoids useful; however, dysphoria may occur.

22. How is dyspnea treated?

One of the most distressing symptoms at the end of life is dyspnea. Treatments include:

- Oxygen.
- Morphine given in concentrated doses sublingually (ex: liquid morphine 20 mg = 1 ml placed on the tongue as needed).
- Nebulized morphine (5–10 mg in normal saline nebulized the same way as a bronchodilator).
- Bronchodilators are useful for symptom relief in some patients.
- Cough is a common concomitant of dyspnea, and is best treated with dextromorphan and/or opioids. If excessive secretions are an issue, the patient may have some relief with an air humidifier, nebulized saline, or anihistamines or anticholinergics.

23. What is terminal dyspnea, and how is it treated?

Terminal dyspnea (called "death rattle" in some literature) is a gurgling noise caused by pooled secretions in patients who are unconscious or too weak to swallow or cough. Patients may be positioned on the side, and anticholinergics may be helpful. Scopolamine hydrobromide 0.4 mg sc q 2-4 hours may help, but may occasionally cause paradoxical excitation. Scopolamine transdermal patches are useful, but the onset of action may be 4-12 hours.

24. What is the difference between euthanasia and physician-assisted suicide? Are they legal?

The ethical issues related to physician-assisted suicide and euthanasia are quite complex and controversial. In the simplest terms, euthanasia is the painless termination of life of someone with a disease that will undoubtedly eventuate in death, even if the death is not imminent. With the exception of the Netherlands, euthanasia is not legal. This is distinct from withholding heroic life-saving treatments from people who are dying; this is sometimes termed passive euthanasia, and is appropriate when a DNR order has been chosen by the family and patient (see below). Physician-assisted suicide is a suicide of a patient accomplished with the help of the physician either by providing medication or a plan to a patient.

Most experts in the palliative care field believe that if patients had access to the best palliation treatment, physician-assisted suicide would be unnecessary. Others believe that there are circumstances that justify physician-assisted suicide. In the United States, only Oregon permits physician-assisted suicide, for adults. In pediatrics, the issue is even more complex due to the fact that adolescents and children are not legally empowered to make such decisions for themselves. Ethically there seems to be no real place for physician-assisted suicide in the care of children.

25. What is "double effect" in relation to analgesia at the end of life?

Double effect means that medication given to prevent suffering may have the unintended effect of shortening life. If the intent is to decrease suffering, and the doses of medication required to do so have the complication of possibly shortening life, it is considered ethically justifiable to treat the patient for the pain and suffering as needed. In most instances, relief of pain and/or dyspnea is achieved without levels of medication that are associated with respiratory depression or respiratory compromise. However, there are situations that require sedating medications that may hasten the dying process. There are some instances that require treatment of the parent; for example, as discussed above, treatment of terminal dyspnea is more for the parents than for the child.

26. What is a DNR order, and why should one never "get" a DNR?

DNR means do not resuscitate. One should not "get" a DNR order, because the decision not to resuscitate should never be coerced. A parent may decide to forego resuscitation that will not meaningfully prolong a child's life if the child is unable to consent or assent. Adolescents may choose to give advance directives concerning his or her wishes regarding resuscitation before they are terminally ill. Conflicts over the appropriateness of resuscitation between patient and parent, between parents, between parents and physicians, or between physicians and other hospital caregivers is not uncommon. The goal should always be the best care—emotional and physical—of the family. Every effort should be made to discuss facts clearly, and to support the family's wishes, and to resolve conflicts.

27. What should one do if there is a conflict in regard to plans regarding resuscitation?

Most often ongoing discussion among the involved parties will ultimately result in resolution of the conflict. Social workers, psychologists, psychiatrists, and pastoral counselors should be involved as needed. All hospitals have ethics boards that are available for the discussion of conflicts.

28. What is hospice care?

Hospice care is either home or in-patient care that is palliative in intent. Hospice caregivers are trained in symptom management and the emotional care of the family and patient. Offering hospice care to a family is difficult, as it signals the transition from intention to cure and palliation. However, when offered compassionately when it is clear that the patient is dying, it is appropriate and most often very comforting to the patient and parent.

29. Should a physician attend a patient's funeral or call or write a patient's family after the patient has died?

If a patient or parent has notified the hospital workers of the funeral or mourning arrangements, and the physician feels comfortable, it is appropriate but not required to attend a patient's funeral. Physicians should always feel that a condolence note or call is appropriate. It is extremely rare for a parent not to appreciate a health care provider's acknowledgment of their loss.

30. What can health professionals do to facilitate the bereavement process?

Parents, siblings, and other involved family and friends should be advised that hospital staff members are available to them should future questions or problems arise. They should be welcome to call to set up a time to speak with the primary physician and other caretakers for further discussion, at a future date. If the patient has had an autopsy, the physician should contact the family when the results are available, and invite them in for a meeting to discuss the results.

31. How long should it take for a parent to recover from the loss of a child?

It is important to acknowledge that the loss of a child will change everyone in the family forever. No parent should be told that they'll get over it, or that they should have another child, etc. It is not uncommon for a parent to say that life is not worth living now (without their child) or that they will never "get over" the loss. It is appropriate and realistic to acknowledge that indeed no parent will ever completely resolve the loss of a child, but that there will come a time when the pain will diminish, and treasured positive memories will be stronger than the pain.

INDEX

Page numbers in **boldface** type indicate complete chapters.